P9-CRM-938

COMPUTERS IN THE DENTAL OFFICE

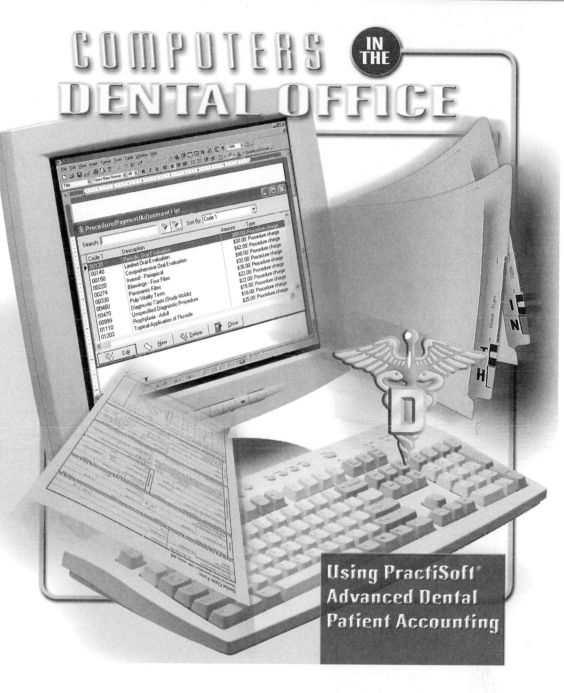

**Using PractiSoft®
Advanced Dental
Patient Accounting**

Cynthia Newby, CPC

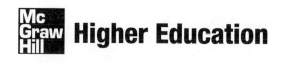

Higher Education

Boston   Burr Ridge, IL   Dubuque, IA   Madison, WI   New York   San Francisco   St. Louis
Bangkok   Bogotá   Caracas   Kuala Lumpur   Lisbon   London   Madrid   Mexico City
Milan   Montreal   New Delhi   Santiago   Seoul   Singapore   Sydney   Taipei   Toronto

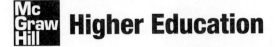

Higher Education

COMPUTERS IN THE DENTAL OFFICE: USING PRACTISOFT® ADVANCED
DENTAL PATIENT ACCOUNTING

Published by McGraw-Hill, a business unit of The McGraw-Hill Companies, Inc., 1221 Avenue of the Americas, New York, NY 10020. Copyright © 2004 by The McGraw-Hill Companies, Inc. All rights reserved. No part of this publication may be reproduced or distributed in any form or by any means, or stored in a database or retrieval system, without the prior written consent of The McGraw-Hill Companies, Inc., including, but not limited to, in any network or other electronic storage or transmission, or broadcast for distance learning.

Some ancillaries, including electronic and print components, may not be available to customers outside the United States.

This book is printed on recycled, acid-free paper containing 10% postconsumer waste.

1 2 3 4 5 6 7 8 9 0 QPD/QPD 0 9 8 7 6 5 4 3

ISBN 0–07–294105-7

Publisher: *David T. Culverwell*
Developmental editor: *Patricia Forrest*
Senior marketing manager: *Roxan Kinsey*
Project manager: *Jane Mohr*
Production supervisor: *Kara Kudronowicz*
Senior media project manager: *Stacy A. Patch*
Coordinator of freelance design: *Michelle D. Whitaker*
Cover and interior designer: *Jessica Wachs*
Cover image: © *Photodisc*
Compositor: *Lithokraft*
Typeface: *11/13.5 Palatino*
Printer: *Quebecor World Dubuque, IA*

All brand or product names are trademarks or registered trademarks of their respective companies.

Dental codes are based on CDT-4, © 2002 American Dental Association.

The Student Data Disk, illustrations, instructions, and exercises in *Computers in the Dental Office* are compatible with the PractiSoft Advanced Dental Patient Accounting software available at the time of publication. Adaptations may be necessary for use with subsequent versions of the software. Text changes will be made in reprints when possible.

All names, situations, and anecdotes are fictitious. They do not represent any person, event, or dental record.

Library of Congress Cataloging-in-Publication Data

Newby, Cynthia.
     Computers in the dental office : using PractiSoft® advanced dental patient
         accounting / Cynthia Newby. — 1st ed.
         p.   cm.
     Includes index.
     ISBN 0–07–294105–7
     1. Dentistry—Data processing. 2. Dental offices. I. Title.

RK240.N49   2004
617.6'00285—dc21   2003046351
                                                     CIP

www.mhhe.com

BRIEF CONTENTS

CONTENTS

PREFACE

Administrative duties in dental offices are becoming more involved with technology. Computers are now used in most dental practices. Students who aim to find an administrative job in the dental care environment will find that computer skills are often a prerequisite for employment.

This text/workbook, *Computers in the Dental Office*, prepares students for administrative tasks in a dental practice. The text/workbook introduces and simulates situations using PractiSoft Advanced Dental Patient Accounting, a widely used dental administrative software program. While progressing through PractiSoft's menus and windows, students learn to input patient information, schedule appointments, and handle billing. In addition, they produce various lists and reports, and learn to handle insurance claims both electronically and on paper. These invaluable skills are important in effective financial management of a dental practice.

Although this text/workbook features PractiSoft Advanced Dental Patient Accounting software, its concepts are general enough to cover most administrative software intended for dental care providers. Students who complete *Computers in the Dental Office* should be able to use other dental administrative software with a minimum of training.

TEXT/WORKBOOK OVERVIEW

Computers in the Dental Office is divided into four parts. The first, "Introduction to Computers in the Dental Office," covers the general flow of information in a dental office, the major dental services that are covered by insurance carriers, and the role that computers play in a dental office. If students have had other courses in computers, instructors may wish to use Chapter 3, "The Role of Computers in the Dental Office," as a review, or they may wish to skim the material and then move on to Part 2.

Part 2, "PractiSoft Advanced Dental Training," teaches students how to start PractiSoft, input data in the program, and then use the program to bill patients, prepare estimates, file claims, record data, print reports, and schedule appointments. The sequence takes the student through PractiSoft in a clear, concise manner. Each chapter includes a number of exercises that are to be done at the computer. These exercises give the student realistic experience using an administrative dental software program.

Part 3, "Applying Your Knowledge," completes the learning process by requiring the student to perform a series of tasks using PractiSoft. Each task is an application of the knowledge required in the dental office.

At the end of the text/workbook, a section of Source Documents (Part 4) gives the student the data needed to complete the exercises. These documents, which include patient information forms and encounter forms, are similar to those used in dental offices.

COMPUTER SUPPLIES AND EQUIPMENT

The Student Data Disk that comes with the text/workbook provides a base of case study information. Other equipment and supplies needed are as follows:

◆ 233 MHz or greater IBM or IBM-compatible processor
◆ 64 MB RAM
◆ 1 gig hard drive
◆ CD-ROM 2X or faster disk drive
◆ Mouse or compatible pointing device
◆ Windows 98, ME, NT, 2000, or XP operating system
◆ PractiSoft Advanced Dental Patient Accounting, Version 7.02 (free to adopters)
◆ One 3.5-inch disk drive
◆ Blank, formatted floppy diskette
◆ Printer

PractiSoft Advanced Dental Patient Accounting is free to schools adopting *Computers in the Dental Office*. Information on ordering and installing the software is located in the *Instructor's Manual* that accompanies the text/workbook.

CHAPTER STRUCTURE

At the beginning of each chapter, students are provided with a preview of what will be studied:

What You Need to Know Describes the basic knowledge required in order to complete the chapter.

Objectives Describes the primary areas of knowledge that can be acquired by studying the chapter and performing the exercises.

Key Terms Presents an alphabetic list of important vocabulary terms found in the chapter. Key terms are printed in bold-faced type and defined when introduced in the text/workbook. Key term definitions also appear in the left margin of the page where they are first used.

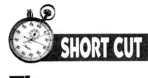

Throughout the instructional chapters, the narrative is supported by numerous figures and tables for reference. These instructional portions of the chapter include Short Cut and Tip features to enhance the learning experience (see icons in left margin). Computer exercises follow the portions of instructional material to reinforce what was just read.

Various types of testing are supplied in the *Chapter Review* at the end of each chapter in Parts 1 and 2. *Using Terminology* and *Checking Your Understanding* test the student's knowledge of the chapter's key terms and content. *Applying Knowledge* and *At the Computer* encourage the student to use critical thinking skills and apply practical knowledge using the computer and the chapter-by-chapter solutions file.

SUPPLEMENTARY MATERIAL

An *Instructor's Manual* provides the instructor with answers to chapter exercises, answers to Chapter Review questions/exercises, teaching suggestions, SCANS and National Health Care Skill Standards (NHCSS) correlations, and information on ordering and installing PractiSoft Advanced Dental Patient Accounting software. The CD contains the ExamView® Pro test generator program and the chapter-by-chapter solutions files.

ACKNOWLEDGMENTS

For insightful reviews, criticisms, helpful suggestions, and information, we would like to acknowledge the following:

Linda Butcher
Cleveland Institute of Dental Medical Assistants
Mentor, OH

Christine Discello
Career Training Academy
New Kensington, PA

Debbie Gilbert
Dalton State College
Dalton, GA

Patty Leary
Mecosta-Osceloa Career Center
Big Rapids, MI

Bonnie Lightner
Western School of Health and Business
Monroeville, PA

Joleen Parker
Davis Applied Technical College
Kaysville, UT

Sherri Steele AST, RMA
Career Training Academy
New Kensington, PA

For special assistance, we thank Dr. Harold Orlow, DDS,
Stamford, CT.

Introduction to Computers in the Dental Office

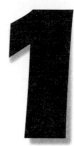

1

The Flow of Information in the Dental Office

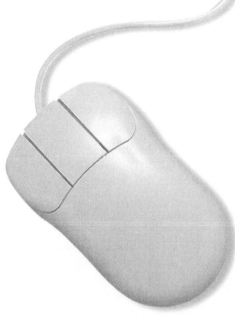

OBJECTIVES

When you finish this chapter, you will be able to:

1. Describe the tasks that are routinely performed in dental offices, including scheduling appointments, gathering and recording patient information, recording procedures, billing patients and filing insurance claims, and reviewing and recording payments.
2. Discuss different types of dental insurance plans.
3. List the steps involved in processing claims and collecting payments.
4. Describe the daily and monthly reports required to balance the practice's accounts receivable.

KEY TERMS

accounting cycle
accounts receivable (AR)
ADA Dental Claim Form
capitation
coinsurance
copayment
Current Dental Terminology (CDT-4)
day sheet
Dentist's Pretreatment Estimate
Dentist's Statement of Actual Services

encounter form
explanation of benefits (EOB)
health maintenance organization (HMO)
HIPAA (Health Insurance Portability and Accountability Act of 1996)
HIPAA Privacy Rule
indemnity plan
insurance carrier
managed care
patient information form
payer

KEY TERMS *(continued)*

policyholder
practice analysis report
preferred provider organization
  (PPO)

premium
procedure code
procedures
remittance advice (RA)

THE TASK CYCLE

From a business standpoint, the key to the financial health of a dental practice is billing and collecting fees for services. Without a steady flow of money coming in, payroll cannot be met, supplies cannot be ordered, and utility bills cannot be paid. To maintain a regular flow of income, certain tasks must be completed in a regular cycle and in a timely manner. These tasks include:

◆ Scheduling patients' appointments

◆ Gathering and recording patient information

◆ Recording procedures and services performed

◆ Billing patients and filing insurance claims

◆ Reviewing and recording payments

◆ Balancing the accounts

SCHEDULING APPOINTMENTS

The cycle begins when a patient requests an appointment. New appointment requests are usually made by telephone; follow-up appointments are typically scheduled when the patient is at the front desk, having just seen the dentist. When new patients phone for appointments, they should be informed of the practice's policy regarding payment.

Many dental offices use computerized scheduling programs to keep track of patient appointments. (Chapter 9 of this text/workbook covers this task in depth.) If the individual requesting an appointment is an established patient of the practice, the dental office assistant searches for an available time slot that is suitable for the patient and books the appointment. If the person is a new patient, basic information (such as the patient's name and phone number) is recorded when the appointment is made. When the new patient arrives at the office for the appointment, additional information is collected. However, in some practices, this additional information is taken over the telephone at the time the appointment is made.

RECORDING PATIENT INFORMATION

Patients who are first visiting the practice are asked to complete two important forms: a patient information form and a patient medical/dental history form.

The Patient Information Form

patient information form
form that includes a patient's personal, employment, and insurance data needed to complete an insurance claim

The **patient information form** contains the personal, employment, and dental insurance information needed to collect payment for the dentist's services. This form is filed in the patient's dental record and is updated when the patient reports a change, such as a new address or a change in insurance carrier. Many offices ask patients to update these forms periodically to ensure that the information is current and accurate.

Some patient information forms also include other information, such as:

◆ Student status
◆ Patient allergies
◆ Referring dentist
◆ Reason for visit
◆ Accident information, if appropriate

As shown in Figure 1-1 on page 6, the patient information form also requires the patient's signature or a parent's or guardian's signature if the patient is a minor, mentally incapacitated, or incompetent. The signature authorizes the insurance carrier or government program to send payments directly to the dentist rather than to the patient. It also gives the dental office permission to release treatment information to the insurance company for the purpose of reimbursement for services provided by the dentist.

HIPAA (Health Insurance Portability and Accountability Act of 1996)
Federal government act that set forth guidelines for standardizing the electronic data interchange of administrative and financial transactions, exposing fraud and abuse in government programs, and protecting the security and privacy of health information.

HIPAA Privacy Rule
Regulations for protecting individually identifiable information about a patient's past, present, or future physical or mental health or payment for health care that is created or received by a health care provider.

HIPAA (Health Insurance Portability and Accountability Act of 1996) governs the conditions under which private information in patients' records may be given to others. Under this law, the **HIPAA Privacy Rule** protects individually identifiable health information. This *personal health information* (PHI) includes information about a patient's past, present, or future physical or mental health or payment for health care. If this information is created or received by a health care provider in any form—oral or recorded—and if it can be used to find out the person's identification, it is protected information.

Collier Family Dental Care
Medical/Dental Arts Building
2890 Palm Avenue
Naples, FL 34104-8756
941-555-8900

PATIENT INFORMATION FORM

PERSONAL INFORMATION

Name (last, first): _____   Sex: ☐ Male

Address: _____   ☐ Female

_____

Date of Birth: _____   Marital Status: ☐ Married   ☐ Single

Social Security No.: _____   ☐ Separated ☐ Divorced

Home Phone No.: (___) _____   ☐ Widowed

(___) _____

Employer: _____

Address: _____

_____

Work Phone No.: (___) _____   Reason for Visit: _____

(___) _____   Name of Referring Dentist: _____

SPOUSE/PARENT INFORMATION   ### EMERGENCY CONTACT

Name (last, first): _____   Name (last, first): _____

Social Security No.: _____   Relationship: _____

Employer: _____   Phone No.: (___) _____

Address: _____

_____   ### INSURANCE INFORMATION

PHYSICIAN INFORMATION   Insurance Company: _____

Policy No.: _____

Name (last, first): _____   Copayment: _____

Specialty: _____   Plan Name/Group No.: _____

Phone No.: (___) _____   Name of Responsible Party: _____

Location/City: _____   Relationship to Patient: _____

_____   ☐ Self   ☐ Spouse   ☐ Child   ☐ Other

PAYMENT INFORMATION

Check all that apply: ☐ Insurance   ☐ Cash   ☐ Check   ☐ Credit Card   ☐ Other

Assignment and Release: I hereby authorize any insurance benefits to be paid directly to the dentist. I am financially responsible for the services provided, regardless of insurance coverage. I also authorize the dentist to release any information required.

_____   _____
Patient's signature/Parent or guardian's signature   Date

Figure 1-1   Patient Information Form

Patient Medical/Dental History Form

Dental practices often also require patients to complete a history of problems and complaints. Some practices ask patients to complete these forms before the first visit. The form may be mailed to the patient soon after the appointment is made, or the patient may be offered the opportunity to complete the form via the Internet. Figure 1-2 is an example of a form that can be completed online.

FAMILY GENTLE DENTAL CARE

| Home | Our Office | Services | Staff | Patient Education | Site Map |

MEDICAL HISTORY

Welcome! We are pleased to welcome you to our practice.
Please fill out this form as completely as you can.
The following information is essential for our staff to provide dental care in a manner that is compatible with your general health. Your cooperation in providing accurate information is necessary to safely and efficiently protect your dental needs. Incorrect information can be dangerous to your health.
If you have any questions, we would be glad to help you. We look forward to working with you in maintaining good dental health.
You may fill it out online; print it out and bring the completed form with you at your next appointment; mail it; or fill it out and fax it to our office.

(WARNING: there is no encryption system protecting the confidentiality of any information from this form you may send to us)

Physician's Name: _____ Phone #: _____

Date of last visit to Dr: _____

1. Are you currently under the care of a physician? Yes__ No__ For: _____
2. Medications you are currently taking: _____
3. List drug/medicine allergies: _____
4. Have you taken other drugs not listed above in the past 6 months, such as steroids, cocaine, any over-the-counter medications or herbal remedies or vitamins?
   Yes__ No__ List: _____
5. Have you had any serious illnesses or operations in the last five years? Yes__ No__
   If yes, please describe: _____
6. Have you ever had a blood transfusion? Yes__ No__ If yes, list dates: _____
7. Have you ever had a bad reaction to local anesthetic? Yes__ No__ If yes, please describe: _____
8. WOMEN ONLY: Are you pregnant? Yes__ No__ Maybe__ Nursing? Yes__ No__
   Are you taking birth control pills? Yes__ No__ Hormone medication? Yes__ No__
9. Do you need antibiotic premedication before dental treatment? Yes__ No__ List the condition: _____
10. Your current physical health is: Good__ Fair__ Poor__

Please click in the ☑ check box if you had or are now having any of the following problems:

☐ AIDS ☐ Anaphylaxis ☐ Anemia ☐ Arthritis, Rheumatism ☐ Artificial heart valves ☐ Artificial Joints ☐ Asthma

☐ Allergies: _____ (☐ Rash ☐ Itching ☐ Rhinitis ☐ Wheezing) ☐ Back problems

☐ Blood disease ☐ Cancer: _____ ☐ Chemotherapy ☐ Circulatory problems ☐ Cold

☐ Cortisone ☐ Congenital heart lesions ☐ Cough, persistent ☐ Cough up blood ☐ Diabetes ☐ Drastic weight loss

☐ Drug dependent ☐ Epilepsy ☐ Excessive bleeding ☐ Fainting ☐ Food allergies ☐ Fen-Phen or Redux used ☐ Heart murmur

☐ Heart problems, describe: _____ ☐ Hemophilia ☐ Herpes ☐ Hepatitis, Type: _____

☐ High blood pressure ☐ HIV positive ☐ Incest/sexual abuse ☐ Jaundice ☐ Kidney disease/malfunction ☐ Liver disease

☐ Latex allergy ☐ Mitral valve prolapse ☐ Nervous problems ☐ Pacemaker ☐ Persistent diarrhea ☐ Psychiatric care

☐ Rapid weight loss ☐ Radiation treatment: _____ ☐ Replacement surgery, Kind: _____

☐ Respiratory disease ☐ Skin rash ☐ Special diet, Kind: _____ ☐ Spina Bifida ☐ Sports, List sports in: _____

☐ Stress ☐ Stroke ☐ Surgical implants, Kind: _____ ☐ Swelling, feet/ankles ☐ Thyroid disease

☐ Tobacco use: ☐ Cigarette ☐ Chew ☐ Pipe ☐ Tonsillitis ☐ Tuberculosis ☐ Ulcer/colitis ☐ Venereal disease

Are you allergic to any of the following drugs?

☐ Aspirin ☐ Codeine ☐ Dental Anesthetics ☐ Erythromycin ☐ Latex ☐ Penicillin ☐ Tetracyclin

Do you have any other conditions, diseases, or problems not listed above? Yes__ No__
   If yes, please describe: _____

Up To Top

Figure 1-2 Medical/Dental History Form

DENTAL HISTORY

Why have you come to the dentist today?

_____
_____
_____
_____
_____
_____
_____

Please click in the ☑ check box if you have had or have in the present any of the following:

☐ Abscess in mouth	☐ Any food traps	☐ Bad breath	☐ Bad tastes	☐ Bite nails/objects	☐ Bleeding gums
☐ Blisters: ☐ Lip ☐ Mouth	☐ Chew on one side	☐ Chew tobacco	☐ Clenching/grinding teeth	☐ Cold Sores	☐ Difficulty chewing
☐ Dry mouth	☐ Gag easily	☐ Infection in gums ☐ Loose teeth		☐ Missing teeth	☐ Pain around ears
☐ Pain jaw joint	☐ Sensitive gums	☐ Sensitive to: ☐ Hot ☐ Cold ☐ Sweets			

☐ Smoke, How many a day: _____   ☐ Chew, How much: _____ Drink alcohol Yes __ No __ If yes, how much a day: _____

☐ Stained teeth ☐ Swelling, Where: _____ ☐ Unusual noises when eat

How often do you see your dentist? ____ 3 months ____ 6 months ____ 9 months ____ Yearly

I have reviewed the information on this questionnaire and it is accurate to the best of my knowledge.
I understand that this information will be used by the dentist and staff to help determine appropriate and healthful dental treatment. If there are any changes in my medical status, I will inform the dentist.
I authorize my insurance company to pay to Family Gentle Dental Care all insurance benefits otherwise payable to me for services rendered.
I authorize the use of this signature on all insurance submissions.
I authorize the release of all information necessary to secure the payment of benefits.
I understand that I am fully financially responsible for ALL charges whether covered or not covered or denied by my insurance company.

Since at each visit treatment plans are presented and the work to be done is explained to me before treatment is begun, I give my consent to perform any needed dental treatment, including the use of local anesthetic as needed.
I also give consent for the use of photographs for patient education purposes.

____ I agree   ____ I disagree

When you arrive for your appointment we will have you sign and date your Medical and Dental History as required by law.

Name: _____   Date: _____

Please fill out Patient Information

Wondering why you have to fill out these forms? Visit Reasons for Dental Forms to find out the reasons.

Submit Medical/Dental History

Up To Top

| Back | Home | Our Office | Services | Staff | Patient Education | Site Map |

Figure 1-2   Medical/Dental History Form

RECORDING PROCEDURES

procedure work that is done by a provider for a patient

encounter form a list of the procedures and charges for a patient's visit

When the patient sees the dentist, the results of the dentist's examination and diagnosis of the patient's condition and any medications prescribed are recorded in the patient's record. The dentist notes the **procedures**—the dental services—that are performed. The dentist also completes an **encounter form**, also known as a superbill (see Figure 1-3 on pages 9–10). The encounter form lists the most common procedures done by the particular specialty of the dental office. It often has a place for office visit charges and payments.

Collier Family Dental Care
Medical/Dental Arts Building
2890 Palm Avenue
Naples, FL 34104-8756
941-555-8900

Patient Name: **Chart Number:**   **Dentist:**   **Date of Service:**

	SERVICE DIAGNOSTIC/PREVENTIVE		FEE
	D1110 Prophylaxis – adult		
	D0120 Periodic oral evaluation		
	D0274 Bitewings – four X rays		
	D1120 Prophylaxis – child		
	D0210 Intraoral – complete series (including bitewings)		
	D0220 Intraoral – first X ray		
	D0230 Intraoral – each additional X ray		
	D0321 TMJ film		
	D0470 Diagnostic casts		
	ENDODONTICS	**Tooth #s**	
	D3310 Root canal 1		
	D3320 Root canal 2		
	D3330 Root canal 3		
	D3110 Pulp cap		
	D3220 Pulpotomy		
	D0460 Pulp vitality test		
	D2940 Sedative filling		
	RESTORATIVE Amalgam Restorations:	**Surface Tooth #s**	
	D2140 One surface, primary or permanent		
	D2150 Two surfaces, primary or permanent		
	D2160 Three surfaces, primary or permanent		
	D2161 Four or more surfaces, primary or permanent		
	Resin-based Composite Restorations Anterior:	**Surface Tooth #s**	
	D2330 One surface		
	D2331 Two surfaces		
	D2332 Three surfaces		
	D2335 Four or more surfaces		
	Posterior:	**Surface Tooth #s**	
	D2391 One surface		
	D2392 Two surfaces		
	D2393 Three surfaces		
	D2394 Four or more surfaces		
	Crown Restorations:	**Tooth #s**	
	D2740 Porcelain		
	D2750 Porcelain–metal		

cont.'d

Figure 1-3   Encounter Form

Collier Family Dental Care
Medical/Dental Arts Building
2890 Palm Avenue
Naples, FL 34104-8756
941-555-8900

Patient Name: Chart Number: Date of Service:

		Tooth #s	
	Crown Restorations:		
	D2920 Recement Crown		
	D2950 Core buildup		
	D2980 Repair		
	PROSTHETICS Complete Dentures:		
	D5110 Upper denture		
	D5120 Lower denture		
	D5130 Immediate upper denture		
	D5140 Immediate lower denture		
	Partial Dentures:		
	D5211 Upper partial denture–resin		
	D5212 Lower partial denture–resin		
	D5213 Upper partial denture–cast		
	D5214 Lower partial denture–cast		
	D5750 Reline full upper denture		
	D6930 Recement fixed partial denture		
	PERIODONTICS/SURGERY	**Tooth/Quad**	
	D4341 Periodontal scaling and root planing, per quadrant		
	Upper right		
	Upper left		
	Lower right		
	Lower left		
	D4210 Gingivectomy		
	D4240 Gingival flap		
	D4260 Osseous surgery		
	Upper right		
	Upper left		
	Lower right		
	Lower left		
	D7111 Extraction–Coronal remnant		
	D7140 Extraction–erupted tooth or exposed root		
	D7210 Surgical extraction		
	ADJUNCTIVE GENERAL SERVICES	**Tooth #s**	
	D9951 Occlusal adjustment–limited		
	OTHER		

Payments: Total charge:

Remarks:

Figure 1-3   Encounter Form

procedure code a code that identifies a dental services

Current Dental Terminology (CDT-4) American Dental Association publication containing a standardized classification system for reporting dental procedures and services

As Figure 1-3 illustrates, procedures are assigned **procedure codes**. Dental procedure codes are five-digit codes that begin with the letter *D*. The American Dental Association (ADA) develops and maintains the dental codes in a publication entitled *Current Dental Terminology*, Fourth Edition. The codes, which were most recently revised in 2003, are referred to as the **CDT-4** codes. The information on encounter forms should be checked annually to be sure that current codes are used.

BILLING PATIENTS AND FILING INSURANCE CLAIMS

During a typical day, dozens of patients visit the dental office. They have a variety of problems and needs, and they receive different services from the dentist. When patients receive services from a dental practice, the costs are paid either by the patient or by the patient's insurance plan.

policyholder a person who buys an insurance plan; the insured

insurance carrier a company that offers financial protection as a result of a specified event

premium the periodic amount of money the insured pays to an insurance company for an insurance plan

Many patients are covered by some type of dental insurance. Dental insurance, one type of health insurance, represents an agreement between a person, known as the **policyholder**, and an **insurance carrier**. Payments made to the carrier by the policyholder for insurance coverage are called **premiums**. In exchange for these payments, the carrier agrees to pay for the insured's dental services according to the terms of the insurance policy.

The ADA Dental Claim Form

ADA Dental Claim Form authorized form for submitting dental insurance claims

To receive payment from patients or insurance plans, most dental practices must complete or produce documents. One kind of document is an insurance claim form. The most common claim form for dental services is the **ADA Dental Claim Form**. The ADA Dental Claim Form is approved and updated by the American Dental Association (see Figure 1-4 on page 12). This form contains sections for patient coverage information, information on the billing dentist, and details about the examination and treatment plan. Practices may submit a claim to an insurance carrier for a patient, or patients may attach the ADA Dental Claim Form dentists complete to their own carriers' claim form.

Dentist's Pretreatment Estimate dentist's estimate of needed dental work that is submitted to an insurance carrier before the service is performed

A dental claim form is used for two purposes: (1) to report the **Dentist's Pretreatment Estimate** to an insurance carrier before the service is performed for an analysis of what will be reimbursed and (2) to submit the **Dentist's Statement of Actual Services** for claim processing and payment.

Dentist's Statement of Actual Services dental claim form that reports the services a dentist has performed for a patient

A Dentist's Pretreatment Estimate may be submitted for a number of reasons. The primary reason is for insurance approval—to find out whether the procedure is covered and the amount of the reimbursement. In addition, this estimate helps to resolve the disagreements that at times arise between a dentist and a carrier about appropriate treatments. Also, dental patients often have choices regarding

ADA Dental Claim Form

HEADER INFORMATION

1. Type of Transaction (Check all applicable boxes)

☐ Statement of Actual Services – OR – ☐ Request for Predetermination/Preauthorization

☐ EPSDT/Title XIX

2. Predetermination/Preauthorization Number

PRIMARY PAYER INFORMATION

3. Name, Address, City, State, Zip Code

OTHER COVERAGE

4. Other Dental or Medical Coverage? ☐ No (Skip 5–11) ☐ Yes (Complete 5–11)

5. Subscriber Name (Last, First, Middle Initial, Suffix)

6. Date of Birth (MM/DD/CCYY)

7. Gender ☐ M ☐ F

8. Subscriber Identifier (SSN or ID#)

9. Plan/Group Number

10. Relationship to Primary Subscriber (Check applicable box) ☐ Self ☐ Spouse ☐ Dependent ☐ Other

11. Other Carrier Name, Address, City, State, Zip Code

PRIMARY SUBSCRIBER INFORMATION

12. Name (Last, First, Middle Initial, Suffix), Address, City, State, Zip Code

13. Date of Birth (MM/DD/CCYY)

14. Gender ☐ M ☐ F

15. Subscriber Identifier (SSN or ID#)

16. Plan/Group Number

17. Employer Name

PATIENT INFORMATION

18. Relationship to Primary Subscriber (Check applicable box) ☐ Self ☐ Spouse ☐ Dependent Child ☐ Other

19. Student Status ☐ FTS ☐ PTS

20. Name (Last, First, Middle Initial, Suffix), Address, City, State, Zip Code

21. Date of Birth (MM/DD/CCYY)

22. Gender ☐ M ☐ F

23. Patient ID/Account # (Assigned by Dentist)

RECORD OF SERVICES PROVIDED

	24. Procedure Date (MM/DD/CCYY)	25. Area of Oral Cavity	26. Tooth System	27. Tooth Number(s) or Letter(s)	28. Tooth Surface	29. Procedure Code	30. Description	31. Fee
1								
2								
3								
4								
5								
6								
7								
8								
9								
10								

MISSING TEETH INFORMATION

34. (Place an 'X' on each missing tooth)

Permanent: 1 2 3 4 5 6 7 8 9 10 11 12 13 14 15 16 / 32 31 30 29 28 27 26 25 24 23 22 21 20 19 18 17

Primary: A B C D E F G H I J / T S R Q P O N M L K

32. Other Fee(s)

33. Total Fee

35. Remarks

AUTHORIZATIONS

36. I have been informed of the treatment plan and associated fees. I agree to be responsible for all charges for dental services and materials not paid by my dental benefit plan, unless prohibited by law, or the treating dentist or dental practice has a contractual agreement with my plan prohibiting all or a portion of such charges. To the extent permitted by law, I consent to your use and disclosure of my protected health information to carry out payment activities in connection with this claim.

X _____
Patient/Guardian signature   Date

37. I hereby authorize and direct payment of the dental benefits otherwise payable to me, directly to the below named dentist or dental entity.

X _____
Subscriber signature   Date

BILLING DENTIST OR DENTAL ENTITY (Leave blank if dentist or dental entity is not submitting claim on behalf of the patient or insured/subscriber)

48. Name, Address, City, State, Zip Code

49. Privider ID

50. License Number

51. SSN or TIN

52. Phone Number (   )   –

ANCILLARY CLAIM/TREATMENT INFORMATION

38. Place of Treatment (Check applicable box) ☐ Provider's Office ☐ Hospital ☐ ECF ☐ Other

39. Number of Enclosures (00 to 99) Radiograph(s) Oral Image(s) Model(s)

40. Is Treatment for Orthodontics? ☐ No (Skip 41–42) ☐ Yes (Complete 41–42)

41. Date Appliance Placed (MM/DD/CCYY)

42. Months of Treatment Remaining

43. Replacement of Prosthesis? ☐ No ☐ Yes (Complete 44)

44. Date Prior Placement (MM/DD/CCYY)

45. Treatment Resulting from (Check applicable box) ☐ Occupational illness/injury ☐ Auto accident ☐ Other accident

46. Date of Accident (MM/DD/CCYY)

47. Auto Accident State

TREATING DENTIST AND TREATMENT LOCATION INFORMATION

53. I hereby certify that the procedures as indicated by date are in progress (for procedures that require multiple visits) or have been completed and that the fees submitted are the actual fees I have charged and intend to collect for those procedures.

X _____
Signed (Treating Dentist)   Date

54. Provider ID

55. License Number

56. Address, City, State, Zip Code

57. Phone Number (   )   –

58. Treating Provider Specialty

©American Dental Association, 2002
J515 (Same as ADA Dental Claim Form)—J516, J517, J518, J519

Figure 1-4   ADA Dental Claim Form

treatments. For example, one type of crown material may look better than another, but it may also be more expensive. If the dental insurance coverage has a set rate for a crown, a patient who desires the more expensive material may have to pay a higher cost.

Charges that are not covered by an insurance carrier are billed to the patient. The patient statement informs the patient of the amount owed for a specific visit. The patient statement lists all services performed, along with the associated charges. Most dental practices have a regular schedule, perhaps daily or weekly, for submitting claims to insurance carriers. For example, some practices bill half the patients on the fifteenth of the month and the other half on the thirtieth.

Overview of Dental Insurance

There are a wide variety of dental insurance plans in the United States. Most policyholders are covered by group policies, often through their employers. A few people, such as those who are self-employed, have individual plans. Insurance coverage may be supplied by a private company, such as Delta Dental, or by a government plan, such as TRICARE, a government program that covers dental expenses for dependents of active duty members of the uniformed services and for retired military personnel. Whether private company or government program, the insurance carrier is called a **payer**. The term *third-party payer* is also used, because the primary relationship is between the dentist and the patient, and the insurance carrier is the third party.

payer private or governmental organization that insures or pays for health care on the behalf of beneficiaries

indemnity plan an insurance company's agreement to reimburse a policyholder for covered losses

Different types of insurance plans can be purchased. In an **indemnity plan**, policyholders are paid back for costs for health care due to illnesses and accidents. Under an indemnity plan, the policy lists the services that are covered and the amounts that are paid. The benefit may be for all or part of the charges. For example, the policy may indicate that 80 percent of charges for periodontal work are covered. The policyholder is responsible for paying the other 20 percent. This amount—the portion of charges that an insured person must pay—is known as **coinsurance**.

coinsurance part of charges that an insured person must pay for health care services after payment of the deductible amount

managed care a type of insurance in which the carrier is responsible for both the financing and the delivery of health care

Another type of insurance system is **managed care**. About one-third of those insured are covered by some form of managed care for dental insurance. Managed care plans control both the financing and the delivery of health care to policyholders. To create a managed care plan, an insurance carrier reaches agreements with dentists and other health care providers to provide their services for fixed fees. The managed care plan sets the fees. The most common type of managed care program is a **preferred provider organization (PPO)**. A PPO is a network of health care providers who agree to perform services for plan members at discounted fees. In most plans, members may receive care from other doctors or dentists outside the network for a higher cost.

preferred provider organization (PPO) managed care network of health care providers who agree to perform services for plan members at discounted fees

health maintenance organization (HMO) a managed health care system in which providers agree to offer health care to the organization's members for fixed periodic payments from the plan

copayment amount that an insured person must pay for each health care encounter

capitation advance payment to a provider that covers each plan member's health care services for a certain period of time

Another common type of managed care system is a **health maintenance organization (HMO)**. In an HMO, patients pay fixed rates at regular intervals, such as monthly. In some HMOs, patients pay a **copayment**—a small fixed fee, such as $10, at the time of the office visit. In HMOs, patients must choose from a specific group of health care providers for care.

In some managed care plans, dentists are paid a fixed amount per month to provide necessary, contracted services to patients who are plan members. This fixed prepayment is referred to as **capitation**. The rate the dentist is paid is based on several factors, including the number of plan members and their ages. The capitated rate is paid to the dentist even if the dentist does not provide any dental services to the patient during the time period covered by the payment. Similarly, the dentist receives the same capitated rate if a patient is treated more than once during the time period.

Processing Claims

For an insurance carrier to pay a claim, certain information about the patient must be shared. The insurance carrier needs to know the procedures the dentist performed while the patient was in the office. The date of the visit and the location of the visit must be indicated. The insurance carrier also requires basic information about the dentist who is providing the treatment, including the provider's name and/or provider identification number. There may be a group number and an individual identification number for a provider who is part of a group practice.

The information needed to create a claim is found on the patient information form and the encounter form. Most insurance claims are submitted electronically by transferring information from a computer in the provider's office to a computer at the insurance company. In some instances, such as when an attachment is required, paper forms are filed. Some offices pay a fee to a clearinghouse to file their claims electronically. A clearinghouse is a service company that receives electronic or paper claims from the provider, checks and prepares them for processing, and transmits them in proper data format to the correct carriers.

When the claim is received by the insurance carrier, it is reviewed and processed. If the patient's insurance is an indemnity plan, the insurance company compares the fees to the schedule of benefits in the patient's policy and determines the amount of benefit to be paid. If the patient's insurance coverage is a managed care plan, the insurance company pays a contracted fee to the provider, and the patient pays the copayment directly to the provider.

REVIEWING AND RECORDING PAYMENTS

remittance advice (RA) an explanation of benefits transmitted by a payer to a provider

explanation of benefits (EOB) document from a payer that shows how the amount of a benefit was determined

After the amount of the benefit is determined, the insurance carrier issues a notification payment. At the same time, it issues a **remittance advice (RA)**, or **explanation of benefits (EOB)**. An RA is used with electronic claims, while an EOB is sent when a paper claim is submitted. An RA or EOB indicates how the amount of benefit was determined. The insurance company sends the payment to the dentist or to the policyholder to whom it is owed.

When the RA arrives at the dentist's office, it is reviewed for accuracy. If an error is found, a request for a review of the claim must be filed with the carrier. If a check is enclosed, the amount of the payment from the insurance carrier is recorded. In some cases, the patient is billed for an outstanding balance. In other circumstances, an account adjustment is made.

BALANCING THE ACCOUNTS

accounting cycle the flow of financial transactions in a business

accounts receivable (AR) monies that are flowing into a business

day sheet a report that lists all transactions for a single day

The **accounting cycle** is the flow of financial transactions in a business—from making a sale to collecting payment for the goods or services delivered. In a dental practice, this is the cycle from seeing and treating the patient to receiving payments for services provided.

Accounting software can be used to track **accounts receivable (AR)**—monies that are coming into the practice—and to produce financial reports. Reports are usually created at the end of each day and at the end of the month, quarter, and year. At the end of each day, a report is generated that lists all charges, payments, and adjustments entered during that day. This report is known as a **day sheet**. To balance out a day, transactions listed on encounter forms (charges and payments) and totals from deposit tickets are compared against the computer-generated day sheet.

practice analysis report a report that shows the total revenue for each procedure performed during a specified time period

At the end of the month, a **practice analysis report** summarizes the financial activity of the entire month. This report lists charges, payments, and adjustments and the total accounts receivable for the month. It is possible to balance out the month by taking all the day sheets for the month, totaling the charges, payments, and adjustments, and then comparing the totals to the amounts listed on the practice analysis report.

It is also good practice to print aging reports on a regular basis. Aging reports list the outstanding balances owed to the practice by insurance companies or patients. There are also reports that provide current information on the status of patient and insurance billing. Regular review of aging reports can alert the billing staff to accounts that require action to collect the amount due. In addition to these reports, most accounting programs provide other useful report tools that offer a clear picture of the practice's financial health at any point in time. Timely printing of reports also helps the office staff meet claim filing deadlines and collect unpaid insurance payments.

CHAPTER REVIEW

USING TERMINOLOGY

Match the terms on the left with the definitions on the right.

1. accounting cycle

2. accounts receivable (AR)

3. ADA Dental Claim Form

4. HIPAA

5. capitation

6. coinsurance

7. copayment

8. *Current Dental Terminology* (CDT-4)

9. day sheet

10. Dentist's Statement of Actual Services

11. Dentist's Pretreatment Estimate

12. encounter form

13. remittance advice (RA)/ explanation of benefits (EOB)

14. health maintenance organization (HMO)

15. indemnity plan

a. A document from an insurance carrier that lists the amount of a benefit and explains how it was determined.

b. The most commonly used dental claim form.

c. A document that contains personal, employment, and dental insurance information about a patient.

d. Regulations for protecting individually identifiable information about a patient's past, present, or future physical or mental health or payment for health care that is created or received by a health care provider.

e. A form listing procedures relevant to the specialty of a dental office, used to record the procedures performed.

f. A claim form that is submitted before dental work is performed.

g. A term used to describe an insurance carrier in the context of the dentist's and the patient's relationship.

h. Services performed by a dentist.

i. Federal government act that set forth guidelines for standardizing the electronic data interchange of administrative and financial transactions, exposing fraud and abuse in government programs, and protecting the security and privacy of health information.

j. An individual who has contracted with an insurance company for coverage.

k. Payments made to an insurance carrier by a policyholder for coverage.

l. A fixed amount that is paid to a dentist in advance to provide medically necessary services to patients.

m. A type of insurance in which the carrier is responsible for the financing and delivery of health care.

16. insurance carrier

17. managed care

18. patient information form

19. HIPAA Privacy Rule

20. payer

21. policyholder

22. practice analysis report

23. preferred provider organization (PPO)

24. premium

25. procedure code

26. procedures

n. A term used to describe money coming in to a business.

o. A claim form that is submitted after dental work is performed.

p. A type of managed care system in which patients pay fixed rates at regular intervals.

q. An insurance plan in which policyholders are reimbursed for health care costs.

r. Under an insurance plan, the portion or percentage of the charges that the patient is responsible for paying.

s. A network of health care providers who agree to provide services to plan members at a discounted fee.

t. A report that summarizes the financial activity of a practice for a period of time, such as a month or a year.

u. A number that represents dental procedures that were performed.

v. The flow of financial transactions in a business.

w. A company that provides insurance coverage to individuals and/or groups.

x. A report that summarizes the financial activity of a practice for a single day.

y. The American Dental Association approved list of dental procedure codes.

z. A small fixed fee paid by the patient at the time of an office visit.

CHECKING YOUR UNDERSTANDING

Write "T" or "F" in the blank to indicate whether you think the statement is true or false.

_____ **27.** Many patient information forms contain a place for the patient to sign to authorize the patient's insurance carrier to send payments directly to a provider.

_____ **28.** CDT-4 codes have eight digits.

_____ **29.** Coinsurance refers to a small fixed fee that must be paid by the patient at the time of an office visit.

_____ **30.** To receive payment for services, most dental offices must create two documents (either paper or electronic)—a patient statement and an insurance claim.

Answer the question below in the space provided.

31. List the five basic categories of administrative tasks in a dental office.

_____

_____

_____

_____

_____

Choose the best answer.

32. A patient information form contains information such as name, address, employer, and:
 a. procedure code
 b. insurance coverage information
 c. charges for procedures performed

33. A health maintenance organization (HMO) is one example of:
 a. an indemnity plan
 b. a government plan
 c. a managed care plan

34. In a managed care plan, a _____ is collected from the patient at the office visit.
 a. deductible
 b. patient statement
 c. copayment

35. The most commonly used system of dental procedure codes is found in the:
 a. CDT
 b. ICD
 c. HCFA-1500

36. Information about a patient's dental procedures that is needed to create an insurance claim is found on the:
 a. remittance advice
 b. patient statement
 c. encounter form

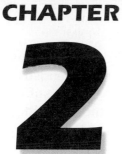

CHAPTER

2

Dental Services

OBJECTIVES

When you finish this chapter, you will be able to:

1. Locate and describe the parts of the mouth and the teeth.
2. Describe the major dental services that are covered by insurance carriers.
3. Discuss the categories of dental codes.

KEY TERMS

canines
cement
dental caries
dentin
enamel
endodontics
gingivae (sing., gingiva)
incisors
mandible
maxilla
maxillofacial surgery
molars
occlusion

oral cavity
oral surgery
orthodontics
palate
periodontics
premolars
prophylaxes
   (sing., prophylaxis)
prostheses
   (sing., prosthesis)
pulp
restorative services
uvula

Specific medical terms are used to describe oral (related to the mouth) anatomy, diagnoses, and treatments. In dentistry, the word elements of roots, combining vowels, prefixes, and suffixes are put together to describe the specific parts of the mouth and teeth as well as the procedures performed.

oral cavity *inner section of the mouth*

gingivae (sing., gingiva) *the gums*

The mouth, shown in Figure 2-1, is at the beginning of the digestive system. It has an outer part, made up of the lips and cheeks, and an inner section, or **oral cavity**, leading to the throat. The oral cavity contains the gums, called **gingivae**; the teeth; the tongue; and the tonsils.

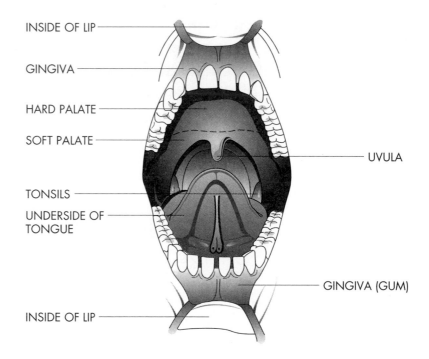

INSIDE OF LIP

GINGIVA

HARD PALATE

SOFT PALATE

UVULA

TONSILS

UNDERSIDE OF TONGUE

GINGIVA (GUM)

INSIDE OF LIP

Figure 2-1   The Mouth

mandible *lower jaw bone*

maxilla *upper jaw bone*

palate *the hard and soft tissues that make up the roof of the mouth*

uvula *the cone-shaped structure at the end of the soft palate*

The mouth's underlying bone structure also has two major parts. The **mandible**, the U-shaped lower jaw bone, has tooth sockets to hold the lower teeth. The upper jaw bone is the **maxilla**. It houses the upper teeth and the **palate**, which is the roof of the mouth. The hard palate is a bony structure that separates the oral cavity from the inner nose, or nasal cavity. The soft palate, made up of muscle tissue, is located behind the hard palate. The soft palate extends downward toward the throat, ending in the cone-shaped **uvula**.

The teeth tear and grind food, which is moistened by saliva from the salivary glands. The three major pairs of salivary glands are the parotid, submandibular, and sublingual. Saliva helps to soften food and contains an enzyme that begins the breakdown, or digestion, of food. When a person swallows, muscles pull the soft palate and uvula upward, closing the opening between the nasal cavity and the pharynx. This keeps food from entering the nasal cavity.

Saliva also helps to clean the cellular and food debris in the mouth and the teeth, to keep the soft parts of the mouth supple, and to buffer the acidity of the oral cavity. Lowered acidity helps to reduce **dental caries** (cavities).

dental caries common term for tooth decay

The 32 permanent teeth that adults have are set in two arches, one in the mandible and the other in the maxilla. Each of the jaws holds four **incisors**, which are the cutting teeth; two **canines**; four **premolars**; and six **molars**. Third molars, commonly called wisdom teeth, usually erupt between the ages of 17 and 21. Sometimes, however, they remain within the bone and do not erupt. These teeth are referred to as impacted, and they may need to be surgically removed.

incisors four of the 32 permanent adult teeth; the cutting teeth

canines two of the 32 permanent adult teeth

premolars four of the 32 permanent adult teeth; before the molars

molars six of the 32 permanent adult teeth; the grinding teeth

The upper and lower jaw bones are connected by a joint. When the jaws close, the contact between the upper and lower teeth is referred to as **occlusion**. The upper incisors are wider than the lower ones, so the lower grinding teeth are usually aligned slightly in front of the upper grinders. This arrangement helps the grinding movement between the upper and lower teeth.

occlusion the contact between the upper and lower teeth

Teeth are held in their sockets by connective tissue called periodontal ligaments. The fibers of the ligaments run from the bone to the cement of the tooth. This allows for some normal movement of teeth during chewing.

Figure 2-2 on page 22 shows the structure of a tooth. Each tooth is covered by an outer coating, the **enamel**, which is not sensitive. A hard material called **dentin**, which is very sensitive, fills up 80 to 90 percent of the tooth, covering the soft core, or **pulp**, which contains nerves and blood vessels. The **cement** is the boneline covering of the neck and root.

enamel the outer coating of the tooth

dentin the hard material that fills 80 to 90 percent of the tooth

pulp the soft core of the tooth containing the nerves and blood vessels

cement hard connective tissue covering the tooth root

A tooth has three main sections: the crown, the neck, and the root. The cavity that contains the pulp is called the root canal. The part that is covered with enamel is the crown. The neck is the section where the tooth meets the gum. The section below the gum line is the root. The gums are attached to the enamel of the tooth somewhere along the crown, but the gum line gradually recedes as people age. In elderly people, it may move far enough that the gum is attached to the cement rather than to the enamel.

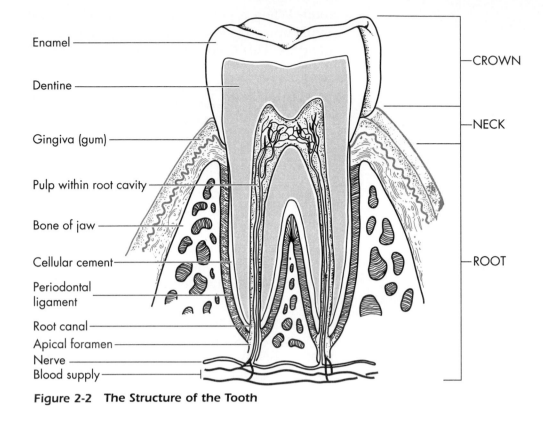

Figure 2-2 The Structure of the Tooth

Labels on figure:
Enamel
Dentine
Gingiva (gum)
Pulp within root cavity
Bone of jaw
Cellular cement
Periodontal ligament
Root canal
Apical foramen
Nerve
Blood supply

CROWN
NECK
ROOT

DENTAL CODES AND SERVICES

In dental insurance claims, the teeth are numbered from a person's right to left, upper to lower, as shown in Figure 2-3.

DENTAL CODE ORGANIZATION

Reporting dental procedures on dental claim forms is done with dental procedure codes. Dental codes begin with the letter *D* to make them different from numbers in other coding systems. The second number of the code indicates the category of dental service. There are twelve categories:

Category of Service	Code Series
I. Diagnostic	D0100 - D0999
II. Preventive	D1000 - D1999
III. Restorative	D2000 - D2999
IV. Endodontics	D3000 - D3999
V. Periodontics	D4000 - D4999
VI. Prosthodontics, removable	D5000 - D5899
VII. Maxillofacial Prosthetics	D5900 - D5999
VIII. Implant Services	D6000 - D6199
IX. Prosthodontics, fixed	D6200 - D6999
X. Oral Surgery	D7000 - D7999
XI. Orthodontics	D8000 - D8999
XII. Adjunctive General Services	D9000 - D9999

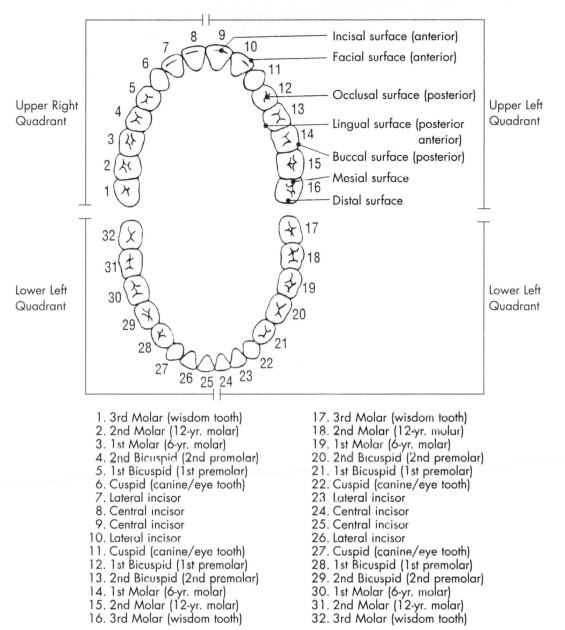

Figure 2-3   The Teeth

1. 3rd Molar (wisdom tooth)
2. 2nd Molar (12-yr. molar)
3. 1st Molar (6-yr. molar)
4. 2nd Bicuspid (2nd promolar)
5. 1st Bicuspid (1st premolar)
6. Cuspid (canine/eye tooth)
7. Lateral incisor
8. Central incisor
9. Central incisor
10. Lateral incisor
11. Cuspid (canine/eye tooth)
12. 1st Bicuspid (1st premolar)
13. 2nd Bicuspid (2nd premolar)
14. 1st Molar (6-yr. molar)
15. 2nd Molar (12-yr. molar)
16. 3rd Molar (wisdom tooth)

17. 3rd Molar (wisdom tooth)
18. 2nd Molar (12-yr. molar)
19. 1st Molar (6-yr. molar)
20. 2nd Bicuspid (2nd premolar)
21. 1st Bicuspid (1st premolar)
22. Cuspid (canine/eye tooth)
23. Lateral incisor
24. Central incisor
25. Central incisor
26. Lateral incisor
27. Cuspid (canine/eye tooth)
28. 1st Bicuspid (1st premolar)
29. 2nd Bicuspid (2nd premolar)
30. 1st Molar (6-yr. molar)
31. 2nd Molar (12-yr. molar)
32. 3rd Molar (wisdom tooth)

DENTAL SERVICES

Dental services that are covered by insurance carriers vary. Some of them include:

◆ Diagnostic Services—Diagnostic procedures, such as X rays and laboratory work, are used by the dentist to evaluate conditions and determine what dental treatment is needed.

◆ Preventive Services—These benefits cover **prophylaxes,** or cleanings, at regular intervals and the application of fluoride treatments to coat the teeth of children.

prophylaxes (sing., prophylaxis) prevention of disease by removal of calculus, stains, and other extraneous materials from the teeth; cleaning of teeth by dentist or dental hygienist

Many dental plans cover routine periodic examinations. For example, some plans cover a routine examination every six months. In order for insurance to cover the charge, the interval between appointments must be no less than six months and one day. For instance, appointments on March 3 and September 3 would be considered two visits in six months, and the second visit would not be covered.

restorative services dental procedures that repair the surface of the tooth

endodontics dental specialty that treats disease and injuries of the pulp

periodontics dental specialty that treats diseases of the supporting and surrounding tissues of the teeth

prostheses (sing., prosthesis) dental bridges and dentures

orthodontics dental specialty that treats malocclusion of the teeth and their surrounding structures

oral surgery surgical procedure related to the face and jaw

maxillofacial surgery surgical procedure related to the face and jaw

◆ Basic Services—Most plans cover **restorative services** such as fillings, crowns, and inlays; **endodontic** procedures such as root canal fillings; and **periodontic** procedures to prevent or treat gum disease.

◆ Prosthodontic Services—These cover the construction of bridges and dentures, called dental **prostheses**, and the repair of existing prosthetic appliances. Most dental contracts limit the number and timing of prosthesis replacements.

◆ **Orthodontic** Services—These cover the use of braces and other devices to straighten teeth. In plans covering orthodontic treatments, dates and months of treatment remaining affects the pro-rated monthly reimbursement made to the dentist.

◆ Oral and Maxillofacial Surgery—**Oral surgery** and **maxillofacial surgery**, which is a surgical procedure relating to the face and jaw, as well as the necessary general anesthesia are covered.

Carriers do not normally pay the same percentage for every type of procedure. For example, many plans cover the cost of prophylaxes and examinations in full, but they may pay from 50 to 90 percent of other procedures.

Note that a series of treatments is one that is planned to be done over a number of appointments. The date of the first visit is important in determining what services are covered when a patient becomes eligible in the middle of an active treatment plan.

CHAPTER REVIEW

USING TERMINOLOGY

Match the terms on the left with the definitions on the right.

1. canines

2. dentin

3. enamel

4. endodontics

5. gingivae

6. incisors

7. mandible

8. maxilla

9. maxillofacial surgery

10. molars

11. occlusion

12. oral cavity

13. oral surgery

14. orthodontics

15. palate

16. periodontics

17. premolars

18. prophylaxes

19. prostheses

20. pulp

21. restorative services

22. uvula

a. The cone-shaped structure at the end of the soft palate.

b. Dental bridges and dentures.

c. Surgical procedure related to the face and jaw.

d. The outer coating of the tooth.

e. Six of the 32 permanent adult teeth.

f. The lower jaw bone.

g. The hard material that fills 80 to 90 percent of the tooth.

h. Branch of dentistry concerned with the diseases of the pulp.

i. Four of the 32 permanent adult teeth; the cutting teeth.

j. The upper jaw bone.

k. Two of the 32 permanent adult teeth.

l. Surgical procedure related to the face and jaw.

m. The soft core of the tooth containing the nerves and blood vessels.

n. Branch of dentistry concerned with correcting irregularities of the teeth.

o. The inner section of the mouth.

p. Four of the 32 permanent adult teeth; before the molars.

q. The contact between the upper and lower teeth.

r. The gums.

s. Branch of dentistry concerned with fillings, crowns, and inlays.

t. Branch of dentistry that deals with diseases of the gums.

u. The roof of the mouth.

v. Dental procedure to clean the teeth.

CHAPTER REVIEW

CHECK YOUR UNDERSTANDING

Choose the best answer.

23. On a dental claim form, a treated tooth is indicated by:
  a. the name of the tooth
  b. the letter of the tooth
  c. the number of the tooth

24. A regular cleaning of the teeth by a dentist to prevent disease is called:
  a. prosthesis
  b. prophylaxis
  c. impaction

25. A set of dentures is a:
  a. prosthesis
  b. prophylaxis
  c. impaction

26. In general, claims for dental treatments require:
  a. diagnostic codes
  b. procedure codes
  c. neither a nor b

27. CDT codes begin with:
  a. a C
  b. an R
  c. a D

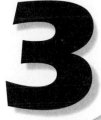

CHAPTER

3

The Role of Computers in the Dental Office

OBJECTIVES

When you finish this chapter, you will be able to:

1. Describe how dental offices use computers to accomplish daily tasks.
2. Discuss common applications of computer systems in the dental office, including scheduling, accounting, records, e-mail, and the Internet.
3. List the advantages that computers offer over traditional paper methods in the dental practice.

KEY TERMS

audit/edit report
clearinghouse
database
e-commerce

electronic funds transfer (EFT)
electronic media claim (EMC)
walkout receipt

INTRODUCTION

In the past, most of the administrative work carried out in the dental office involved paper. Appointments were recorded in scheduling books, insurance claims were printed on paper forms, and dentists' schedules were often prepared with handwritten notes. All this paper had to be filed and stored.

Today, the trend is to use computers for the storage, retrieval, and transmission of health information. Most dental offices use computers to perform a variety of administrative tasks. Information is entered into a computer program that is structured as a collection of related facts called a **database**. A dental office computer database stores information about the practice's dentists, patients, insurance carriers, procedure codes, charges, and payments. Computers are used to verify insurance eligibility, produce insurance claims, store and retrieve dental records, create financial reports, accept electronic payments, schedule appointments, handle payroll, prepare referral letters, and other tasks. Computer literacy has become a basic requirement for employment in an administrative position in a dental office.

database a collection of related facts

A TYPICAL DAY IN A COMPUTERIZED DENTAL PRACTICE

To understand the role that computers play in today's dental office, consider a typical day in a computerized dental office. At the beginning of each day, the computer is used to print a listing of that day's appointments for each dentist in the practice (see Figure 3-1). New appointments are booked during the day using an electronic scheduling program. As each patient arrives, new or revised data on patient information forms, such as patients' addresses, insurance plans, and allergies, are keyed into the computer. Insurance eligibility is verified over the Internet or directly with the carrier via modem.

As the dentists see patients, procedures and services are recorded on computer-generated encounter forms. Some dentists record clinical notes as they work, and the notes are transferred to the computer later. When an office visit is completed, information from the encounter form is entered into the computerized billing program. If the patient has made a payment, the computer prints a **walkout receipt**, which lists the charges and the amount paid by the patient (see Figure 3-2).

walkout receipt a completed form a patient receives after an encounter that lists the services provided, fees, and payments received and due

Collier Family Dental Care   Monday, November 12, 2007

Miller, Harold

Time	Name	Phone	Length	Notes
8:00a	Staff Meeting		60	
				Every week on Mon
11:00a	Sanchez, Melanie SANCHME0	(941)777-6666	30	
1:45p	Louise Grass	(941)555-3604	30	
2:30p	Barlow, Daniel H BARLODA0	(941)444-2222	60	
3:30p	Elllison, John ELLISJO0	(941)444-4444	30	
4:00p	Rossi, Sheila ROSSISH0	(941)777-5555	15	
4:15p	Klinger, Russell R KLINGRU0	(941)777-1111	30	

Figure 3-1   Sample computerized appointment schedule

Collier Family Dental Care
Medical/Dental Arts Building
Naples, FL 34104-8756
(941)555-8900

Statement Date	Page
9/6/2007	1

Jack M. Spacek
75 Northford Blvd.
Naples, FL 34102

Chart Number
SPACEJA0

Date	Document	Description	Case Number	Amount
Date of Last Payment: 9/6/2007		Amount: -15.00	Previous Balance:	0.00
Patient: Jack M. Spacek		Chart #: SPACEJA0	Case Description: Preventive	
9/6/2007	0709060000	prophylaxis--adult	31	60.00
9/6/2007	0709060000	bitewings--four X rays	31	25.00
9/6/2007	0709060000	Sunshine Copayment	31	15.00
9/6/2007	0709060000	Cash copayment $15	31	-15.00

Figure 3-2   Sample walkout receipt

Insurance claims are created in a billing program, and the dental office assistant uses the computer to electronically transmit the claims to insurance carriers for payment or to print paper claims. Once a claim has been processed by the insurance company, payment is transmitted electronically to the practice's bank account or mailed to the practice. Claim information is also sent from the carrier to the practice and recorded in the computer. The patient is then billed for any remaining balance. At the end of the day, reports are printed showing the daily activity of the practice—the number of patient visits, the diagnosis and procedure codes used, the fees charged, and the payments received. At the end of the month, financial reports are created and analyzed.

DENTAL OFFICE APPLICATIONS

The tasks listed in Table 3-1 are performed on a regular basis in most dental offices. In each instance, the task can be completed more efficiently with the use of a specialized computer application. Each computer application is discussed separately in the following sections.

Table 3-1   Computer Applications in a Dental Office

TASK	COMPUTER APPLICATION
Scheduling	Scheduling application: Scheduling appointments and producing recall notices
Dental Records	Recording and storing chart notes, procedures, etc.
Accounting	Billing/accounting application: Entering transactions, creating and processing pretreatment estimates and actual claims, billing patients, receiving electronic payments, generating financial reports
Correspondence	Written documents or e-mail: Sending referral letters, patient recall notices, etc.
Inventory/Supplies	E-commerce: Ordering office and dental supplies and equipment

SCHEDULING Computers are often used to keep track of dentists' schedules. Appointments can easily be canceled or moved to a different day. Computers can also print a daily list of appointments for each provider in the practice. Recurring appointments can be booked for future dates, such as once a week for the next six weeks. In addition, patient recall appointment notices can be generated on a timely basis.

One of the major advantages of computerized scheduling is the ability to easily locate scheduled appointments. For example, suppose a patient calls to ask when his or her next appointment is scheduled. Instead of searching page by page in a schedule book, the dental office assistant enters the patient's name in a search box, and the computer locates the appointment.

Computer scheduling also simplifies the entry of repeated appointments. Rather than looking through an appointment book for acceptable dates and times, the computer performs the search and displays available dates and times. Computer scheduling programs are also used to store information about time reserved for surgeries, seminars, appointments, and days out of the office.

DENTAL RECORDS Patients' dental records may be stored in a computer instead of on paper, offering substantial benefits to the practice. One of the most important aspects of an electronic dental record is instant access to data. A patient's entire dental history, including dentist notes, extractions, test results, and X rays, is part of an electronic dental record.

Storing patient records on the computer also raises the issue of computer security and the confidentiality of patient records. Everyone working in a dental office is responsible for maintaining patient confidentiality. The federal law known as HIPAA (the Health Insurance Portability and Accountability Act) requires all health care providers, including dental practices, to protect confidential patient records. This is important because dental records also contain other pertinent medical information about patients.

ACCOUNTING Like other businesses, dental offices keep track of accounts receivable, or payments coming in from patients and insurance carriers, and accounts payable, or amounts owed to suppliers and staff. Keeping accurate financial records is critical to a practice's survival. Not only are accurate records needed to meet financial obligations, but they are also required for tax reporting purposes. As in any business, accurate financial reports let management know whether the dental office is profitable.

Computerized accounting programs perform the tasks that were accomplished manually in the past. Dental offices may use different computerized accounting systems to keep track of their finances, but all accounting systems require certain types of information:

◆ **Patient Data** Personal information about the patient, as well as information on the patient's insurance coverage, is extracted from the program's patient database.

◆ **Transaction Data** Transaction information is taken from the encounter form and keyed into the computer program. It includes the date of the visit, procedure codes, and payments.

From these sources of information, patient statements are generated, insurance claims are created, and reports on the financial health of the practice are produced.

Insurance Claims

One of the major uses of computer technology in the dental office is to create insurance claims. A computerized system automatically generates completed insurance forms. The forms can be printed or transmitted electronically. By comparison, when a manual system is used, the dental office assistant must first compile all the needed resources and then key all the data on the claim form. This process takes longer and is more likely to create processing errors.

PractiSoft, the computerized dental billing system used in *Computers in the Dental Office*, is one example of a computer program used in the dental office to process insurance claims. Processing information to create completed insurance claim forms is one of the main functions of programs such as PractiSoft. Three major steps are followed to create insurance claims using PractiSoft: (1) setting up the practice, (2) entering transaction information, and (3) creating and transmitting the completed insurance claim form.

Before a dental practice opens its doors to patients, a lot of preparation must be done. Equipment, supplies, staff, and procedures all need to be readied. Similarly, before PractiSoft is used to store information about patients and their visits, basic facts about the practice itself are entered. The information includes dentists' names, tax identification numbers, the practice name, the address, and phone numbers. Often a computer consultant or an accountant helps set up PractiSoft's records about the practice. Then the provider database is entered, including descriptions of each dentist's office hours and facts about referring dentists and lab services. Finally, the insurance carrier database is entered. It contains information about the carriers that most patients use. Each database in PractiSoft is linked, or related, to each of the others by having at least one fact in common.

When a patient visits a dentist, information about the visit is collected on the patient information form and the encounter form. After analyzing and checking the data, the dental office assistant enters each element in the computer program. A new record must be created for a new patient, and information on established patients may need to be updated. Next, the appropriate insurance carrier for the visit is selected. Then the purposes of the visit and the procedure codes are entered, with the appropriate charges.

When all transaction information has been entered and checked, the dental office assistant issues the command to PractiSoft to create an insurance claim form. The format for the claim—usually the ADA Dental Claim Form—is also designated. PractiSoft organizes the necessary databases and selects the data from each database to produce a complete claim form. The program follows the instructions to print or transmit the form electronically to the designated receiver.

Electronic Processing

electronic media claim (EMC) an insurance claim that is sent by a computer over data communication lines

An **electronic media claim (EMC)** is an insurance claim that is sent by a computer over a telephone line using a modem. Electronic claim filing has several advantages. First, filing and processing claims electronically takes less time than processing paper forms. In addition, filing electronically costs less; the costs of paper forms, envelopes, and postage are higher than the costs of transmission over phone lines. Chances of error or omission are reduced because information is entered once, not twice. In the case of paper forms, information also has to be entered into the insurance company's computer when the forms arrive by mail.

electronic funds transfer (EFT) a system that transfers monies electronically from one account to another

Usually, EMCs are paid more quickly than paper claims. Another advantage for the practice of submitting an EMC is **electronic funds transfer (EFT)**. This capability, which is an optional part of most EMC processing systems, allows for payments to be deposited directly into the provider's bank account.

Problems with EMCs usually result when transmission failures occur as a result of power outages. Transmission problems may also result from the breakdown of computer equipment. In these cases, the remedy is to retransmit missing claims after the problem is solved.

clearinghouse a service company that receives electronic/paper claims from providers and transmits them in proper data format to carriers

Electronic media claims can be sent directly to an insurance carrier, or they can be sent to a **clearinghouse**. A clearinghouse is a service bureau that collects electronic insurance claims from many different dental practices and forwards them to payers. Clearinghouses translate claim data to fit the setup of each carrier's claims processing department. Many dental practices choose to use a clearinghouse instead of transmitting claims directly to insurance carriers.

audit/edit report response from a receiver to a sender regarding the status and completeness of a transmitted claim

When a clearinghouse receives a claim, it checks to see that all necessary information is included. An **audit/edit report** is used to inform the dental office of problems that need to be corrected (see Figure 3-3 on page 35). This reduces the number of claim rejections by insurance carriers and speeds the processing and payment of claims.

CORRESPONDENCE

Like other businesses, dental offices use computers to produce written correspondence, reports, forms, and other documents. These documents can be printed and mailed, or they can be sent via e-mail. Correspondence that normally took several days can now be transmitted in a matter of seconds. Documents are stored electronically, which greatly reduces the amount of storage space required. Once again, practices that use e-mail must have security measures in place to safeguard patient confidentiality.

INVENTORY/ SUPPLIES

e-commerce the exchange of monies over the Internet

The Internet is being used by some practices to order dental supplies and equipment. **E-commerce**—the exchange of funds over the Internet—allows offices to purchase supplies online at a discount from the standard price, since there is no middleman or distributor in the transaction. These discounts can save the practice a significant amount of money over the course of a year.

ADVANTAGES OF COMPUTERS

In a dentist's practice, there are a number of advantages to performing tasks with a computer instead of on paper. First, with a computer database, all the information is located in one place. Pieces of paper and forms are not located in different file cabinets in the office; they are all stored on one computer system.

In addition, computer data can be used by more than one person at a time. If an office has more than one computer, the computers can be linked together in a network, which allows them to share files in the central database. In an office without a computer database, it is difficult for someone to update a document if another person is working on it.

Another advantage of computer databases is the simplicity of conducting a search for information. Instead of having to look in different file cabinets and folders, a search can be conducted by just entering a few keystrokes. In a very short time, the information is retrieved and displayed on the computer screen.

Computers also eliminate the need for large amounts of physical storage space, since much of the information is stored in the computer, not on paper.

Computer databases are more efficient than manual filing systems. Computers save enormous amounts of time in a dental practice. For example, when dental records are stored electronically, a staff member does not have to pull patient charts at the start of each day and refile them at the end of the day.

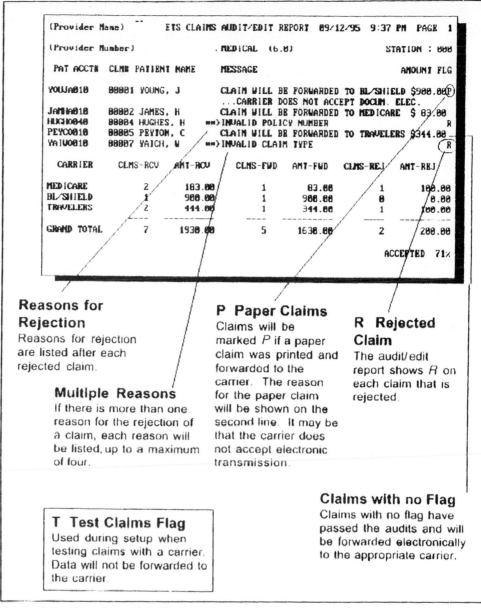

Figure 3-3 Sample audit/edit report

From an administrative perspective, the most significant use of the computer in the dental office is to create and process insurance claim forms. When preparing patients' claims, the computer selects information from its databases to create an electronic file of the information needed to complete the claim forms. Those claim forms can then be printed or transmitted electronically.

Bringing computers into the dental office has greatly increased productivity, primarily because computers are much more efficient at processing large amounts of data than human beings. Tasks that would take minutes for a person to complete can be done by the computer in a matter of seconds. For example, suppose a dental practice has four dentists and hundreds of patients. The phone rings, and a patient would like to know the amount owed on an account. With a computerized billing program in place, the dental office assistant might simply key the first few letters of the patient's last name into the computer, causing the patient's account to appear on the screen. The outstanding balance could then be communicated to the patient.

In another example, suppose the wrong procedure code has been entered on an insurance claim form, and the claim has been rejected by the insurance carrier. To resubmit the claim without the use of a computer might require the entire form to be completed again by hand. However, if the dental office uses a computerized billing program, the error can be quickly corrected and a new form either printed or submitted electronically.

Computers not only make the dental office more efficient, they also reduce errors. Information is entered once, then used over and over. If the information is entered correctly the first time, it will be correct every time it is used. For example, information such as the patient's address and insurance policy number is entered in the computer once. The computer stores the information, and when the information is needed to fill out a claim form, the computer locates it and uses it to complete the task, such as printing a completed claim form. The next time a claim needs to be created, the computer goes through the same process, using the same information. Without a computer, someone would have to enter all the information on an insurance form each time a claim was being submitted for the patient. Not only does this consume more time, but it introduces the possibility of error every time the information has to be rekeyed.

While computers do increase the efficiency of the dental office and reduce errors, they are not more accurate than the individual entering the data. If human errors occur while entering the information, the data coming out of the computer will be incorrect. Computers are very precise, but may be very unforgiving. If a computer operator accidentally enters a name as "ORourke" instead of "O'Rourke," a person might know what is meant; the computer does not. It would probably respond with a message such as "No such patient exists in the database."

Most human errors occur during data entry, such as pressing the wrong key on the keyboard, or because of the lack of computer literacy—not knowing how to use a program to accomplish the tasks. For this reason, proper training in data-entry techniques and the use of computer programs is essential for dental office personnel who are working with computers.

CHAPTER REVIEW

USING TERMINOLOGY

Match the terms on the left with the definitions on the right.

1. audit/edit report

2. clearinghouse

3. database

4. e-commerce

5. electronic funds transfer (EFT)

6. electronic media claim (EMC)

7. walkout receipt

a. An insurance claim that is sent by a computer over a telephone line using a modem.

b. A system that transfers money electronically from one account to another.

c. The exchange of funds over the Internet.

d. A service bureau that collects electronic insurance claims and forwards them to the appropriate insurance carriers.

e. A report from a clearinghouse that lists errors that need to be corrected before a claim can be submitted to the insurance carrier.

f. A document listing charges and payments that is given to a patient after an office visit.

g. A collection of related facts.

CHECKING YOUR UNDERSTANDING

Write "T" or "F" in the blank to indicate whether you think the statement is true or false.

_____ **8.** Computerized scheduling makes it easier to reschedule appointments in a dental office.

_____ **9.** Online databases store personal information on patients.

_____ **10.** A federal law, HIPAA, protects the privacy of a patient's dental records.

_____ **11.** Electronic media claims are usually paid in about the same number of days as claims submitted on paper forms.

_____ **12.** Clearinghouses perform audits of claim data before transmitting them to insurance carriers.

Answer the question below in the space provided.

13. List two advantages of using computers in the dental office.

_____

_____

Choose the best answer.

14. Electronic remittance advice (ERA) is:
   a. the electronic transfer of funds from one bank account to another
   b. a report from a clearinghouse listing any errors in a claim
   c. an electronic explanation of benefits

15. E-commerce allows dental practices to:
   a. track changes in computer data by individual users
   b. purchase supplies over the Internet
   c. safeguard confidential patient dental records that are stored on a computer

PractiSoft
Advanced
Training

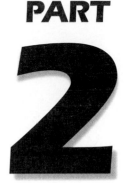

PART
2

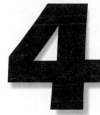

CHAPTER 4

Introduction to PractiSoft

WHAT YOU NEED TO KNOW

To use this chapter, you need to know how to:

◆ Start your computer and Microsoft Windows version 98 or later.
◆ Use the keyboard and mouse.

OBJECTIVES

When you finish this chapter, you will be able to:

1. Start PractiSoft.
2. Restore the backup file on the Student Data Disk to the hard drive.
3. Move around the PractiSoft menus.
4. Use the PractiSoft toolbar.
5. Enter, edit, and save data in PractiSoft.
6. Delete data.
7. Use PractiSoft's Help feature.
8. Make a backup copy of the database files while exiting PractiSoft.

KEY TERMS

backup data
knowledge base
MMDDCCYY format

status bar help
transactions

WHAT IS PRACTISOFT?

PractiSoft is a dental patient accounting software program. Information on patients, providers, insurance carriers, and patient and insurance billing is stored and processed by the system. Programs such as PractiSoft are widely used by dental practices throughout the United States. They are typically used to accomplish the following daily work in a dental office:

- Enter information on new patients, and change information on established patients as needed.
- Enter transactions, such as charges, to patients' accounts.
- Record payments and adjustments from patients and insurance companies.
- Print walkout receipts and statements for patients.
- Submit insurance claims to carriers.
- Print standard reports, and create custom reports.
- Schedule appointments.

Many of the general working concepts used in operating PractiSoft are similar to those in other software programs. Thus, you should be able to transfer many skills taught in this book to other dental patient accounting programs.

HOW PRACTISOFT DATA ARE ORGANIZED AND STORED

Information entered into PractiSoft is stored in databases. As defined in Chapter 3, a database is a collection of related pieces of information.

PRACTISOFT DATABASES

PractiSoft stores these major types of data:

- **Provider Data** The provider database has information about the dentist(s) as well as the practice, such as its name and address, phone number, and tax identification number.
- **Patient Data** Each patient information form is stored in the patient database. The patient's unique chart number and personal information—name and address, phone number, birth date, Social Security number, gender, marital status, and employer—are examples of information stored in this database.
- **Insurance Carriers** The insurance carrier database contains the names, addresses, and other data about each insurance carrier used by patients, such as the type of plan. Usually, this database also contains information on each carrier's electronic media claim (EMC) submission.

- **Procedure Codes** The procedure code database contains the data needed to create charges. The *Current Dental Terminology* (CDT) codes most often used by the practice are selected for this database. The practice's encounter form is often a good source document for these codes. Other claim data elements, such as the charge for each procedure, are also stored in the procedure code database.

- **Transactions** The transaction database stores information about each patient's visits and procedures, as well as received and outstanding payments. **Transactions** in the form of charges, payments, and adjustments are also stored in the transaction database.

transactions *charges, payments, and adjustments*

Within PractiSoft, each database is linked, or related, to each of the others by having at least one fact in common. For example, information entered in the patient database is shared with the transaction database, linking the two. Information is entered only once; PractiSoft selects data from each database as needed.

THE STUDENT DATA DISK

The Student Data Disk located inside the back cover contains a set of database files for Collier Family Dental Care, the dental practice used in the examples and exercises throughout this book. Before a dental office begins using PractiSoft, basic information about the practice and its patients must be entered in the computer. This preliminary work has been done for you on the Student Data Disk. The files have been compressed into a backup file that will be restored to the hard drive in Exercise 4-1.

MAKING A COPY OF THE STUDENT DATA DISK

Before you begin using the Student Data Disk, make a copy of it for safekeeping following the instructions below. When you are finished making the disk copy, store the original Student Data Disk in a safe place. You may need to use the original disk to restore the database files if your working files are accidentally damaged or lost.

NOTE: These instructions assume that Windows 98 or a later version is installed on your computer.

1. Turn on the computer and monitor.

2. After the Windows desktop is displayed, insert the Student Data Disk in the 3 1/2" floppy drive (drive A).

3. Double-click the My Computer icon on the desktop. The My Computer window is displayed.

4. Click the icon labeled "3 1/2 Floppy (A:)."

5. On the File menu, click Copy Disk. The Copy Disk dialog box is displayed.

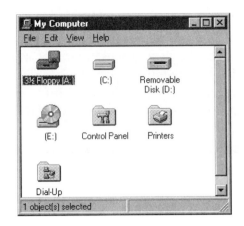

6. The Copy From and Copy To windows should both have "3 1/2 Floppy (A:)" highlighted. If they are not highlighted, click 3 1/2 Floppy (A:) in both the Copy From and Copy To windows.

7. Click the Start button. The computer begins reading the files on the source disk. You can monitor the computer's progress by viewing the bar above the words "Reading source disk."

8. When the system prompts you to insert the disk you want to copy to (the destination disk), eject the Student Data Disk from the drive.

9. Insert a blank disk in the floppy drive, and click the OK button. The files are copied to the destination disk. Again, you can monitor the progress by looking at the bar above the words "Writing to destination disk."

10. When the copy is completed, the message "Copy completed successfully" is displayed. Eject the disk from the drive, and label it "Working Copy Collier Backup File."

11. Close the Copy Disk dialog box by clicking the Close button.

12. Close the My Computer dialog box by clicking the Close button (in this case, the X in the upper right corner).

The following exercise takes you through the steps of starting the PractiSoft program and restoring the backup file of the Collier Family Dental Care database from the Student Data Disk onto the hard drive for future use.

EXERCISE 4-1

The following steps should only be followed the first time PractiSoft is used with this text. The exercise is designed to start the program, create a new directory and data set name for the Collier Family Dental Care files on the hard drive, and restore the backup file to the new directory.

TIP . . . PractiSoft is programmed to open whatever database files it used during the previous session automatically. Therefore, in all subsequent exercises, you can start PractiSoft simply by double-clicking the PractiSoft Advanced Dental Patient Accounting icon on the desktop and the required data set will load automatically.

1. While holding down the F7 key, Click Start, Programs, PractiSoft, PractiSoft Advanced Dental Patient Accounting to start PractiSoft. When the Find PractiSoft Database dialog box appears, release the F7 key. (The F7 key bypasses any starting directions that may have been left in the program by a previous user.) This dialog box asks you to enter the PractiSoft data directory.

2. Click the bar that reads "Find PractiSoft Database" at the top of the dialog box to make the dialog box active. (If you do not do so, your keystrokes will not appear in the white box.) Key *C:\PractiData* in the space provided. The dialog box should now look like the one shown below on the left.

3. Click the OK button. An Information dialog box appears with the following message, "This is not an existing root data directory. Do you want to create a new one?"

4. Click Yes. The Create Data dialog box is displayed.

Find PractiSoft Database

Cannot connect to the PractiSoft data directory. Enter the PractiSoft data directory.

C:\PractiData

✓ OK
Browse
✗ Cancel

Create Data

Do you want to

Create a new set of data

Convert existing MediSoft Data

☐ Add tutorial data to list

✗ Cancel

5. Click the Create a New Set of Data button. The Create a New Set of Data dialog box appears. In the upper box, key *Collier Family Dental Care*. In the lower box, key *Collier*. The dialog box should now look like this:

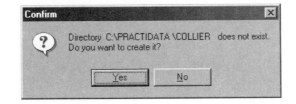

6. Click the Create button. A Confirm dialog box is displayed.

7. Click the Yes button. The Practice Information dialog box appears. In the Practice Name box, key *Collier Family Dental Care*. For the purposes of this text, the remaining boxes can remain blank. The dialog box should now look like this:

8. Click the Save button. The main window of the PractiSoft program is displayed. Your screen should look similar to this:

Note: If a side bar menu with four options appears on the left side of the screen, press CTRL + S to close it, as it is not required for the purposes of this text.

9. Insert the working copy of the Student Data Disk in the floppy drive. (This is usually the A: drive; if your computer uses a different letter to represent the floppy drive, please substitute that letter for "A:" whenever it appears in these instructions.)

10. Open the File menu (the first option on the menu bar at the top of the screen) and locate the Restore Data option.

11. Click Restore Data. A Warning dialog box is displayed.

12. Click the OK button. The Restore dialog box is displayed. In the top box, key A:\Collier.mbk. The Restore dialog box should now look like this:

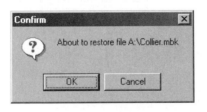

13. Click the Start Restore button. A Confirm dialog box is displayed.

14. Click the OK button. After the program restores the database to the hard drive, an information dialog box is displayed, indicating that the restore is complete. Click OK.

15. You are returned to the main PractiSoft window. To open the newly restored data, open the File menu and click the Open Practice option.

16. The Open Practice dialog box is displayed, with the Collier Family Dental Care practice name listed.

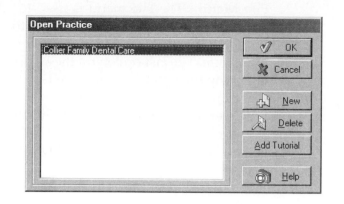

17. To open the Collier database files, click the OK button.

18. The main PractiSoft window is displayed again. The database is now ready for use. (*Hint:* If the main PractiSoft window does not fill the screen, click the Maximize button to expand it. The Maximize button is the middle of the three small buttons displayed in upper-right corner of the window.)

19. For now, keep the PractiSoft program open, as it is required to complete the remaining exercises in the chapter.

THE BASICS OF USING PRACTISOFT

To begin using PractiSoft, it is necessary to have a basic understanding of how to:

♦ Use the PractiSoft menu bar
♦ Use the PractiSoft toolbar
♦ Enter, edit, save, and delete data
♦ Use the PractiSoft Help feature
♦ Back up PractiSoft data while exiting the program
♦ Restore a backup file if required.

THE PRACTISOFT MENU BAR

PractiSoft offers choices of actions through a series of menus. Commands are issued by clicking an option on the menu bar or by clicking a shortcut button on the toolbar. The menu bar lists the names of the menus in PractiSoft: File, Edit, Activities, Lists, Reports, Tools, Window, and Help (see Figure 4-1). Beneath each menu name is a pull-down menu of one or more options.

File Edit Activities Lists Reports Tools Window Help

Figure 4-1   PractiSoft menu bar.

File Menu   The File menu is used to enter information about the dental office practice. It is also used to back up data, restore data, change program options, set security options, and change the program date. The last option on the File menu, Exit, provides one way of exiting the PractiSoft program (see Figure 4-2).

Edit Menu   The Edit menu contains the basic commands needed to move, change, or delete information (see Figure 4-3). These commands are Cut, Copy, Paste, and Delete.

Activities Menu   Most dental office data collected on a day-to-day basis are entered through options on the Activities menu (see Figure 4-4). This menu is used to enter financial transactions, create insurance claims, enter and manage dentists' pretreatment estimates, view summaries of patient account information, calculate billing charges, access Office Hours, PractiSoft's built-in appointment scheduler, and manage credit card payments. Financial transactions include charges, payments, and adjustments.

Lists Menu   Information on new patients, such as name, address, and employer, is entered through the Patients/Guarantors and Cases option on the Lists menu (see Figure 4-5). If information needs to be changed for an established patient, it is also updated through this option. The Lists menu also provides access to lists of patient treatment plans, codes, insurance carriers, providers, and contacts. These lists may be updated and printed when necessary.

Reports Menu   The Reports menu is used to print reports about patients' accounts and practice reports (see Figure 4-6). PractiSoft comes with a number of standard report formats, such as day sheets, aging reports, and patient ledgers, as well as a superbill option and a variety of custom reports. Custom reports range from a patient recall list, to insurance forms, to a patient birthday list and labels. Practices may also create their own report formats using the Design Custom Reports and Bills option.

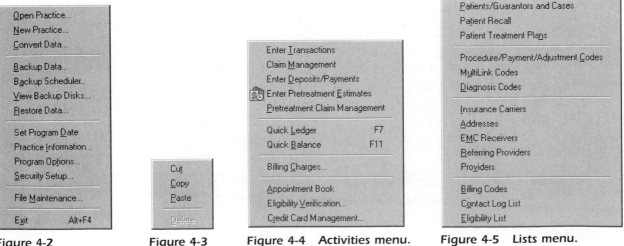

Figure 4-2
File menu.

Figure 4-3
Edit menu.

Figure 4-4   Activities menu.

Figure 4-5   Lists menu.

Tools Menu   The built-in calculator is accessed through the Tools menu. Other options on the Tools menu can be used to view the contents of a file as well as a profile of the computer system (see Figure 4-7). There is also an option for customizing the menu bars. By default, PractiSoft displays the menu bar and toolbar. A blue side bar can also be displayed containing five options. Each option groups similar tasks, for example, patient management, into a submenu that opens up to the right. Any of the three menu bars can be customized through the Tools menu. The side bar can be turned on or off by clicking the Show Side Bar option on the Window Menu.

Window Menu   When more than one window is open at a time, the Window menu can be used to close or minimize all open windows with a single keystroke. The Window menu also contains options for changing the arrangement of open windows—windows can be tiled horizontally or vertically. Other options are used to reset all closed windows to their default positions or to toggle the side bar on or off. Using the Window menu, it is also possible to switch back and forth between several open windows. For example, if the Transaction Entry dialog box and the Patient List dialog box were both open, the Window menu would look like the menu in Figure 4-8.

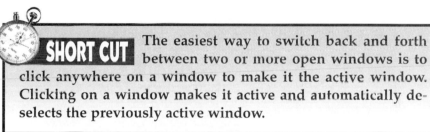

SHORT CUT   The easiest way to switch back and forth between two or more open windows is to click anywhere on a window to make it the active window. Clicking on a window makes it active and automatically deselects the previously active window.

Help Menu   The Help menu, shown in Figure 4-9, is used to access PractiSoft's built-in Help feature. It also provides a link to MediSoft support on the World Wide Web. MediSoft is the company that produces and supports PractiSoft. Another option on the Help menu is used to obtain free online program updates.

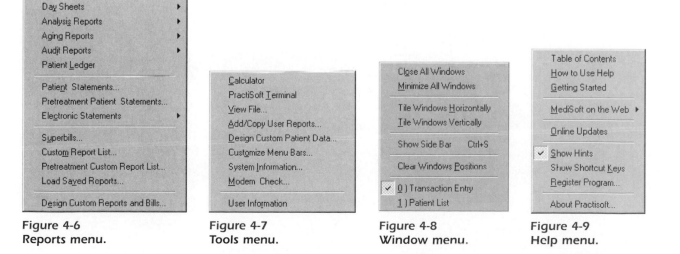

Figure 4-6
Reports menu.

Figure 4-7
Tools menu.

Figure 4-8
Window menu.

Figure 4-9
Help menu.

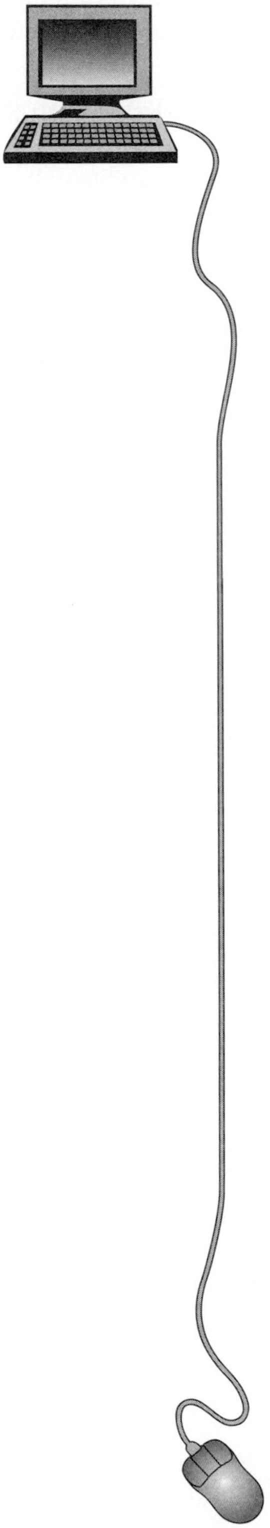

Practice using the PractiSoft menus.

1. If it is not already open, start the PractiSoft program.

2. Click the Lists menu on the menu bar.

3. Click Patients/Guarantors and Cases. The Patient List dialog box is displayed (see Figure 4-10).

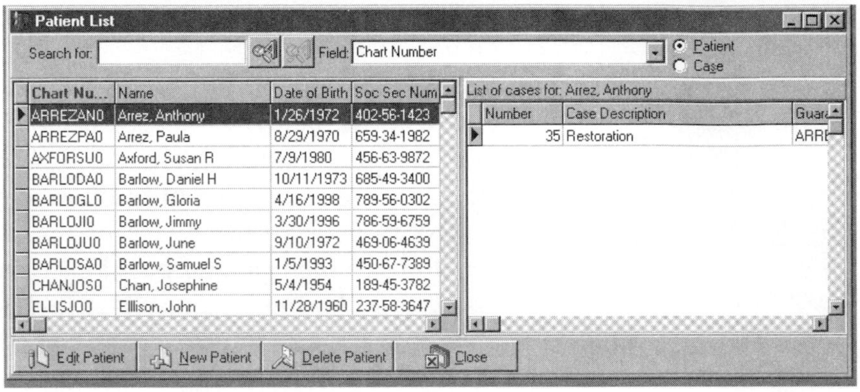

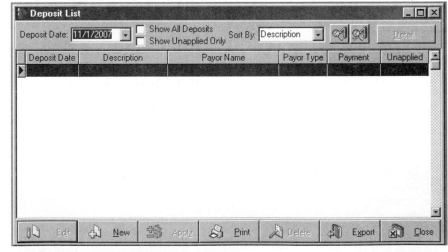

Figure 4-10   Patient List dialog box.

4. Click the Close button at the bottom of the dialog box.

5. Click the Activities menu.

6. Click Enter Deposits/Payments. The Deposit List dialog box is displayed (see Figure 4-11).

Figure 4-11   Deposit List dialog box.

7. Click the Close button.

THE PRACTISOFT TOOLBAR

Located below the menu bar, the toolbar contains a series of icons that represent the most common activities performed in PractiSoft. These buttons are shortcuts for frequently used menu commands. The toolbar displays 21 icons (see Figure 4-12 and Table 4-1).

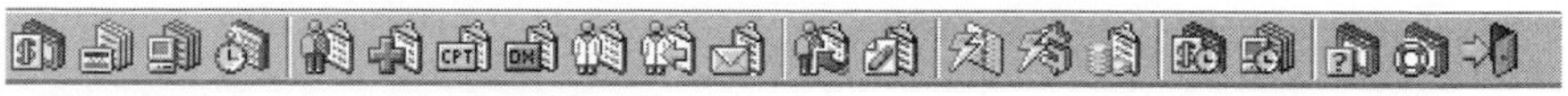

Figure 4-12   PractiSoft toolbar.

Table 4-1   Toolbar Buttons

BUTTON	BUTTON NAME	ASSOCIATED FUNCTION	ACTIVITY
	Transaction Entry	Transaction Entry dialog box	Enter transactions.
	Credit Card Management	Credit Card Management dialog box	Process credit card transactions.
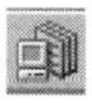	Claim Management	Claim Management dialog box	Create and send insurance claims.
	Appointment Book	Office Hours	Schedule appointments.
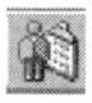	Patient List	Patient List dialog box	Enter and edit patient information.
	Insurance Carrier List	Insurance Carrier List dialog box	Add, edit, or delete insurance carriers.
	Procedure Code List	Procedure/Payment/ Adjustment List dialog box	Add, edit, or delete procedure, payment, and adjustment codes.
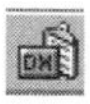	Diagnosis Code List	Diagnosis List dialog box	Add, edit, or delete diagnosis codes.
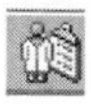	Provider List	Provider List dialog box	Add, edit, or delete providers.
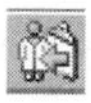	Referring Provider List	Referring Provider List dialog box	Add, edit, or delete referring providers.
	Address List	Address List dialog box	Add, edit, or delete addresses.
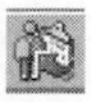	Patient Recall Entry	Patient Recall dialog box	Add a patient to the recall list.
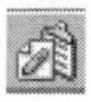	Custom Report List	Open Report dialog box	Display or print reports.

Table 4-1 Toolbar Buttons *(cont.)*

BUTTON	BUTTON NAME	ASSOCIATED FUNCTION	ACTIVITY
	Quick Ledger	Quick Ledger dialog box	View data in patient ledger.
	Quick Balance	Quick Balance dialog box	View patient account balance.
	Enter Deposits and Apply Payments	Deposit List dialog box	Enter deposits and apply payments.
	Pretreatment Transaction Entry	Pretreatment Plan/ Estimate dialog box	Prepare a pretreatment estimate.
	Pretreatment Claim Management	Claim Management— Pretreatment Plan/Estimate dialog box	Prepare a pretreatment claim.
	Show/Hide Hints	Balloon help	Turn the Hints feature on or off.
	Help	Contents dialog box	Access PractiSoft's built-in help files.
	Exit Program	Exit	Exit the PractiSoft program.

EXERCISE 4-3

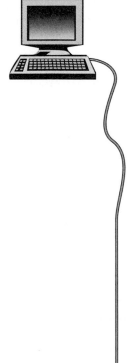

Practice using buttons on the toolbar.

1. **Click the Provider List button. The Provider List dialog box is displayed (see Figure 4-13).**

2. **Click the Close button to close the dialog box.**

Code	Name	Credentials	License Number	Medicare Part	Last Name
APS	Singh, Asha P			False	Singh
HSM	Miller, Harold S	DDS	5240	False	Miller
JDW	Wu, Josephine D	DDS	56388-T	False	Wu

Provider List — Search for: Field: Code

Edit   New   Delete   Close

Figure 4-13 Provider List dialog box.

3. **Click the Procedure Code List button. The Procedure/Payment/Adjustment List dialog box is displayed (see Figure 4-14).**

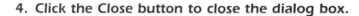

Code 1	Description	Amount	Type Description
ADJ	Adjustment	$0.00	Adjustment
AETADJ	Aetna Adjustment	$0.00	Insurance Adjustment
AETDED	Aetna Deductible	$0.00	Deductible
AETPAY	Aetna Payment	$0.00	Insurance payment
AETWIT	Aetna Withhold Adjustment	$0.00	Insurance Withhold Adju
BCBADJ	BCBS Adjustment	$0.00	Insurance Adjustment
BCBDED	BCBS Deductible	$0.00	Deductible
BCBPAY	BCBS Payment	$0.00	Insurance payment
BCBWIT	BCBS Withhold Adjustment	$0.00	Insurance Withhold Adju
CACOPAY15	Cash copayment $15	$0.00	Cash co-payment

Figure 4-14   Procedure/Payment/Adjustment List dialog box.

4. **Click the Close button to close the dialog box.**

ENTERING AND EDITING DATA

All data, whether patients' addresses or charges for procedures, are entered into PractiSoft by using the menus on the menu bar or the icons on the toolbar. Selecting an option from the menus or toolbar brings up a dialog box. The Tab key is used to move between text boxes within a dialog box. In some dialog boxes, information is entered by keying data into a text box. For example, a patient's name would be keyed directly into a text box. At other times selections are made from a list of choices already present. For example, when entering the name of the provider a patient is seeing, the provider is selected from a drop-down list of providers already in the system.

SHORT CUT To make a selection from a drop-down list, either of these techniques can be used: the scroll bars can be used to scroll up or down the list until the desired entry is displayed, or, the first few letters of the desired entry can be keyed in the text box next to the drop-down list. When characters are keyed, the system displays the entry in the list that most closely matches the characters keyed. When the desired entry appears highlighted, the Enter key is pressed. In most instances, the latter method is much quicker than using the scroll bars to locate the desired entry. Imagine a practice with 3000 patients. To locate a patient named Yates using the scroll method would require scrolling down a very long list. Keying in the first few letters of the patient's chart number, in this case, "YAT," would cause the system to display the first entry beginning with those letters. (Chart numbers are discussed in Chapter 5.)

Dates

PractiSoft is a date-sensitive program. When transactions are entered in the program, the dates must be accurate, or the data entered will be of little value to the practice. Many times, date-sensitive information is not entered into PractiSoft on the same day that the event or transaction occurred. For example, because of time constraints, Friday afternoon's office visits may not be entered into the program until Monday. If the PractiSoft Program Date is not changed to Friday's date before entering the data, all the information entered on Monday will be stored as Monday's transactions. For this reason, it is important to know how to change the PractiSoft Program Date.

For the purposes of this book, when you carry out many of the exercises, you will need to change the PractiSoft Program Date to a specific date. The date will be listed at the beginning of each exercise, when applicable. The following steps are used to change the PractiSoft Program Date:

1. Click Set Program Date on the File menu, or click the date displayed on the program's status bar. A pop-up calendar is displayed. (See Figure 4-15.)

2. Click the name of the month that is currently displayed. A pop-up menu appears. Click the desired month on the pop-up menu.

3. Select the desired year by clicking the year that is currently displayed. A pop-up menu appears. Click the desired year on the pop-up menu.

4. Select the desired date by clicking on that date in the calendar.

5. After you click on a date, the pop-up calendar disappears, and the changes made to the PractiSoft Program Date are automatically saved. The new date will remain in effect until you set a different date or until the program is turned off.

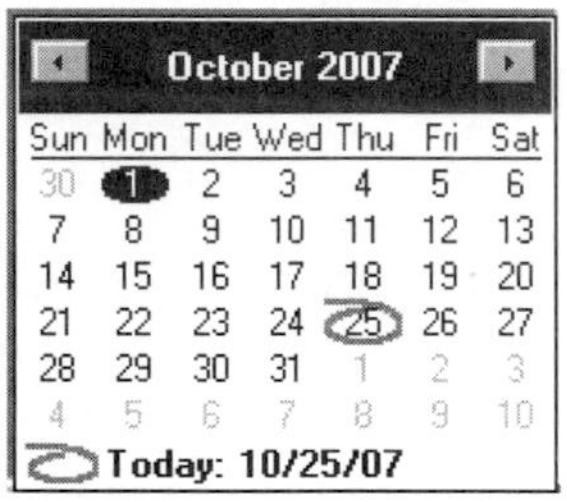

Figure 4-15
Pop-up calendar.

Note: The date displayed at the bottom of the calendar labeled "Today" is the Windows system date—the current date on the computer you are using. If you decide not to change the PractiSoft Program Date or if you want to return it to today's date, click Today at the bottom of the calendar.

In most PractiSoft dialog boxes, dates are entered in the MMDD-CCYY format. The **MMDDCCYY format** is a specific way in which dates must be keyed. "MM" stands for the month, "DD" stands for the day, "CC" represents century, and "YY" stands for the year. Each day, month, century, and year entry must contain two digits and no punctuation. For example, the date of February 1, 2007, would be keyed as *02012007*.

MMDDCCYY format   a specific way in which dates must be keyed, in which "MM" stands for month, "DD" stands for day, "CC" stands for century, and "YY" stands for year

SHORT CUT In most PractiSoft dialog boxes, when a date is required in a particular text box, the date can either be keyed in the text box or selected from a pop-up calendar. The pop-up calendar appears when the triangle button to the right of the text box is clicked. You can use the pop-up calendar to change the date as described above.

EXERCISE 4-4

Practice changing the program date to November 1, 2007. Then correct an error in a pretreatment estimate.

1. To change the PractiSoft program date to November 1, 2007, open the File menu and click Set Program Date, or click the date displayed on the program's status bar.

2. A pop-up calendar appears.

3. To change the month to November, click the name of the month that is currently displayed on the calendar. On the pop-up menu of months that appears, click November.

4. To change the year to 2007, click the year that is currently displayed. A pop-up menu appears. Click 2007.

5. To change the date to November 1, click 1 in the calendar.

6. The pop-up calendar disappears, and the program date, as shown in the status bar, is now set to November 1, 2007.

7. To correct an error in James Smith's pretreatment estimate for an upper partial denture, the estimate must be pulled up in the Pretreatment Plan/Estimate dialog box and edited. To access the Pretreatment Plan/Estimate dialog box, open the Activities menu and click Enter Pretreatment Estimates.

8. The Pretreatment Plan/Estimate dialog box is displayed.

9. Click the triangle button in the Chart box. The Chart drop-down list is displayed (see Figure 4-16). To select James Smith, key the first two letters of his chart number (SMITH-JAØ): *SM*

Chart Number	Name	Date of Birth
ARREZANO	Arrez, Anthony	1/26/1972
ARREZPA0	Arrez, Paula	8/29/1970
AXFORSU0	Axford, Susan R	7/9/1980
BARLODA0	Barlow, Daniel H	10/11/1973
BARLOGL0	Barlow, Gloria	4/16/1998
BARLOJI0	Barlow, Jimmy	3/30/1996
BARLOJU0	Barlow, June	9/10/1972
BARLOSA0	Barlow, Samuel S	1/5/1993

Figure 4-16 Chart drop-down list.

Notice that when *SM* was keyed, the system went to the entry for the first patient whose chart number begins with "SM," in this case James Smith.

10. Press the Enter key.

11. James Smith's account data appears in the top section of the dialog box, and the pointer moves to the next box, Case, with the most recent case for James Smith displayed (Pretreatment Estimate). In the transaction data for this case, the estimated amount for procedure D5213 (upper partial denture—cast) that was entered in the database on 9/6/07 needs to be changed from $1,400 to $1,300.

12. Notice in the Document box that a document number has automatically been assigned based on today's date (YYMMDD, followed by four zeros). This is the correct document number to use for a new transaction. However, to locate an earlier transaction, the document number for that transaction needs to be displayed in the Document box. To locate the required document number, click the ellipses to the right of the Document box.

13. A Search box opens, listing all document numbers for the selected case. Notice that Document number 070906000, based on the date 9/6/07, is displayed. Click the OK button to display the associated transaction data.

14. All charges associated with this document number are displayed. The estimated amount for procedure D5213 is $1,400. To change the amount to $1,300, click the Amount box.

15. The current amount, $1400.00, is highlighted.

16. Key *1300* and press the Enter key.

17. The amount displayed changes to $1300. The system automatically adds the decimal point (see Figure 4-17). The system also saves the change automatically.

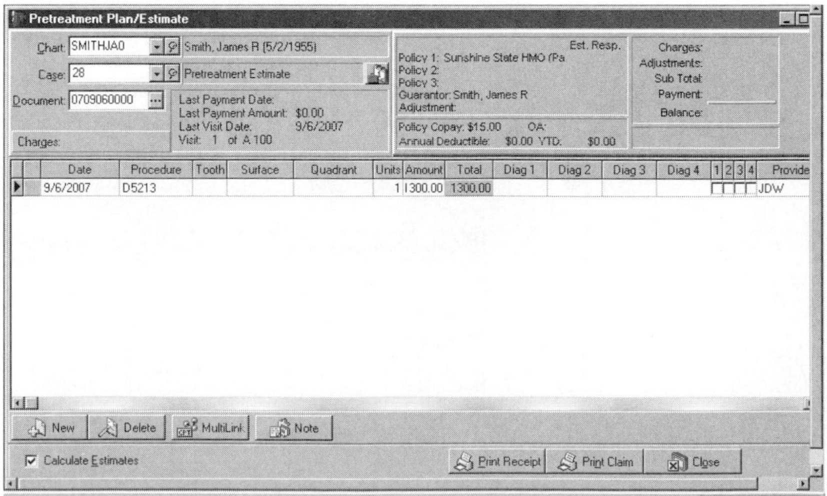

Figure 4-17 Pretreatment Plan/Estimate dialog box with data displayed.

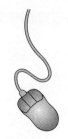

18. Press the Tab key repeatedly and watch as the cursor moves from box to box.

19. Exit the Pretreatment Plan/Estimate dialog box by clicking the Close button in the lower right corner of the dialog box.

20. The main PractiSoft window is displayed again.

SAVING DATA

In the Pretreatment Plan/Estimate dialog box, and similarly in the Transaction Entry dialog box, as a safeguard, changes are saved automatically. For this reason, there is no Save button in either transaction dialog box. However, in all other dialog boxes in PractiSoft, information that is entered must be saved by clicking a Save button inside the dialog box.

DELETING DATA

In most PractiSoft dialog boxes, there are buttons for the purpose of deleting data. For example, to delete an insurance carrier, the entry for the carrier is clicked in the Insurance Carrier List dialog box. Then the Delete button is clicked. PractiSoft will ask for a confirmation before deleting the data.

In some situations, the right mouse button can also be used to delete data. While working with transactions, for example, the entry to be deleted can be selected by clicking it; when the right mouse button is clicked, a shortcut menu with a Delete option is displayed. Again, PractiSoft will ask for confirmation before deleting the data.

USING PRACTISOFT HELP

PractiSoft offers users three different types of help.

Status Bar Help   Status bar help is information provided through a series of messages that appear on the status bar as the mouse pointer is moved to certain items on the screen. The status bar is located at the bottom of the screen. The messages display text that explains the purpose of the particular item (see Figure 4-18).

status bar help   information provided in a series of messages that appear on the status bar as the mouse pointer is moved to certain items on the screen

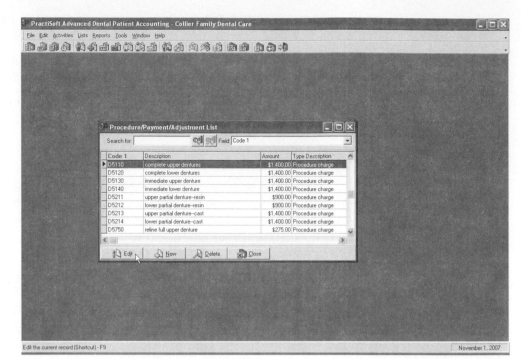

Figure 4-18 **Example of status bar help.**

Built-in Help   For more detailed help, PractiSoft has an extensive help feature built into the program itself, which is accessed through the Help menu.

Online Help   The Help menu also provides access to PractiSoft help available on the MediSoft corporate Web site, www.medisoft.com. The Web site contains a searchable **knowledge base**, which is a collection of up-to-date technical information about all MediSoft products.

knowledge base *a collection of up-to-date technical information*

EXERCISE 4-5

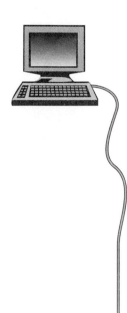

Practice using PractiSoft's built-in help feature.

1. Click the Help menu.

2. Click Table of Contents. In the left panel of the Help screen, PractiSoft displays a list of topics for which help is available.

3. Scroll down the list and click Contact Log Entry. In the right panel of the Help screen, read through the first few paragraphs to learn what a contact log entry is and how to use it.

4. Any Help topic can also be printed. Click the Print button at the top of the dialog box to print the information currently displayed in the right Help window. The Print dialog box is displayed.

5. Click the OK button to print.

6. To exit Help, click the Close button (X) in the upper right corner of the Help screen or click File on the Help menu bar and then click Exit.

7. The main PractiSoft window is displayed. To avoid the inconvenience of exiting and restarting PractiSoft many times during a day when the computer is needed for other programs, PractiSoft can be made temporarily inactive by using the Minimize button, the first of the three small buttons displayed in the upper-right corner of the window. Click the Minimize button.

8. The PractiSoft program temporarily disappears from the screen. The PractiSoft button that appears on the Windows taskbar (see Figure 4-19) indicates the program is still running in the background. To reactivate PractiSoft, you would click this button. For now, until you have completed the following exercise, leave the program in its minimized state.

| Start | PractiSoft Advanced ... | 10:03 AM |

Figure 4-19   Sample Windows taskbar with PractiSoft button.

EXERCISE 4-6

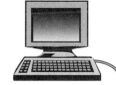

Practice using PractiSoft's online help.

1. Access the World Wide Web, and go to MediSoft's Web site, www.medisoft.com

2. Using the blue side bar menu, click the Support link.

3. Click the word "Support" from the list of options on the left side of the screen. Then click Knowledge Base.

4. Four steps are required to search for a topic. Under Step 1 (Select Product to Search . . .), click PractiSoft.

5. Under Step 2, use the default setting, All Words - Any Order.

6. Under Step 3, key *transactions* in the Search box.

7. Under Step 4, click the Search button.

8. Review the results of the search.

9. Click the entry, "Why are there two Transaction Entry icons in PractiSoft?" Review the information displayed. Notice that you also have the option to print or e-mail the information.

10. To exit the knowledge base, click the Close button in the upper right corner of the window. Terminate your Internet connection, if appropriate.

11. Click the PractiSoft button on the Windows taskbar to reactivate the PractiSoft program.

MAKING A BACKUP FILE WHILE EXITING PRACTISOFT

backup data   a copy of data files made at a specific point in time that can be used to restore data to the system

Data are periodically saved on removable magnetic media, such as diskettes or tapes, through a process known as backing up. **Backup data** is an extra copy of data files made at a specific point in time that can be used to restore data to the system in the event the data in the system are accidentally lost or destroyed. Backups are performed on a regular schedule, determined by the dental practice. Many practices back up data at the end of each day.

In an instructional environment, files are also backed up regularly to store each student's work securely and separately. If you are a student working in a computer lab setting, it is important to make a backup copy of your work after each PractiSoft session. This ensures that you can restore your work during the next session and be sure of using your own data, in the event another student uses the computer during the interim or if, for any reason, the data on the hard drive have been changed or corrupted.

In PractiSoft, the Backup Data option on the File menu can be used to make a backup copy of the active database at any time. By default, PractiSoft also displays a Backup Reminder dialog box every time the program is exited. The Backup Reminder dialog box gives you the opportunity to backup your work every time you exit PractiSoft. To perform the backup, the Backup Data Now button is clicked. To continue to exit the program without making a backup, the Exit Program button is clicked. The following exercise provides practice.

EXERCISE 4-7

Practice backing up your work on exiting PractiSoft.

1. To exit PractiSoft, click Exit on the File menu or click the Exit button on the toolbar.

TIP . . . To learn the function of any button on the toolbar, move the mouse pointer over it. The name of the button appears near it as well as on the status bar.

2. The Backup Reminder dialog box appears, displaying three options: Backup Data Now, Exit Program, or Cancel (see Figure 4-20). For the purposes of this text, it is recommended you back up your work to the Student Data Disk in Drive A: each time you exit the program. The current backup file will overwrite the previous backup file (A:\Collier.mbk) on the disk. To begin the backup, make sure your working copy of the Student Data Disk is inserted in Drive A: . Then click Backup Data Now.

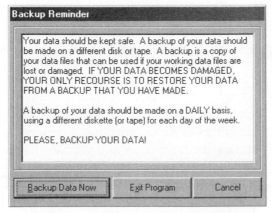

Figure 4-20   Backup Reminder dialog box.

3. The PractiSoft Backup dialog box is displayed (see Figure 4-21). Depending on the last time the dialog box was accessed, the Destination File Path and Name box may already contain the entry A:\Collier.mbk. If the box is blank, or if it contains something other than this, key *A:\Collier.mbk* in the Destination File Path and Name box.

```
┌─────────────────────────────────────────────────────┐
│ PractiSoft Backup                              ☒      │
├─────────────────────────────────────────────────────┤
│ Destination File Path and Name                        │
│ ┌──────────────────────────────────┐    ┌──────┐     │
│ │ A:\Collier.mbk                   │    │ Find │     │
│ └──────────────────────────────────┘    └──────┘     │
│ Existing Backup Files                                 │
│ ┌──────────────────────────────────────────────┐     │
│ │ Collier.mbk                                    │     │
│ │                                                │     │
│ │                                                │     │
│ │                                                │     │
│ └──────────────────────────────────────────────┘     │
│ Password:                                             │
│ ┌──────────────────────────────────────────────┐     │
│ │                                                │     │
│ └──────────────────────────────────────────────┘     │
│ ┌──────────────────────┐  ┌───────────────────┐      │
│ │ Source Path          │  │   Start Backup    │      │
│ │ C:\PractiData\Collier\│ └───────────────────┘      │
│ │                      │  ┌───────────────────┐      │
│ │ Backup Progress      │  │ ☒    Close        │      │
│ │ ┌──────────────────┐ │  └───────────────────┘      │
│ │ │      0%          │ │  ┌───────────────────┐      │
│ │ └──────────────────┘ │  │ ◎    Help         │      │
│ │ File Progress        │  └───────────────────┘      │
│ │ ┌──────────────────┐ │                             │
│ │ │      0%          │ │                             │
│ │ └──────────────────┘ │                             │
│ └──────────────────────┘                             │
│ ┌──────────────────────────────────────────────┐     │
│ │                                                │     │
│ └──────────────────────────────────────────────┘     │
└─────────────────────────────────────────────────────┘
```

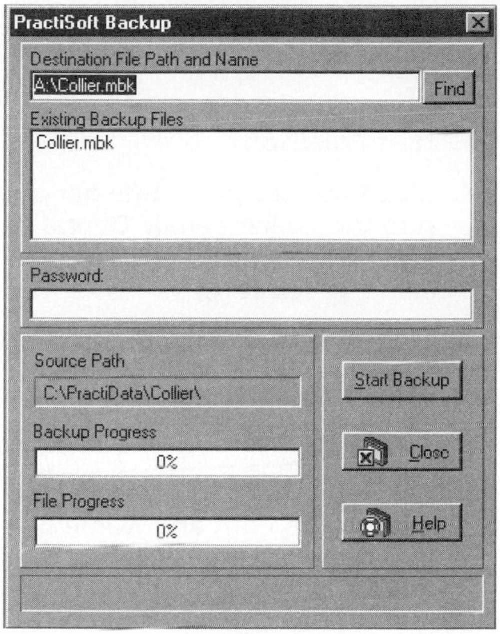

Figure 4-21   PractiSoft Backup dialog box.

4. PractiSoft displays the location of the database files to be backed up in the Source Path box in the lower half of the dialog box automatically. Click the Start Backup button.

5. The program backs up the latest database files to the disk in Drive A:, and displays an Information dialog box indicating the backup is complete. Click OK to continue.

6. The PractiSoft Backup dialog box disappears, and the PractiSoft program closes.

RESTORING THE BACKUP FILE

Whenever a new PractiSoft session begins, the following steps can be used to restore the backup file if required. A restore is only necessary in the event someone else has altered the database files on the hard drive between sessions. If you share a computer in an instructional environment, it is recommended you perform a restore before each new session to be sure you are working with your own data.

These are the steps to restore A:\Collier.mbk to C:\PractiData\Collier.

1. **Start PractiSoft.**

2. **Check the program's title bar at the top of the screen to make sure the Collier Family Dental Care data set is the active data set. (If it is not, use the Open Practice option on the File menu to select it.)**

3. **Insert your working copy of the Student Data Disk in Drive A:.**

4. **Open the File menu and click Restore Data.**

5. **When the Warning box appears, click OK.**

6. **The Restore dialog box appears (see Figure 4-22). In the Backup File Path and Name box at the top of the dialog box (if the following filename is not already displayed), key A:\Collier.mbk.**

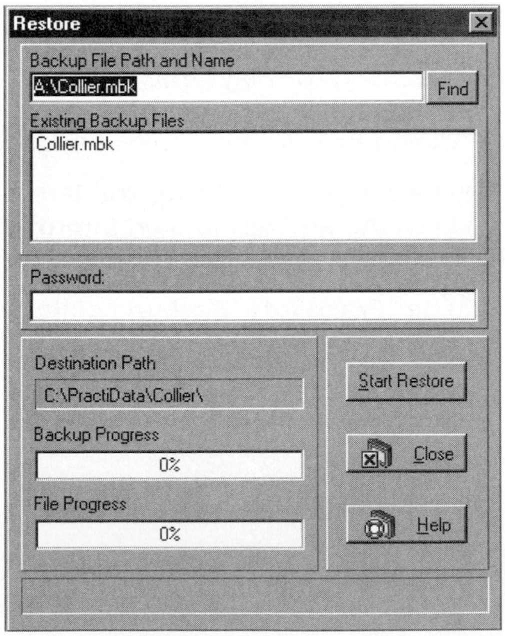

Figure 4-22   Restore dialog box.

7. The Destination Path at the bottom of the box should already say C:\PractiData\Collier. Leave this as it is.

8. Click the Start Restore button.

9. When the Confirm box appears, click OK.

10. An Information dialog box appears indicating the restore is complete. Click OK to continue.

11. The Restore dialog box disappears. You are ready to begin the next session.

CHAPTER REVIEW

USING TERMINOLOGY

Match the terms on the left with the definitions on the right.

_____ **1.** backup data

_____ **2.** status bar help

_____ **3.** knowledge base

_____ **4.** MMDDCCYY format

_____ **5.** transactions

a. Instructional messages that appear at the bottom of the PractiSoft window.

b. A searchable collection of up-to-date technical information.

c. In PractiSoft, charges, payments, and adjustments.

d. A way in which dates must be keyed.

e. A copy of data files made at a specific point in time that can be used to restore data to the system.

CHECKING YOUR UNDERSTANDING

Answer the questions below in the space provided.

6. Describe two ways of issuing a command in PractiSoft.

_____

_____

7. What are two ways data are entered in a box?

_____

_____

8. What three types of PractiSoft help are available?

_____

_____

_____

9. Which menu provides access to Office Hours, PractiSoft's scheduling features?

_____

10. What is the purpose of the buttons on the toolbar?

_____

11. What is the format for entering dates in PractiSoft?

_____

12. Describe two ways of exiting PractiSoft.

_____

_____

APPLYING KNOWLEDGE

13. Use PractiSoft's built-in help to look up information on the following topics:
- How to enter information on a new insurance carrier in the practice's database
- How to print a procedure code list from the practice's database

AT THE COMPUTER

Answer the following questions at the computer:

14. How many options are there in the Reports menu?

_____

15. What is the first choice on the Lists menu?

_____

16. List the options on the Activities menu.

_____

_____

_____

17. Set the PractiSoft Program Date to October 3, 2007; then exit PractiSoft without making a backup file.

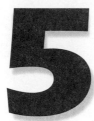

CHAPTER

5 Entering Patient Information

WHAT YOU NEED TO KNOW

To use this chapter, you need to know how to:

◆ Start PractiSoft.
◆ Move around the PractiSoft menus.
◆ Use the PractiSoft toolbar.
◆ Enter and edit data in PractiSoft.
◆ Exit PractiSoft.

OBJECTIVES

When you finish this chapter, you will be able to:

1. **Use the PractiSoft Search feature.**
2. **Assign a chart number for a new patient.**
3. **Enter personal and employer information for a new patient.**
4. **Locate and change information for an established patient.**

KEY TERMS

chart number
guarantor

HOW PATIENT INFORMATION IS ORGANIZED IN PRACTISOFT

Figure 5-1
Patient List
shortcut button.

Patient information is accessed through the Patient List dialog box. The Patient List dialog box is displayed when Patients/Guarantors and Cases is clicked on the Lists menu or when the corresponding shortcut button is clicked on the toolbar (see Figure 5-1).

The Patient List dialog box (see Figure 5-2) is divided into two primary sections. The left side of the window displays information about patients, and the right side of the window contains information about cases. Cases are covered in Chapter 6. At the top right side of the Patient List dialog box, there are two radio buttons: Patient and Case. When the Patient radio button is clicked, the left side of the window becomes active. Correspondingly, when the Case radio button is clicked, the right side of the window becomes active. The command buttons at the bottom of the dialog box vary, depending on which side of the window is active.

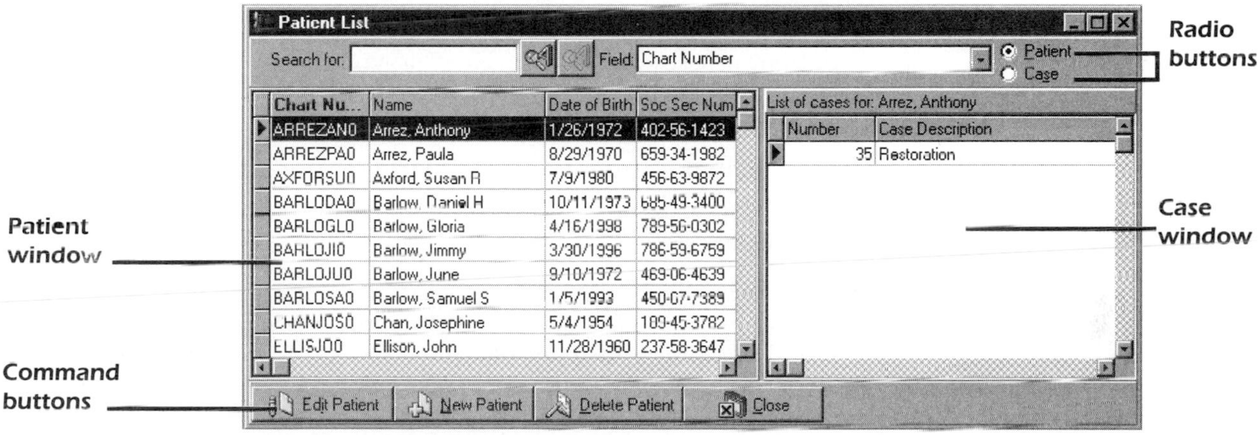

Figure 5-2 Patient List dialog box.

The Patient window contains the following data: Chart Number, Name, Date of Birth, Social Security Number, Patient ID #2, Patient Type, Phone 1, Provider, Last Name, Billing Code, and Patient Indicator. There is not enough room in the Patient window to display all this information, so only a portion is visible at one time. To view the rest of the patient information, use the scroll bars. Scrolling to the right displays information in the additional columns, including Social Security Number, and all the way to Patient Indicator. Scrolling down the Patient window displays additional chart numbers and patient names (see Figure 5-3 on page 70). There are command buttons at the bottom of the screen for editing a patient's information, adding information for a new patient, deleting a patient's information, and closing the Patient List dialog box.

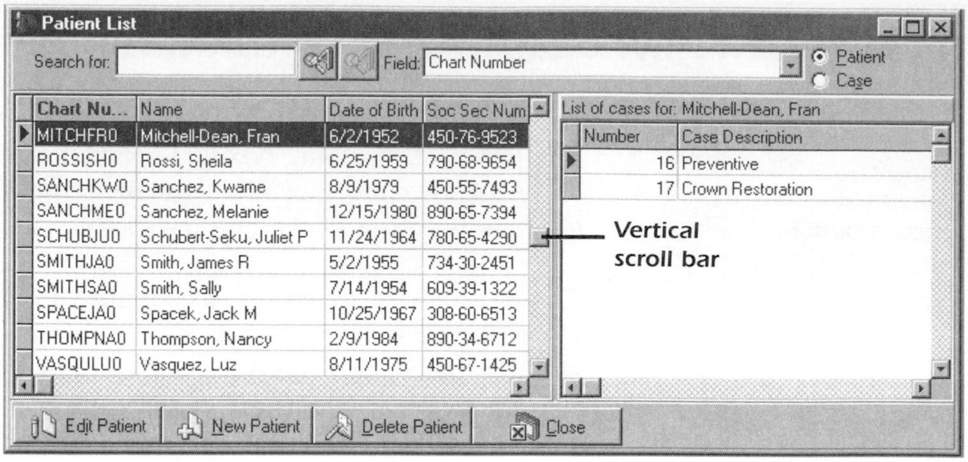

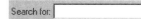

Figure 5-3 Patient List dialog box with vertical scroll bar in use.

SEARCHING FOR PATIENT INFORMATION

A patient who comes to a dental practice for the first time fills out a patient information form. The information on this form needs to be entered into the PractiSoft patient/guarantor database before any insurance claims can be submitted. However, before information on a patient is entered into the system, it is important to search the database to be certain that the patient does not already exist in the database.

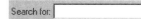

Figure 5-4
Search For box.

PractiSoft's Search feature is used to look for information on patients, insurance carriers, diagnosis codes, and procedure codes, as well as the names and addresses of employers and providers. Searches for information on patients are conducted using the Search box in the upper left corner of the Patient List dialog box (see Figure 5-4).

In a search, PractiSoft locates the name or number that most closely matches the letters and/or numbers entered in the Search box. For example, if the letters *ABB* are entered in the Search box, PractiSoft will match the first patient with a last name beginning with "ABB."

TIP . . . It does not matter whether capital letters or lower-case letters are entered in the Search box. For example, keying *ABBOTT, Abbott,* or *abbott* will all locate the first patient in the database with the last name of Abbott.

EXERCISE 5-1

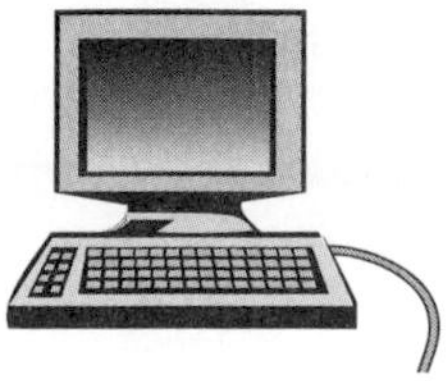

Use the Search feature to locate information on Jack Spacek.

1. **Start PractiSoft.**

2. **On the Lists menu, click Patients/Guarantors and Cases or click the corresponding shortcut button. The Patient List dialog box is displayed, and the cursor is blinking in the Search box.**

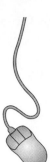

3. Enter the first letter of the patient's last name. Notice that when you keyed *S*, the arrow on the left side of the Patient window moved down to the first patient whose name begins with the letter *S*, Sanchez, Kwame. Continue entering the patient's last name. As soon as you key the next letter, *p*, the arrow points to Jack Spacek. Spacek is the only patient whose name begins with *Sp*.

4. Click the Close button to exit the Patient List dialog box.

ENTERING NEW PATIENT INFORMATION

New Patient

Figure 5-5
New Patient button.

Information on a new patient is entered in PractiSoft by clicking the New Patient button at the bottom of the Patient List dialog box (see Figure 5-5). This action opens the Patient/Guarantor dialog box (see Figure 5-6). The Patient/Guarantor dialog box contains two tabs: the Name, Address tab and the Other Information tab.

Name, Address tab ——

—— Other Information tab

Figure 5-6   Patient/Guarantor dialog box.

NAME, ADDRESS TAB

The Name, Address tab is where basic patient information is entered.

Chart Number

chart number   a unique number that identifies a patient

The **chart number** is a unique number that identifies a patient. In PractiSoft, a chart number links together all the information about a patient that is stored in the different databases, such as name, address, charges, and insurance claims. Each patient is assigned an eight-character chart number. If the chart number box for a patient is left blank, the system will assign a chart number.

Dental practices may use different methods for assigning chart numbers, although these general guidelines must be followed:

◆ The chart number must start with a letter but can contain a combination of letters and numbers.

◆ No special characters, such as hyphens, periods, or spaces, are allowed.

◆ No two chart numbers can be the same.

For the purposes of this book, the following method will be used for assigning chart numbers:

◆ The first five characters of the chart number are the first five letters of a patient's last name. If the patient's last name is less than five characters, add the beginning letters of the patient's first name.

◆ The next two characters are usually the first two letters of a patient's first name. (If the first two letters of the first name were used to complete the first five letters, the next two letters of the patient's first name are used.)

◆ The last character is always a zero, displayed in this book with the symbol "Ø."

For example, the chart number for John Ellison would begin with the first five letters of his last name (ELLIS), followed by the first two characters of his first name (JO), followed by a zero (Ø). John's complete chart number would be ELLISJOØ. Following the same rules, John's wife Ruby would have a chart number of ELLISRUØ.

EXERCISE 5-2

Create a chart number for each of these patients.

Lus Vasquez _____

Josephine Schweikert _____

Joel Hart _____

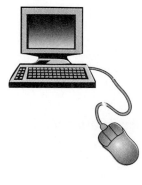

Personal Data

In addition to the chart number, personal information about a patient is entered in the Name, Address tab.

Name, Address, and Phone Numbers The boxes for name, address, and phone numbers contain basic information about a patient. There are two boxes for phone numbers. The box on the left is for the primary phone number; the one on the right is for an alternate phone number or a fax number. It is not necessary to enter parentheses or hyphens with phone numbers and fax numbers, as the program adds these for you. Simply enter the numbers.

Birth Date   The patient's birth date is entered in the Birth Date box using the MMDDCCYY format. Although the program does not display the zeros preceding numbers such as 02, the zeros should be keyed to avoid mistakes between the month and year. Alternatively, the pop-up calendar can be used to enter the birth date. Click the triangle button in the Birth Date box to display the pop-up calendar.

Sex   This drop-down list contains choices for the patient's gender, male or female.

Social Security Number   The nine-digit Social Security number should be entered with hyphens to make the number easier to read. The program will accept the number if entered without hyphens; however, unlike the way it handles phone numbers, the program will not add them for you.

OTHER INFORMATION TAB   The Other Information tab within the Patient/Guarantor dialog box contains facts about a patient's employment and other miscellaneous information (see Figure 5-7).

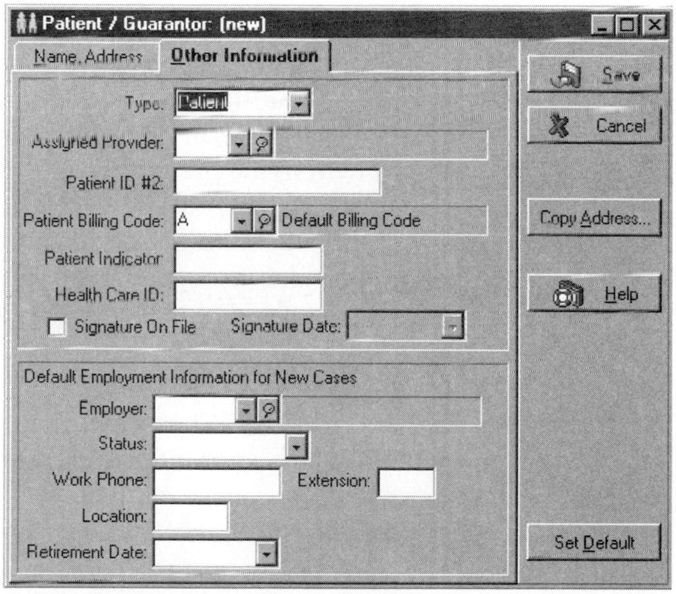

Figure 5-7   Other Information tab.

Type The Type drop-down list is used to designate whether, for billing purposes, an individual is a patient or guarantor (see Figure 5-8).

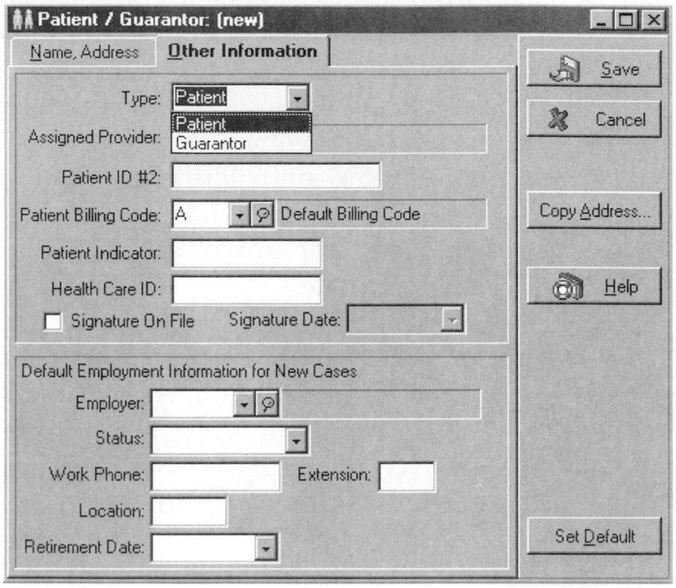

Figure 5-8   Other Information tab with Type drop-down list displayed.

In the PractiSoft Patient/Guarantor dialog box, individuals are classified into two categories: patient and guarantor. *Patient* is used to refer to an individual who is a patient of the practice, whether or not the person is also the insurance policyholder. For the purposes of this dialog box, the term **guarantor** refers only to an individual who is not a patient of the practice, but who is the insurance policyholder for a patient of the practice. For example, a parent who is not a patient of the practice but whose insurance policy provides coverage for a child who is a patient of the practice is listed in the Patient/Guarantor dialog box as a guarantor.

guarantor an individual who is a policyholder for a patient of the practice

Information about the patient is always entered in PractiSoft in the Name/Address tab. When the patient is not the policyholder, information about the guarantor must also be entered in the PractiSoft database for insurance claims to be processed. This information is collected from the patient information or patient update form.

Assigned Provider The Assigned Provider drop-down list contains codes assigned to the doctors in the practice (see Figure 5-9). The code for the specific doctor who provides care to this patient is selected.

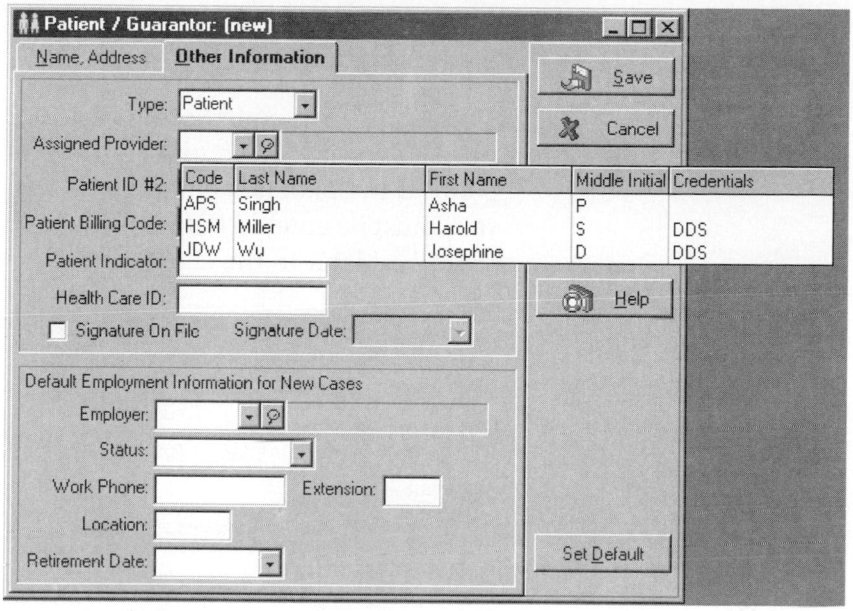

Figure 5-9 Other Information tab with Assigned Provider drop-down list displayed.

Patient ID #2 The Patient ID #2 box is used by some dental practices as a second identification system in addition to chart numbers.

Patient Billing Code The Patient Billing Code is an optional field used to categorize patients according to the billing codes that the practice has set up in PractiSoft. For example, Billing Code A might be for patients with insurance coverage, and B for cash patients. Some practices use billing codes to classify patients according to a billing cycle—for example, patients with Billing Code A are billed on the first of the month, and those with code B are billed on the fifteenth of the month. The Billing Code field is not used in the exercises in this book. All patients have the same billing code, Billing Code A, which is the program's default setting.

Patient Indicator The Patient Indicator is an optional field that practices can use to classify types of patients, such as workers' compensation patients, cash patients, and diabetic patients.

Health Care ID As part of the HIPAA compliance effort, various identifiers have been added to each set of data fields in PractiSoft, including patient data. In the Patient/Guarantor dialog box, the Health Care ID box has been added in anticipation that one day each patient will be assigned a unique health care identification number. Until specific legislation is passed that will protect the use of this code, however, use of the ID is on hold.

Signature on File A check mark in the Signature on File check box means that the patient's signature is on file for the purpose of submitting insurance claims. This box must be completed. If it is not, insurance claims will not be accepted and processed by any insurance carrier.

Signature Date The date keyed in the Signature Date box is the date the patient signed the insurance release form.

Employer The code for the patient's employer is selected from the drop-down list of employers that are in the database (see Figure 5-10). If the patient's employer is not in the database, this information must be entered before the code can be selected. (This process is described later in the chapter.)

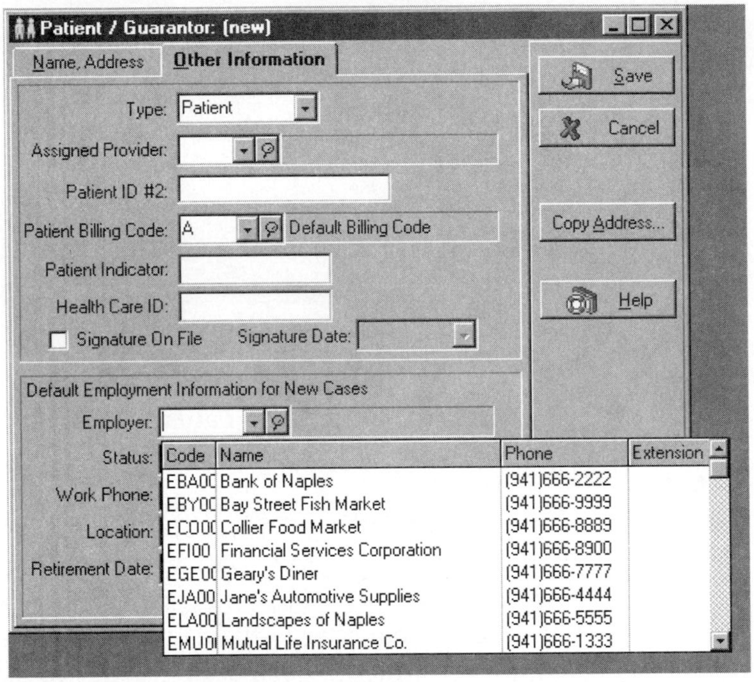

Figure 5-10 Other Information tab with Employer drop-down list displayed.

Status The Status drop-down list displays the following choices for the patient's employment status: Not employed, Full time, Part time, Retired, and Unknown (see Figure 5-11).

Work Phone and Extension As with other phone numbers, work phone numbers may be entered without parentheses or hyphens. The program will add them as needed.

Location Some companies have multiple locations. If the patient supplies information on the specific company location, it is entered in this box.

Retirement Date The Retirement Date box is filled in only if the patient is already retired. Retirement dates should be keyed directly using the MMDDCCYY format or selected from the pop-up calendar. The pop-up calendar is displayed by clicking the triangle button inside the Retirement Date box.

Patient / Guarantor: (new)

| Name, Address | **Other Information** |

Type: `Patient`

Assigned Provider: `[    ]`

Patient ID #2: `[                    ]`

Patient Billing Code: `A` Default Billing Code

Patient Indicator: `[                    ]`

Health Care ID: `[                    ]`

☐ Signature On File   Signature Date: `[          ]`

Default Employment Information for New Cases

Employer: `[       ]`

Status: `[       ]`

Work Phone: `Not employed` | `Full time` | `Part time` | `Retired` | `Unknown`   xtension: `[    ]`

Location:

Retirement Date:

Save

Cancel

Copy Address...

Help

Set Default

Figure 5-11 Other Information tab with Status drop-down list displayed.

When all the fields in the Name, Address tab and the Other Information tab have been filled in, entries should be checked for accuracy. If any of the information needs to be changed, it can easily be corrected. Once the information has been checked and any necessary corrections made, data are saved by clicking the Save button.

EXERCISE 5-3

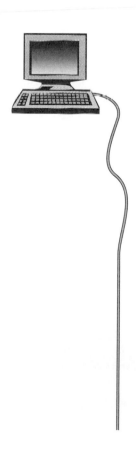

Using Source Document 1 (located in Part 4 of this book), complete the Patient/Guarantor dialog box for Hannah Wilson, a new patient of Dr. Miller's.

Date: October 1, 2007

1. On the Lists menu, click Patients/Guarantors and Cases, or click the corresponding shortcut button on the toolbar.

2. Scroll down the list of patients to make sure Hannah Wilson is not already in the patient database.

3. Click the New Patient button.

4. Create a chart number for this patient. Click the Chart Number box, and enter the chart number.

5. Click the Last Name box, and fill in the patient information. Fill in the rest of the boxes on the Name, Address tab, pressing the Tab key to move from box to box.

6. Click the Other Information tab, and fill in the appropriate boxes. Be sure to select an Assigned Provider (Dr. Miller is Wilson's assigned provider), or subsequent exercises in this chapter will not work. The Patient ID #2, Patient Indicator, and Health Care ID boxes should be left blank. Accept the default entry in the Patient Billing Code box. Check the Signature on File box and enter the signature date. (*Note:*

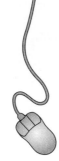

Since Wilson's employer is not in the database, leave the employer boxes blank for now.)

7. Check your entries for accuracy, and make corrections if necessary.

8. Click the Save button to save the data on Wilson. (*Note:* If a Warning box appears with the message, "The Signature Date you have entered is in the future," click OK, and then click the Save button again.)

9. Verify that Wilson has been added to the list in the Patient List dialog box.

10. Close the Patient List dialog box.

ADDING AN EMPLOYER TO THE ADDRESS LIST

If the patient's employer does not appear on the Employer drop-down list in the Other Information tab, it must be entered. Addresses can be entered in one of two ways: by clicking the Addresses command on the Lists menu, or by clicking once in the Employer box on the Other Information tab and then pressing function key F8. The F8 key shortcut enables users to enter data in another part of the program without leaving the current dialog box. Once the F8 key is pressed, the dialog box for new addresses is opened, with the Patient/Guarantor dialog box still open in the background.

When the Addresses command is clicked on the Lists menu, the Address List dialog box is displayed (see Figure 5-12). Clicking the New button at the bottom of the Address List dialog box displays the Address dialog box (see Figure 5-13), just as when clicking F8 in the Employer box of the Other Information tab. Although the Patient/Guarantor dialog box can remain open in the background with either method, notice that by clicking F8, the Address List dialog box is bypassed, saving a keystroke.

Code	Name	Phone	Type	Extension
EBA00	Bank of Naples	(941)666-2222	Employer	
EBY00	Bay Street Fish Market	(941)666-9999	Employer	
ECO00	Collier Food Market	(941)666-8889	Employer	
EFI00	Financial Services Corporal	(941)666-8900	Employer	
EGE00	Geary's Diner	(941)666-7777	Employer	
EJA00	Jane's Automotive Supplies	(941)666-4444	Employer	
ELA00	Landscapes of Naples	(941)666-5555	Employer	
EMU00	Mutual Life Insurance Co.	(941)666-1333	Employer	
ENA00	Naples Realty	(941)666-2828	Employer	
EOU00	Outdoor Furniture Showroo	(941)666-3333	Employer	

Figure 5-12   **Address List dialog box.**

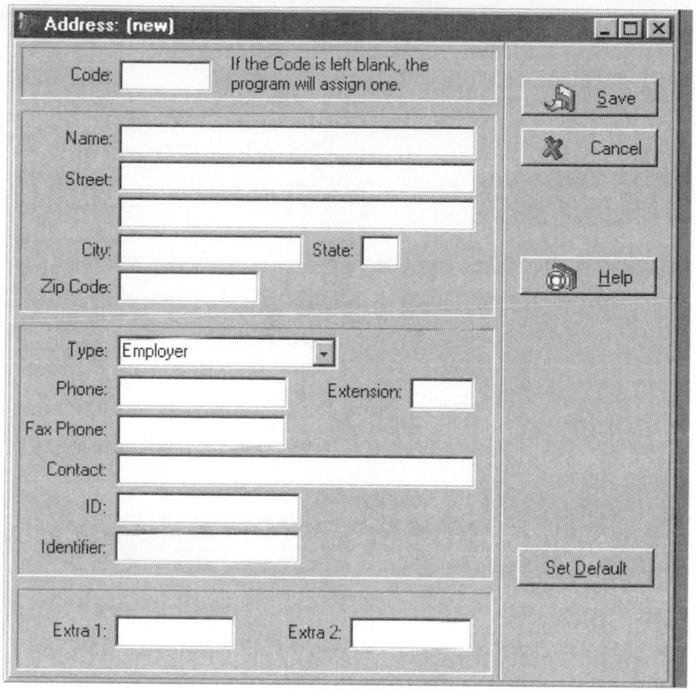

Figure 5-13 Address dialog box.

The Address dialog box contains the following boxes:

Code   The code for an employer should begin with the letter *E*, to indicate that this is an employer. Codes can be a combination of letters and numbers, up to a maximum of five characters, and can be designed according to any system you desire. In this book, employer codes begin with the letter *E*, followed by the first two letters of the employer's name, followed by two zeros. If a code is not assigned, the system will assign one.

Name and Address   The employer's name is entered in the Name box. This field allows up to 30 characters. The employer's street, city, state (two characters only), and Zip code are entered in the boxes provided.

Type   The Type drop-down list displays a list of kinds of addresses: Attorney, Employer, Facility, Laboratory, Miscellaneous, and Referral Source. For example, when the address being entered is that of an employer, "Employer" is selected.

Phone, Extension, Fax Phone   In the Phone box, the employer's phone number is entered without parentheses or hyphens. If there is an extension, it is entered in the Extension box. The employer's fax number is entered in the Fax Phone box.

Contact   The Contact box is used to enter the name of an individual at the place of employment. If there is no contact person, the box is left blank.

ID If there is an identification number for the employer, it is entered in the ID box.

Identifier The Identifier box is used to report the Employer Identification Number (EIN) supplied by the IRS. This box has been added to PractiSoft to ensure HIPAA compliance.

Extra 1, Extra 2 The Extra 1 and Extra 2 boxes are available to keep track of any additional information that needs to be recorded and stored for future reference.

When all the information on the employer has been entered, it is saved by clicking the Save button.

EXERCISE 5-4

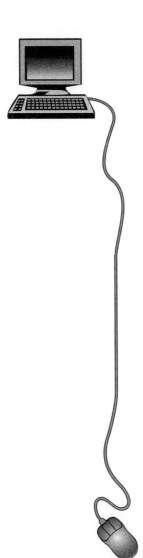

Practice entering information about an employer by adding Hannah Wilson's employer to the Address List.

Date: October 1, 2007

1. Click Addresses on the Lists menu. The Address List dialog box is displayed.

2. Click the New button at the bottom of the dialog box. The Address dialog box is displayed.

3. In the Code box, key *EEA00* for East Collier County Schools ("E" for employer, followed by the first two letters of the employer's name, followed by two zeros.) Press the Tab key.

4. Key *East Collier County Schools* in the Name box. Press the Tab key.

5. Complete the Street, City, State, and Zip Code boxes.

6. Verify that Employer is displayed in the Type box. If it is not, click Employer in the drop-down list and press the Tab key.

7. Complete the Phone box. Press the Tab key.

8. Since there is no extension or fax phone listed, leave the corresponding boxes blank.

9. Since there is no information about a contact, an ID, an identifier (EIN), or any extra information, leave the corresponding boxes blank.

10. Click the Save button to store the information you have entered.

11. Click the Close button to exit the Address List dialog box.

EDITING INFORMATION ON AN ESTABLISHED PATIENT

From time to time, established patients notify the practice that they have moved, changed jobs or insurance carriers, or made other changes. When this happens, information needs to be updated in PractiSoft's patient/guarantor database. The process of changing information on an established patient is similar to that of entering information for a new patient. The patient information is accessed through the Patient List dialog box. This is displayed either by pressing the Patient List toolbar button or by selecting the Patients/ Guarantors and Cases command from the Lists menu. A search is usually performed first to locate the name or chart number of the patient whose record needs to be updated. Data can be edited either by pressing the Enter key or by clicking the Edit Patient button at the bottom of the dialog box. This displays the Patient/Guarantor dialog box with the information to be edited on the screen, where changes can be made. Clicking the Save button stores the changes.

EXERCISE 5-5

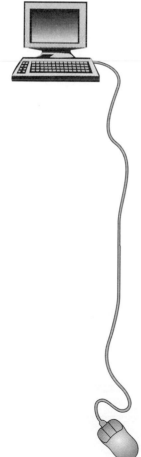

Practice searching for and editing information on Hannah Wilson.

Date: October 1, 2007

1. Open the Patient List dialog box.

2. Search for Hannah Wilson by keying her chart number, WILSOHA0. When the search is done, the selection arrow should be pointing to Wilson, Hannah.

3. Click the Edit Patient button. Now that Hannah Wilson's employer has been added to the database, her employment information can be completed.

4. Click the Other Information tab.

5. Click the triangle button in the Employer box. Click East Collier County Schools on the drop-down list.

6. Select Full time from the Status drop-down list.

7. Verify that her work phone number appears in the Work Phone box. If the number does not appear, enter it (941-555-1001).

8. Click the Save button to store the information you have entered.

9. Close the Patient List dialog box.

10. Exit PractiSoft.

CHAPTER REVIEW

USING TERMINOLOGY

Define the terms in the space provided.

1. chart number

_____

_____

2. guarantor

_____

_____

CHECKING YOUR UNDERSTANDING

Answer the questions below in the space provided.

3. To search for Melanie Sanchez, can you key either "Melanie" or "Sanchez"? Explain.

_____

_____

4. Create a chart number for a patient with the name of Stanley Liebler.

_____

5. A patient of the practice, Sam Wu, is covered by his wife's insurance policy. However, his wife is not a patient of the practice. How would you indicate this in the Patient/Guarantor dialog box?

_____

_____

6. A patient is moving and calls to let you know her new address and phone number. What is the name of the dialog box and tab in which the new information should be recorded?

_____

_____

7. In PractiSoft, how would you key the phone number (555) 340-8112?

_____

APPLYING KNOWLEDGE

Answer the following question in the space provided.

8. A patient in the office named Tim Gabriel cannot remember if he gave you the name and address of his new employer. What should you do?

_____

_____

_____

AT THE COMPUTER

Answer the following questions at the computer.

9. How many patients in the database have the last name of Smith?

_____

10. List the name of the patient who is found when you search for the letters "JO."

_____

11. What is Josephine Chan's chart number?

_____

12. What is Mary Rose Hersen's date of birth? What steps did you take in PractiSoft to locate the information?

_____

_____

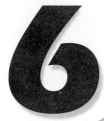

CHAPTER

6 Working with Cases

To use this chapter you need to know how to:

◆ Use the PractiSoft Search feature.

◆ Enter new patient information.

◆ Locate and change information about an established patient.

OBJECTIVES

When you finish this chapter, you will be able to:

1. Determine when to create a new case.
2. Set up a new case.
3. Enter information on a patient's insurance policy.
4. Enter information on an accident or illness.
5. Add a new referring provider to the database.
6. Add a new insurance carrier to the database.
7. Edit information in an existing case.
8. Close a case.
9. Delete a case.

KEY TERMS

capitated plan

cases

chart

record of treatment and
    progress

referring provider

WHAT IS A CASE?

cases *groupings of transactions for visits to a dentist's office organized around a particular condition*

Cases are groupings of transactions for visits to a dentist's office, organized around a particular condition. When a patient comes for treatment, a case is created.

Cases are set up to contain the transactions that relate to a particular condition. For example, all treatments and procedures for a root canal would be stored in a case called "Root Canal." Services performed and charges for those services are entered in the system and linked to the root canal case.

WHEN TO SET UP A NEW CASE

New cases should be set up each time a patient comes to see the dentist for a new condition or when there is a change in the provider or insurance carrier. For example, suppose a patient has been seeing a dentist regularly for acute gingivitis. All the transactions for this treatment would be contained in one case. Then suppose the patient comes in for treatment of a broken tooth. The broken tooth is a new condition. A new case would be set up in PractiSoft for the treatment of the broken tooth.

In addition, when a patient changes insurance carriers, a new case should be set up, even if the same condition is being treated under the new carrier. This makes it easier to submit insurance claims to the appropriate carrier. Transactions that took place while the previous policy was in effect must be submitted under that policy. Transactions that occur after the change in policies must be submitted to the new carrier. By opening a new case, transactions for the two insurance carriers can be kept separate. The information needed to submit claims to the previous carrier is still intact, while information for claims under the new policy is current.

A patient may require more than one case per office visit if treatment is provided for two or more unrelated conditions. For example, a patient who visits the dentist complaining of pain in the jaw may also end up receiving periodontal services such as a scaling. Since the two conditions are unrelated, two cases would need to be created: one for the pain in the jaw, and one for the periodontal services (scaling). In contrast, a patient who is treated for pain in a particular tooth and also complains of sinus pain near the tooth would require one case, provided the dentist determines that the two complaints are related to the same diagnosis.

It is not uncommon for patients to have more than one case open at any one time. Some cases are for chronic conditions and remain open a long time. Other cases, such as a case for a simple filling, may be of short duration. Cases are closed when the patient is no longer being treated for the condition, when the insurance policy in a case is no longer in effect, or when the patient leaves the practice.

CASE COMMAND BUTTONS

In PractiSoft, cases are created, edited, and deleted from within the Patient List dialog box (see Figure 6-1). The Patient List dialog box is accessed by choosing Patients/Guarantors and Cases from the Lists menu. When the Case radio button in the Patient List dialog box is clicked, the following command buttons appear at the bottom of the Patient List dialog box: Edit Case, New Case, Delete Case, Copy Case, and Close (see Figure 6-2).

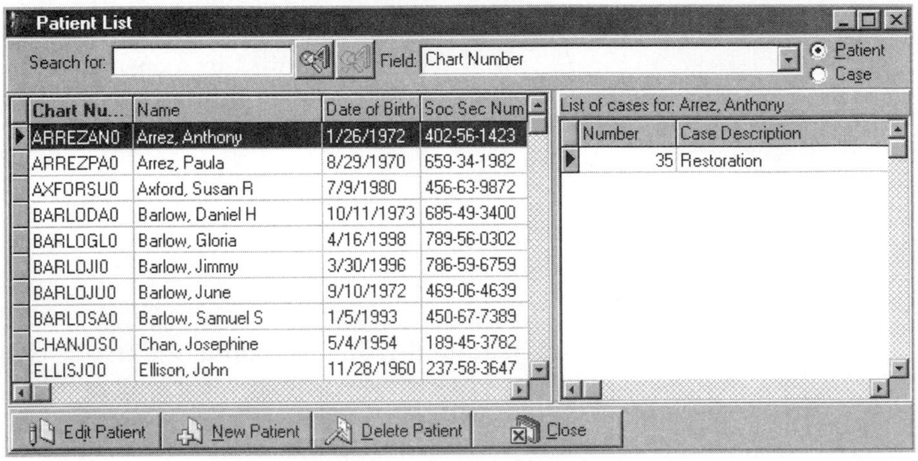

Figure 6-1   Patient List dialog box.

Case command buttons

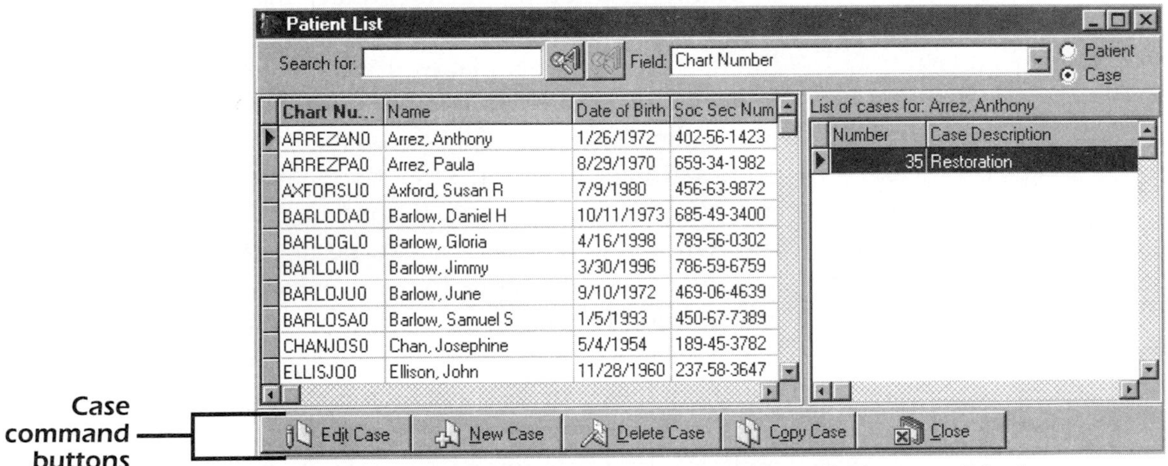

Figure 6-2   Patient List dialog box with Case radio button clicked.

Edit Case

The Edit Case button is used to add, delete, or change information in an existing case. When the Edit Case button is clicked, the Case dialog box is displayed. Case information to be updated is contained in nine different tabs. For example, if a patient changes insurance carriers, information needs to be updated in the Policy 1, 2, or 3 tab. The only item in the Case dialog box that cannot be changed is the Case Number. All other boxes are edited by moving the cursor to the box and making the change, whether this means rekeying, selecting and deselecting a check box, or clicking a different option on a drop-down list.

SHORT CUT When the Patient List dialog box is opened, the Patient radio button is automatically selected. To switch modes from patient information to case information, you must first remember to click the Case radio button. Then select the case to be edited, and click the Edit Case button. Alternatively, as a short cut, cases can be edited by double-clicking the desired case number/description in the Patient List dialog box. The Case radio button will be selected automatically, and the case to be edited will appear in the Case dialog box.

New Case

The New Case button creates a new case.

Delete Case

The Delete Case button deletes a case from the system if the case has no open transactions. Open transactions are charges that have not been fully paid by the insurance carrier or the policyholder. The Delete Case button should be used with caution; once deleted, information cannot be retrieved. Cases should be deleted only when it is definite that the patient's records will never be needed again. Dental offices usually have policies about when a patient's records are deleted. In most instances, it is more appropriate to close a case than to delete it from the system. Cases are closed by clicking the Case Closed box in the Personal tab of the Case dialog box.

When the Delete Case button is clicked, the cases are deleted in the Patient List dialog box. With the Case radio button clicked, the specific case to be deleted is selected by clicking the line that displays the case number and description. The case is then deleted by clicking the Delete Case button at the bottom of the dialog box. The system will ask, "Are you sure you want to delete this case?" Clicking the Yes button deletes the case from the system.

Copy Case

The Copy Case button copies all the information from an existing case into a new case. This feature is useful when creating a new case for a patient who already has a case in the system. Rather than reenter the information in all nine tabs, the information in the existing case is copied into a new case. Then the information that needs to be changed can be edited to reflect the data relevant to the new case. Sometimes the new case requires few changes; other times data must be changed in all the tabs of the Case folder. For this reason, it is important when copying a case to check each tab to make sure the copied information is accurate for the new case. The information that remains the same from the previous case can be left as is.

Save

After the information in all nine tabs has been checked for accuracy and edited as necessary, the case must be saved. Data recorded in the Case dialog box are stored by clicking the Save button on the right side of the Case dialog box (see Figure 6-3). Clicking the Cancel button exits the Case dialog box without saving the newly entered information. The boxes that had new data entered will clear, and the screen will redisplay the Patient List dialog box.

Close

The Close button closes the Patient List dialog box

ENTERING CASE INFORMATION

Clicking the New Case button or the Edit Case button brings up the Case dialog box. Information about a patient is entered in nine different tabs within the Case dialog box:

◆ Personal

◆ Account

◆ Diagnosis

◆ Condition

◆ Miscellaneous

◆ Policy 1

◆ Policy 2

◆ Policy 3

◆ Medicaid and Medical

chart *a folder that contains all records pertaining to a patient*

record of treatment and progress *a record containing a dentist's notes about a patient's condition and diagnosis*

The information required to complete the nine tabs comes from documents found in a patient's chart. The **chart** is a folder that contains all records pertaining to a patient. The new patient information form supplies basic information such as name and address as well as information about insurance coverage, allergies, whether the condition is related to an accident, and the referral source. The **record of treatment and progress** contains the dentist's notes about a patient's condition and diagnosis. The encounter form is a list of services performed and charges for these procedures.

PERSONAL TAB   The Personal tab contains basic information about a patient and his or her employment (see Figure 6-3).

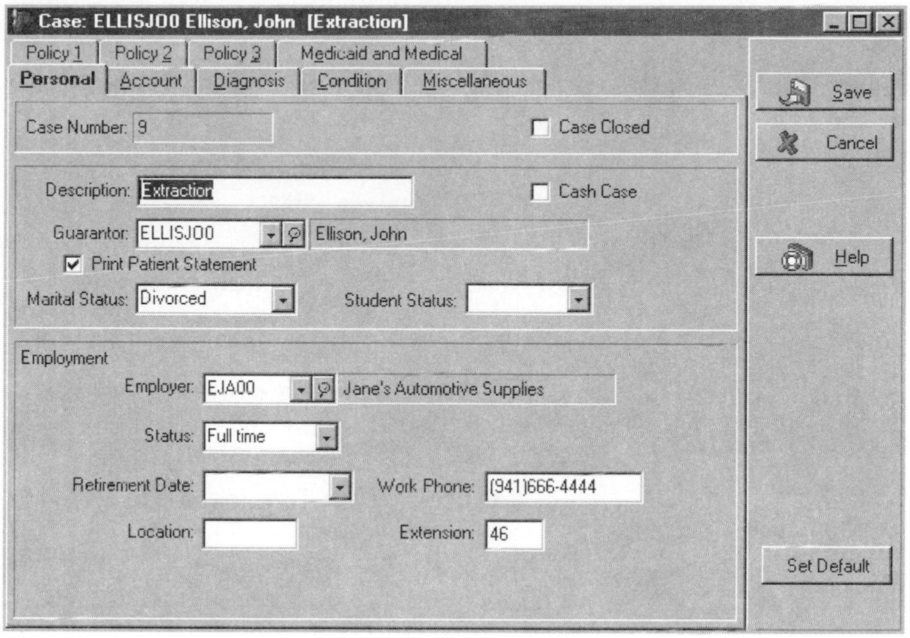

Figure 6-3   Personal tab of the Case dialog box.

Case Number   The case number is a sequential number assigned by PractiSoft. To avoid confusion, case numbers are unique; no two patients ever have the same case number.

Case Closed   A case is marked as closed by placing a check mark in the Case Closed box. At times it is appropriate to close a case. Closing a case indicates that no more data will be entered into the case. When is it appropriate to close a case? Policies vary from practice to practice, but generally cases are closed when a patient changes insurance carriers, completes a treatment plan, or is no longer a patient at the practice.

Description   Information entered in the Description box indicates a patient's complaint, or reason for seeing a dentist. For example, if a patient comes to see a dentist in the practice for a periodic oral evaluation, the Description box would read "Preventive." Other examples of entries are Root canal, Extraction, Restorative (fillings), or Periodontal scaling and root planing. The patient's reason for seeing the dentist can be found in his or her chart.

Cash Case   If the Cash Case box is checked, the patient is paying cash and has no insurance coverage.

Guarantor   The Guarantor box lists the name of the person responsible for paying the bill. The drop-down list contains the chart numbers and names of all potential guarantors in the database.

Print Patient Statement   If this box is checked, a statement for the patient is automatically printed when statements are printed for the practice.

Marital Status   The drop-down list provides the following choices to indicate a patient's marital status: Divorced, Legally separated, Married, Single, Unknown, or Widowed.

Student Status   The Student Status drop-down list is used to indicate whether a patient is a full-time student, a part-time student, or a non-student. If a patient's status is not known, the box should be left blank.

Employer   The Employer box contains the default employer information that has been entered in the Patient/Guarantor dialog box. If it is necessary to change the employer, the default can be overridden by clicking another employer code on the drop-down list.

Status   The Status box lists a patient's employment status as it is recorded in the Patient/Guarantor dialog box. To change the selection that appears in the Status box, another selection is clicked on the drop-down list. The options are Not employed, Full-time, Part-time, Retired, and Unknown.

Retirement Date   The Retirement Date box should be filled in only when a patient is already retired. There are two ways of entering the retirement date. The date can be entered in the Retirement Date box, or it can be selected from the pop-up calendar that appears when the triangle button at the right of the box is clicked.

Location   If a patient has supplied a specific work location, such as "5th Avenue Branch," it is entered in the Location box.

Work Phone   The Work Phone box contains a patient's work phone number.

Extension   The Extension box lists a patient's work phone extension.

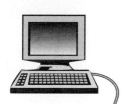

EXERCISE 6-1

Create a new case for patient Hannah Wilson, and enter information in the Personal tab. The information needed to complete this exercise is found on Source Document 1.

Date: October 1, 2007

1. Start PractiSoft. Change the PractiSoft Program Date to the date listed above, October 1, 2007.

2. On the Lists menu, click Patients/Guarantors and Cases. The Patient List dialog box is displayed.

3. Search for Hannah Wilson by keying *WI* in the Search box. The arrow should point to the entry line for Hannah Wilson.

4. Click the Case radio button to activate the case portion of the Patient List dialog box.

5. Click the New Case button. The dialog box labeled "Case: WILSOHA0 Wilson, Hannah (new)" is displayed. The Personal tab is the current active tab. Notice that some information is already filled in.

6. Wilson is seeing the dentist because she needs two teeth pulled. Therefore, in the Description box, key *Extraction*.

7. Choose the correct entry for Wilson's marital status from the drop-down list in the Marital Status box. The Student Status box can be left blank.

8. Notice that the information on Wilson's employment is already filled in. The system copies the information entered in the Patient/Guarantor dialog box to the case file for you.

9. Check your entries for accuracy.

10. Click the Save button to save the case information you just entered. The Patient List dialog box redisplays. Notice that the case you just created is listed in the area of the dialog box labeled "List of cases for: Wilson, Hannah."

11. Do not close the Patient List dialog box.

ACCOUNT TAB

The Account tab includes information on a patient's assigned provider, referring provider, and referral source, as well as other information that may be used in some dental practices but not others (see Figure 6-4 on page 92).

Assigned Provider The Assigned Provider box is automatically filled in with the code number and name of the assigned provider listed in the Patient/Guarantor dialog box. The drop-down list provides a complete list of providers in the practice. If necessary, the Assigned Provider selection can be changed by clicking another provider on the list.

referring provider *a dentist who recommends that a patient see another specific dentist*

Referring Provider A **referring provider** is a dentist who recommends that a patient see another specific dentist. The Referring Provider box contains the name of the dentist who referred the patient to the practice. The referring provider's name and code are selected from the drop-down list. If the referring provider is not listed on the drop-down list, he or she will need to be added to the Referring Provider list, which is found on the Lists menu. It is not necessary to close the Case dialog box to add a referring provider to the database. When Referring Providers is clicked on the Lists menu, the Referring Provider List dialog box opens in front of the other dialog boxes displayed on the screen. Instructions for adding a referring provider to the database are covered later in this chapter.

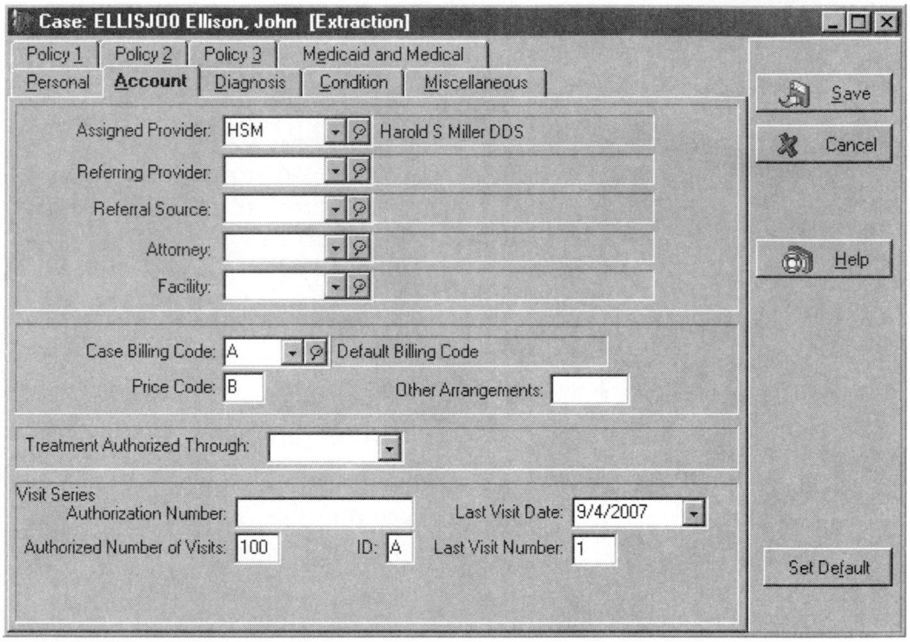

Figure 6-4 Account tab.

Referral Source If known, the source of a patient's referral is selected from the drop-down list of choices.

Attorney The Attorney box is used for accident cases. If a patient has an attorney, the name of the attorney should be selected from the drop-down list. If the attorney is not listed, he or she will need to be added to the system by clicking Addresses on the Lists menu and entering information.

Facility The Facility box lists the place where a patient is receiving treatment. A facility is selected from the drop-down list. When necessary, facilities can be added to the database by clicking Addresses on the Lists menu and entering the necessary information.

Case Billing Code The Case Billing Code box is a one- or two-character box used by some practices to classify and sort patients for billing purposes by insurance carrier, diagnosis, billing cycle, and other criteria.

Price Code The Price Code box determines which set of fees is used when entering transactions for this case. The Price Code fees are entered and stored in the Amounts tab of the Procedure/Payment/Adjustment dialog box, accessed through the Lists menu. Up to 26 different fee schedules can be created (A to Z). In the Collier Family Dental Care database used in the exercises in this text, two fee schedules are used. Fee schedule A is used by the two indemnity plans in the database, BCBS of Florida and Aetna. Fee schedule B is used by the three managed care plans, Sunshine State HMO, DeltaDental PPO, and CIGNA PPO. For the purposes of the Collier Family Dental Care database, fee schedule B was calculated at 80 percent of fee schedule A.

Other Arrangements If a special arrangement is made for billing, it is indicated in the Other Arrangements box.

Treatment Authorized Through A date can be entered in this box if the insurance carrier has authorized treatment only through a certain date.

Visit Series Information in the Visit Series section of the Account tab is used to record an authorization number, if the insurance company has issued one. This section also stores information on the authorized number of visits and the date and number of the last visit.

EXERCISE 6-2

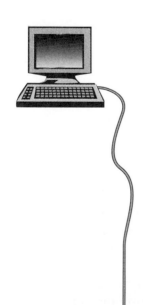

Complete the Account tab for Hannah Wilson. The information needed to complete this exercise is found on Source Document 1.

Date: October 1, 2007

1. In the Patient List dialog box, click the line with Hannah Wilson's name. Then click the Case radio button.

2. Click the Edit Case button to add information to Wilson's case file. The Case dialog is displayed, with the Personal tab active.

3. Make the Account tab active. The word *Account* should now be displayed in boldface type, and the boxes on the Account tab should be visible.

4. Notice that the Assigned Provider box is already filled in with the name of Wilson's assigned provider, Harold S. Miller. The system copies this information from data stored in the Patient/Guarantor dialog box.

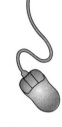

5. Click the name of Wilson's referring provider on the Referring Provider drop-down list.

6. Notice that the entry in the Price Code box is "A." In the Collier Family Dental Care database, schedule A is used by indemnity plans and schedule B is used by managed care plans. Since Wilson's insurance carrier is CIGNA PPO, a managed care plan, change the entry in the Price Code box from A to B.

7. Check your work for accuracy.

8. Save the changes. The Patient List dialog box is redisplayed.

9. Close the Patient List dialog box.

ADDING A REFERRING PROVIDER TO THE DATABASE

If a referring provider is not listed in the Referring Provider drop-down list in the Account tab, he or she will need to be added to the database. To add a referring provider, click Referring Providers on the Lists menu. The Referring Provider List dialog box is then displayed (see Figure 6-5). Clicking the New button brings up the Referring Provider dialog box, which is where information on a new referring provider is entered (see Figure 6-6). The Referring Provider dialog box contains two tabs: Address and Default Pins.

Code	Name	Credentials	License Number	Medicare Part	Last Name
BAT00	Battistone, Salvatore I	DDS	3290088	False	Battistone
LOP00	Lopez, Sheila R	DDS	765410	False	Lopez

Search for: ____ Field: Code

Edit   New   Delete   Close

Figure 6-5   Referring Provider List dialog box.

Address Tab

The Address tab includes various information, such as a provider's name, address, license number, and specialty (see Figure 6-7).

Code The Code box contains a unique identification code assigned to a referring provider. It can have up to five characters. If a code is not entered in the Code box, the system will assign one.

Name, Address, and Phone Numbers The Last Name, Middle Initial, First Name, Street, City, State, Zip Code, Phone, and Fax boxes list basic information about a referring provider.

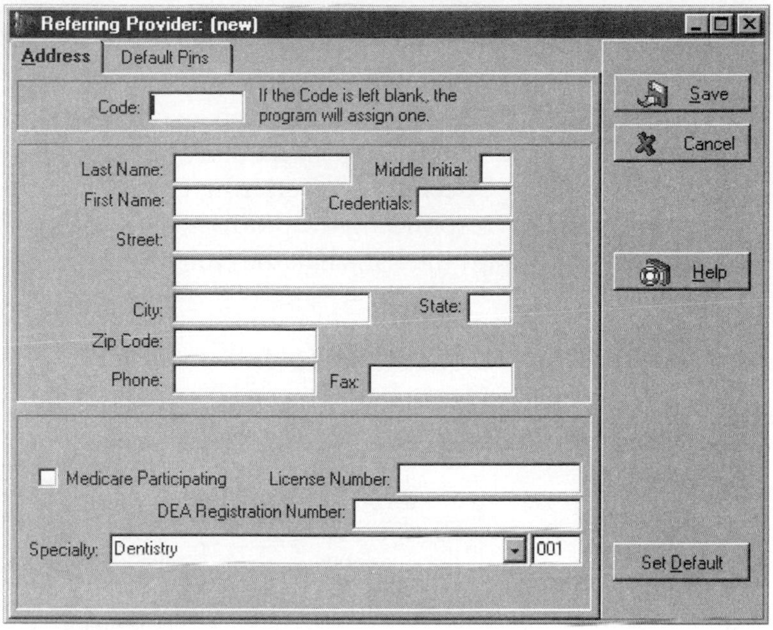

Figure 6-6 Referring Provider dialog box.

Credentials   The Credentials box lists a referring provider's professional credentials, such as MD, DDS, DMD, and RN. This box can be up to three characters long.

Medicare Participating   If a referring provider is a participating Medicare provider, the Medicare Participating box is checked.

License Number   A referring provider's license number is listed in the License Number box.

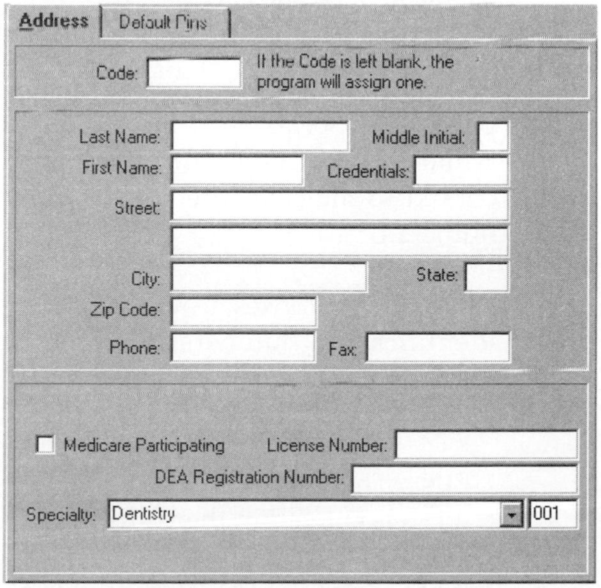

Figure 6-7 Address tab.

DEA Registration Number A referring provider's DEA registration number, the number supplied by the Drug Enforcement Administration (DEA) to track the dispensing of prescription drugs, is listed, if one has been assigned.

Specialty A referring provider's specialty is selected from the corresponding drop-down list. If the specialty is not one of the choices on the list, click the category "All other."

Default Pins Tab

The Default Pins tab contains identification numbers assigned to a referring provider (see Figure 6-8).

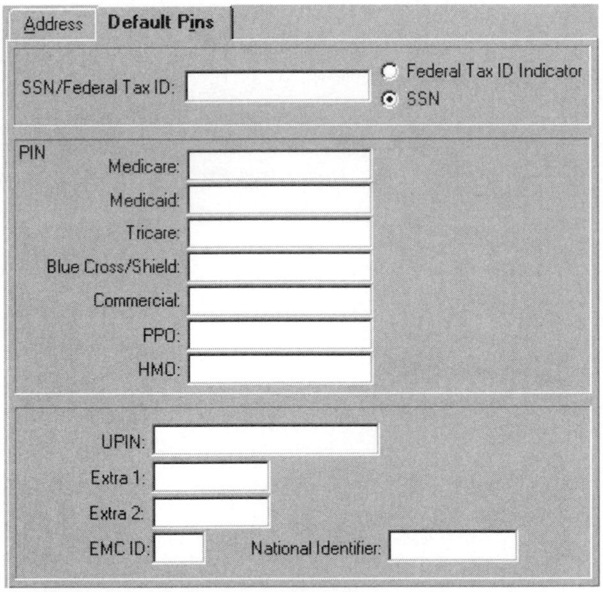

Figure 6-8   Default Pins tab.

SSN/Federal Tax ID The SSN/Federal Tax ID box contains a provider's Social Security number or federal Tax Identification Number (TIN). The corresponding radio button should also be clicked to indicate whether the number listed is a Social Security number or a TIN.

PINs In the boxes listed, a referring provider's PINs (provider identification numbers) are entered for each insurance type: Medicare, Medicaid, Tricare, Blue Cross/Shield, Commercial, PPO, and HMO.

UPIN The provider's Unique Personal Identification Number (UPIN) is entered in the UPIN box.

Extra 1, Extra 2 These boxes can be used to enter any additional information about the referring provider.

EMC ID The EMC ID box contains the identification number assigned to a provider by the EMC clearinghouse.

National Identifier The national identifier box has been added to the PractiSoft program as part of its HIPAA compliance effort. The national identifier is an eight- to ten-digit alphanumeric code to be provided and administered through the CMS (Centers for Medicare and Medicaid Services, formerly HCFA). It is expected that the national identifier will be assigned to a provider for life.

When all the information about the referring provider has been entered and checked for accuracy, it is saved by clicking the Save button in the Referring Provider dialog box.

EXERCISE 6-3

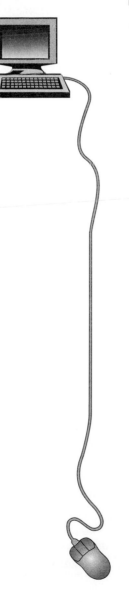

Add Dr. Shelly Zurich to Collier Family Dental Care's list of referring providers. The information needed to complete this exercise is found on Source Document 2.

Date: October 1, 2007

1. Open the Lists menu and click Referring Providers.

2. The Referring Provider List dialog box appears with the names of the two current referring providers displayed, Battistone and Lopez. Notice the codes for each provider. In the Collier Family Dental Care database, a provider code consists of the first three characters of the provider's last name followed by two zeros.

3. To add Dr. Shelly Zurich to the list, click the New button.

4. The Referring Provider dialog box appears, with the Address tab active. Create a code for Dr. Zurich, and enter it in the Code box.

5. In the top section of the Address tab, enter Dr. Zurich's full name, credentials, address, phone number, and fax number.

6. In the lower section of the tab, enter Dr. Zurich's license number and specialty. Leave the remaining boxes blank.

7. Check your work for accuracy.

8. Make the Default Pins tab active. Enter Dr. Zurich's Social Security number. Leave the remaining boxes blank.

9. Click the Save button to save the new information.

10. The Referring Provider List dialog box redisplays. Check to see that Dr. Zurich's name has been added to the list.

11. Click the Close button to close the Referring Provider List dialog box and return to the main PractiSoft window.

DIAGNOSIS TAB The Diagnosis tab contains a patient's diagnosis, information about allergies, and electronic media claim (EMC) notes (see Figure 6-9). In many instances, completing this information is not required.

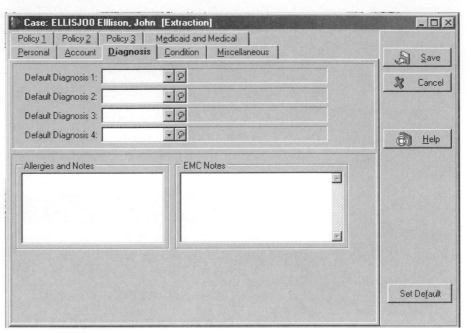

Figure 6-9   Diagnosis tab.

Diagnosis 1 through Diagnosis 4   A patient's diagnosis is selected from the drop-down list of diagnoses.

Allergies and Notes   If a patient has allergies or other special conditions that need to be recorded, they are entered in the Allergies and Notes box.

EMC Notes   If a patient's claim requires special handling when submitted electronically, notes about the procedure, such as an explanation about the charges for supplies, are listed in this box.

CONDITION TAB The Condition tab stores information about a patient's general condition. This includes data relative to a patient's illness, accident, type of insurance, insurance eligibility, and orthodontics and prosthesis information (see Figure 6-10). This information is used by insurance carriers to process claims.

Injury/Illness Date   The date of a patient's injury or illness is entered in the Injury/Illness Date box. (For an illness, the date when the symptoms first appeared is entered.)

Medical Plan Coverage   The Medical Plan Coverage check box is used to indicate whether the patient has medical insurance.

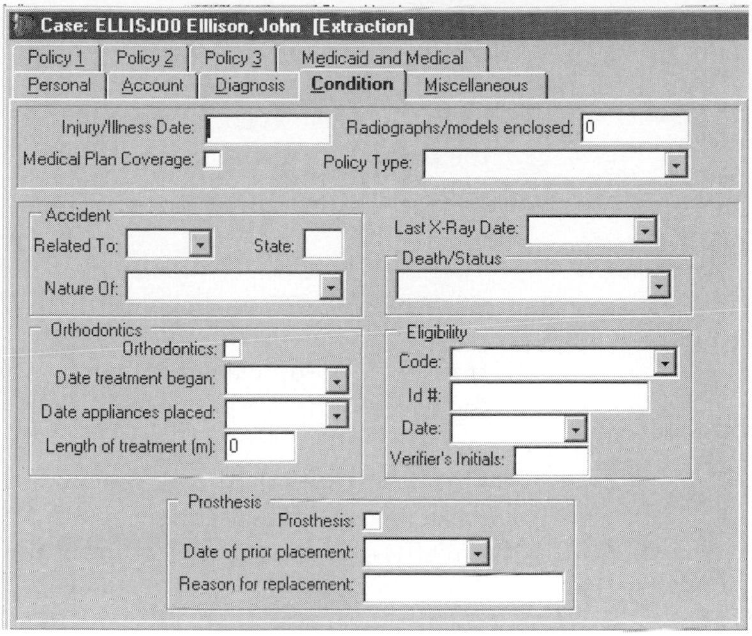

Figure 6-10　Condition tab.

Radiographs/Models Enclosed　If an insurance claim is accompanied by radiographs or models, the number of articles is indicated in the Radiographs/Models Enclosed box.

Policy Type　The Policy Type box is used to indicate the type of insurance policy the patient has. There are three options on the drop-down list: Group policy with employer, Group policy without employer, and Private policy (non-group).

Accident—Related To　The Accident—Related To box indicates whether a patient's condition is related to an accident. The drop-down list offers three choices: Auto, if it is related to an automobile accident; No, if it is not accident-related; and Yes, if it is accident-related but not an auto accident. If a patient's condition is accident-related, the State and Nature Of boxes should also be completed.

Accident—State　The abbreviation for the state in which the accident occurred is entered in this box.

Accident—Nature Of　This box provides additional information about the type of accident. The following choices can be selected from the drop-down list: Injured at home, Injured at school, Injured during recreation, Work injury/Self employed, Work injury/Non-collision, and Motorcycle injury.

Last X-Ray Date　The Last X-Ray Date box is used when the insurance carrier requires the practice to report the date of the last X rays for the current condition.

Death/Status   The Death/Status box indicates a patient's condition; it is usually left blank.

Orthodontics   A check mark in the Orthodontics box indicates that the patient is receiving orthodontic services, such as the application of braces.

Orthodontics—Date Treatment Began   The date the orthodontic treatment began is listed in the Orthodontics—Date Treatment Began box. The date can be entered directly, or it can be selected from the pop-up calendar that appears when the triangle button at the right of the box is clicked.

Orthodontics—Date Appliances Placed   The date the orthodontic appliances were placed is listed in this box. The date can be entered directly, or it can be selected from the pop-up calendar that appears when the triangle button at the right of the box is clicked.

Orthodontics—Length of Treatment (m)   This box is used to indicate the length of the orthodontic treatment in months.

Eligibility   If the patient is eligible for insurance benefits, the eligibility section is used to record the details of how and when proof of eligibility was obtained.

Prosthesis   If a patient is receiving a prosthetic appliance, such as a bridge, the Prosthesis check box should be clicked.

Prosthesis—Date of Prior Placement   If the patient already received a prosthetic appliance, the date of the prior placement should be listed in the Prosthesis—Date of Prior Placement box. This information is required by insurance companies as most dental plans limit the number and timing of dental prostheses. The date can be entered directly or it can be selected from the pop-up calendar that appears when the triangle button at the right of the box is clicked.

Prosthesis—Reason for Replacement   If the present treatment involves a replacement for a prosthesis, the reason for the replacement should be stated in this box.

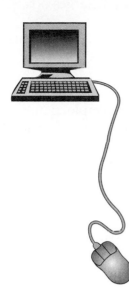

EXERCISE 6-4

Complete the Condition tab for Hannah Wilson. The information needed to complete this exercise is found on Source Document 3.

Date: October 1, 2007

1. Open the Patient List dialog box to edit the case for Hannah Wilson.

2. In the Case dialog box for Wilson, make the Condition tab active.

3. Enter the date of Hannah Wilson's last X rays.

4. Leave the other boxes in the Condition tab blank.

5. Save the new information.

6. Do not close the Patient List dialog box.

MISCELLANEOUS TAB

The Miscellaneous tab records a variety of miscellaneous information about the patient and his or her treatment (see Figure 6-11).

Figure 6-11   Miscellaneous tab.

Outside Lab Work   If the Outside Lab Work box is checked, the lab work was performed by a lab other than the dentist's office. If the lab bills the provider rather than the patient, then the provider bills the patient for the lab work even though it was performed by an outside lab.

Lab Charges   The charges for lab work, whether performed inside or outside the practice, are entered in the Lab Charges box.

Local Use A and B   These boxes may be used by some dental practices to record information specific to the local office.

Indicator   If an indicator code is used to categorize patients or services, it is entered in the Indicator box. For example, patients might be categorized according to their primary diagnoses. Services might be divided into such categories as lab work, consultations, and office visits.

Prior Authorization Number   Before some services are performed, prior authorization must be obtained from the appropriate insurance carrier. If an insurance carrier has issued an authorization number for treatment that has not yet occurred, the number is entered in the Prior Authorization Number box.

Extra 1, 2, 3, and 4   The Extra 1, 2, 3, and 4 boxes are used for various purposes, usually to meet special requirements by insurance carriers, as determined by the dental practice.

Primary Care Provider Outside of This Practice   If a patient is covered by a managed care plan and the patient's primary care provider is outside the practice, the name of the provider is selected from the drop-down list in this box.

Date Last Seen   The Date Last Seen box lists the date a patient was last seen by the outside primary care provider.

POLICY 1 TAB

The Policy 1 tab is where information about a patient's primary insurance carrier and coverage is recorded (see Figure 6-12).

Insurance 1   The Insurance 1 box lists the code number and name of the insurance carrier. The drop-down list provides a list of carriers already in the system. If the carrier is not listed, it must be added to the database. It is not necessary to close the Case dialog box to add an insurance carrier to the database. When Insurance Carriers is clicked on the Lists menu, the Insurance Carrier List dialog box is displayed in front of the other dialog boxes on the screen. Instructions for adding an insurance carrier to the database are covered later in this chapter.

Policy Holder 1   The Policy Holder box lists the person who is the insured for a particular policy. For example, if the patient is a child covered under his or her parent's insurance plan, the parent's chart number would be entered in this box. The insured's chart number is selected from the choices on the drop-down list. (If the insured is not a patient of the practice, he or she must be entered as a guarantor in PractiSoft, and a chart number must be established.)

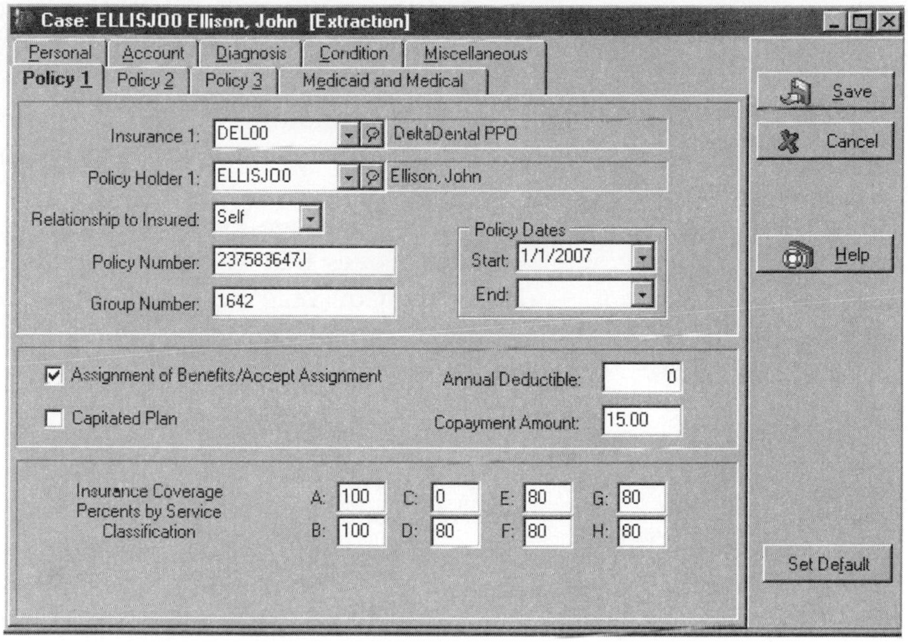

Personal | Account | Diagnosis | Condition | Miscellaneous
Policy 1 | Policy 2 | Policy 3 | Medicaid and Medical

Insurance 1: DEL00 DeltaDental PPO

Policy Holder 1: ELLISJOO Ellison, John

Relationship to Insured: Self

Policy Number: 237583647J

Group Number: 1642

Policy Dates
Start: 1/1/2007
End:

☑ Assignment of Benefits/Accept Assignment   Annual Deductible: 0

☐ Capitated Plan   Copayment Amount: 15.00

Insurance Coverage
Percents by Service
Classification
A: 100   C: 0   E: 80   G: 80
B: 100   D: 80   F: 80   H: 80

Save | Cancel | Help | Set Default

Figure 6-12   Policy 1 tab.

Relationship to Insured   This box describes a patient's relationship to the individual listed in the Insured 1 box. The drop-down list offers the following choices: Self, Spouse, Child, and Other.

Policy Number   A patient's policy number is entered in the Policy Number box.

Group Number   The group number for a patient's policy is entered in the Group Number box.

Policy Dates—Start/End   The date a patient's insurance policy went into effect is entered in the Policy Dates—Start box. If the date is not known, the date the patient first came to the practice for treatment can be entered. If the policy has ended, such as when the carrier changes or when the coverage expires, the date on which coverage terminated is entered in the Policy Dates—End box.

Assignment of Benefits/Accept Assignment   For dentists who are participating in an insurance plan, a check mark in the Assignment of Benefits/Accept Assignment box indicates that the dentist accepts payment directly from the insurance carrier.

capitated plan   a managed care insurance plan in which payments are made for patients on a regular basis to primary care providers regardless of the number of patients' visits

Capitated Plan   In a **capitated plan**, payments are made to providers from managed care companies for patients who select the provider as their primary care provider, regardless of whether they visit the provider or not. A check mark in this box indicates that this insurance plan is capitated.

Annual Deductible The dollar amount of the insured's insurance plan deductible is entered in this box.

Copayment Amount The dollar amount of a patient's copayment per visit is entered in the Copayment Amount box.

Insurance Coverage Percents by Service Classification The percentage of fees that an insurance carrier covers is entered in the Insurance Coverage Percents by Service Classification box. Some dental insurance plans pay different percentages of charges based on the type of service provided. For example, a plan may pay 100 percent of a preventive procedure such as a regular cleaning, but only 60 percent of a restorative procedure such as a crown buildup. A practice can assign a different category of service to each of the letters A through H. For example, "A" could represent basic dental services, "B" could represent preventive procedures, "C" diagnostic services, "D" orthodontic services, and so on. With some managed care plans, 100 percent is entered in boxes A through H, because the patient is required to pay a copayment only, not a percentage of the charges.

ADDING AN INSURANCE CARRIER TO THE DATABASE

If an insurance carrier is not listed in the Insurance drop-down list in the Policy 1, 2, or 3 tabs, it needs to be added to the database. To add an insurance carrier, click Insurance Carriers on the Lists menu. The Insurance Carrier List dialog box lists all the carriers already in the system (see Figure 6-13). Clicking the New button brings up the Insurance Carrier (new) dialog box, where information on a carrier is entered (see Figure 6-14). The Insurance Carrier (new) dialog box contains five tabs: Address; Options; EMC, Codes; Allowed; and PINs.

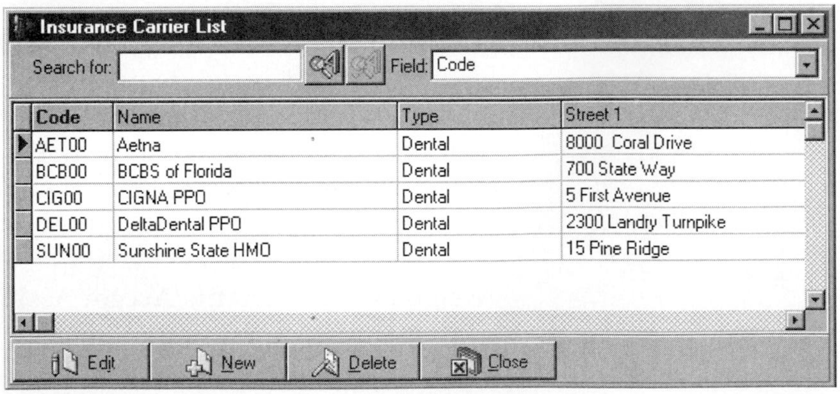
Insurance Carrier List
Search for:
Field: Code
Code
Name
Type
Street 1
AET00
Aetna
Dental
8000 Coral Drive
BCB00
BCBS of Florida
Dental
700 State Way
CIG00
CIGNA PPO
Dental
5 First Avenue
DEL00
DeltaDental PPO
Dental
2300 Landry Turnpike
SUN00
Sunshine State HMO
Dental
15 Pine Ridge
Edit
New
Delete
Close

Figure 6-13 Insurance Carrier List dialog box.

Address Tab

The Address tab contains basic information about an insurance carrier (see Figure 6-14).

Code The code is a unique identification number assigned to an insurance carrier. It can be up to five characters long. If a code is not entered in the Code box, the system will assign one.

Name, Address, and Phone Numbers   The Name, Street, City, State, Zip Code, Phone, Extension, and Fax boxes list basic information about a carrier.

Contact   If there is a specific person at the insurance carrier who is assigned to handle the practice's claims, that person's name is entered in the Contact box.

Practice ID   The Practice ID box lists the identification number assigned to the practice by the insurance carrier.

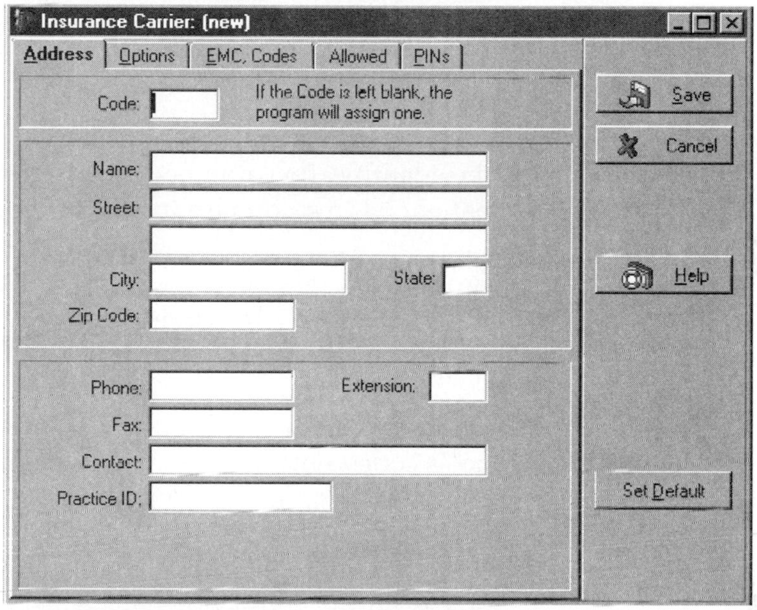

Figure 6-14   Insurance Carrier (new) dialog box.

Options Tab

The Options tab records detailed information about an insurance carrier (see Figure 6-15).

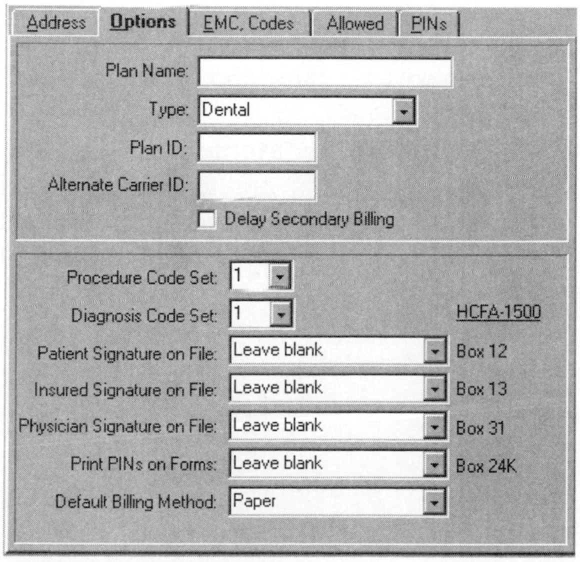

Figure 6-15   Options tab.

Plan Name   The name of the insurance plan is entered in the Plan Name box.

Type   The type of insurance plan is selected from a drop-down list of choices, such as Dental, Medicare, Blue Cross/Shield, Group, HMO, and PPO.

Plan ID   To facilitate HIPAA compliance of the PractiSoft program, the Plan ID box has been added to the Options tab. The Plan ID box is designed to record a ten-digit Health Plan Identifier, which will be administered by insurance carriers. The ID will identify a contract between a provider and an insurance carrier indicating that their health plan transactions comply with HIPAA requirements.

Alternate Carrier ID   The Alternate Carrier ID box is used to list the identification number of an alternate insurance carrier, if the patient has a secondary insurance carrier.

Procedure Code Set   If a practice uses more than one set of procedure codes, enter the code number for the set used by the particular insurance carrier.

Diagnosis Code Set   If a practice uses more than one set of diagnosis codes, enter the code number for the set used by the particular insurance carrier.

Patient, Insured, or Physician Signature on File   The three Signature on File boxes control whether a patient's, insured's, or physician's signature is printed on an insurance claim form to indicate that he or she has authorized payment to be sent directly to the provider. The choices on the drop-down list are Leave blank (prints nothing), Signature on file (prints "Signature on File" if this has been activated in the patient and provider records), and Print name (prints the party's name).

Print PINs on Forms   The Print PINs on Forms box indicates whether the provider name and/or PIN are to be printed on claim forms.

Default Billing Method   The Default Billing Method box indicates whether claims are to be submitted electronically or on paper. Although electronic claim submission for dental claims is prevalent, for the purposes of this book, the default method is paper submission.

EMC, Codes Tab

The third tab in the Insurance Carrier (new) dialog box is the EMC, Codes tab. This tab contains information on electronic media claims (see Figure 6-16).

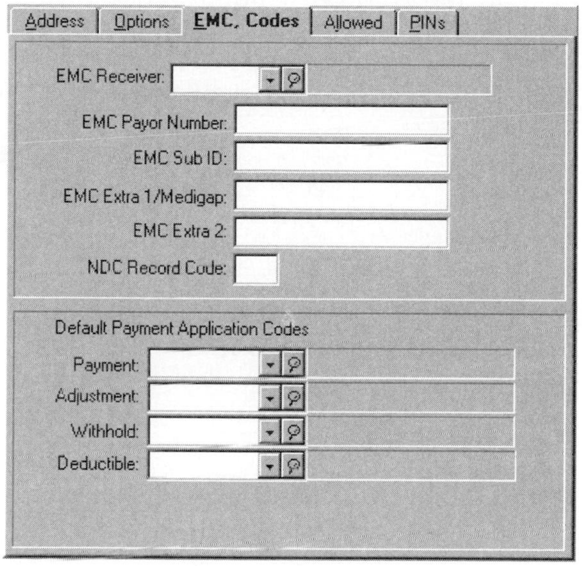

Figure 6-16   EMC, Codes tab.

EMC Receiver   The EMC Receiver box contains the name of the receiver of electronic media claims for a particular insurance carrier.

EMC Payor Number   The payor identification number assigned by the clearinghouse is entered in the EMC Payor Number box.

EMC Sub ID   The EMC Sub ID box contains the sub ID number assigned by the clearinghouse.

EMC Extra 1/Medigap and EMC Extra 2   The EMC Extra 1/Medigap and EMC Extra 2 boxes can be used to enter additional information about the EMC setup.

NDC Record Code   The record code assigned by the clearinghouse is entered in the NDC (National Data Corporation) Record Code box.

Allowed Tab

The next tab in the Insurance Carrier (new) dialog box is the Allowed tab (see Figure 6-17). This tab lists all procedure codes in the PractiSoft database and this insurance carrier's allowed amount for each procedure. The program automatically completes the boxes in the Allowed column when insurance payments are applied to procedures (this is covered in Chapter 8).

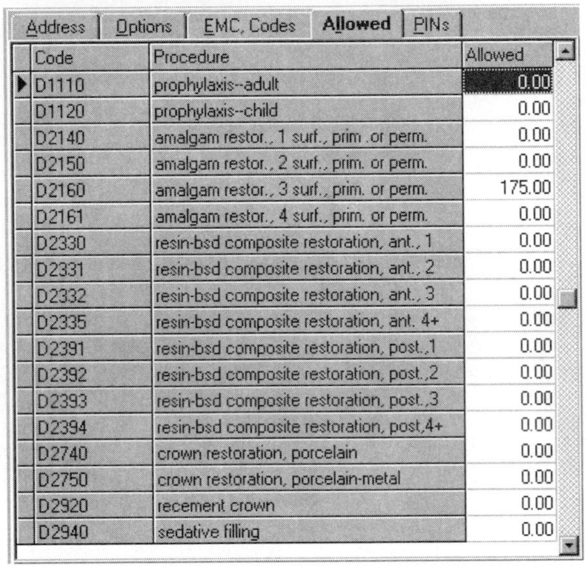

Code	Procedure	Allowed
D1110	prophylaxis--adult	0.00
D1120	prophylaxis--child	0.00
D2140	amalgam restor., 1 surf., prim .or perm.	0.00
D2150	amalgam restor., 2 surf., prim. or perm.	0.00
D2160	amalgam restor., 3 surf., prim. or perm.	175.00
D2161	amalgam restor., 4 surf., prim. or perm.	0.00
D2330	resin-bsd composite restoration, ant., 1	0.00
D2331	resin-bsd composite restoration, ant., 2	0.00
D2332	resin-bsd composite restoration, ant., 3	0.00
D2335	resin-bsd composite restoration, ant. 4+	0.00
D2391	resin-bsd composite restoration, post.,1	0.00
D2392	resin-bsd composite restoration, post.,2	0.00
D2393	resin-bsd composite restoration, post.,3	0.00
D2394	resin-bsd composite restoration, post,4+	0.00
D2740	crown restoration, porcelain	0.00
D2750	crown restoration, porcelain-metal	0.00
D2920	recement crown	0.00
D2940	sedative filling	0.00

Figure 6-17   Allowed tab.

PINs Tab

The last tab in the Insurance Carrier (new) dialog box is the PINs tab (see Figure 6-18). This tab lists the insurance carrier's assigned PIN and Group ID for each provider in the practice.

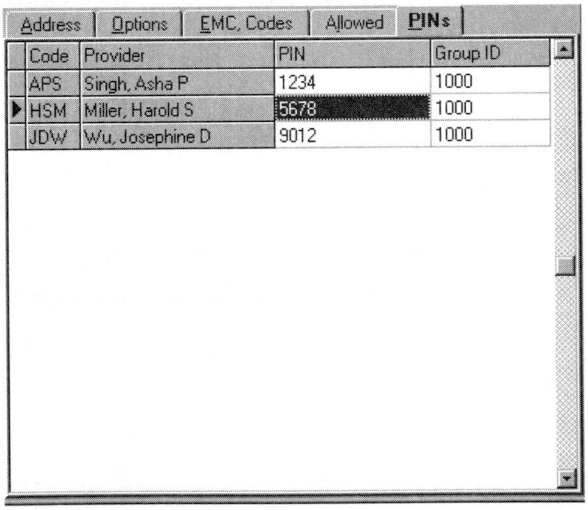

Code	Provider	PIN	Group ID
APS	Singh, Asha P	1234	1000
HSM	Miller, Harold S	5678	1000
JDW	Wu, Josephine D	9012	1000

Figure 6-18   PINs tab.

When all the information about an insurance carrier has been entered and checked for accuracy, it is saved by clicking the Save button.

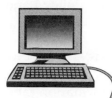

EXERCISE 6-5

Complete the Policy 1 tab for Hannah Wilson. The information needed to complete this exercise is found on Source Document 1.

Date: October 1, 2007

1. Edit the case for Hannah Wilson.

2. Make the Policy 1 tab active.

3. Select Wilson's primary insurance carrier from the drop-down list in the Insurance 1 box.

4. Select the chart number and name of the person who should be entered in the Policy Holder 1 box from the list of choices in the drop-down list.

5. Notice that the Relationship to Insured box already has "Self" entered. If this is correct, do not make any changes. If it is incorrect, make another selection from the drop-down list.

6. Enter Wilson's insurance policy number in the Policy Number box.

7. Enter Wilson's group number in the Group Number box.

8. In the Policy Dates—Start box, key *09012007* as the start date of the policy.

9. Dr. Miller accepts assignment for this carrier, so click the Assignment of Benefits/Accept Assignment box.

10. The insurance plan is not capitated, so do not check the Capitated Plan box. There is no annual deductible, so do not enter an amount in the Annual Deductible box.

11. Key *20* in the Copayment box if it does not already appear in the box.

12. Key *100* in the first Insurance Coverage Percents by Service Classification box (Box A). (According to Wilson's managed care plan, the patient pays a $20 copayment for each visit and the insurance carrier pays 100 percent of charges for covered services.) It is not necessary to change the entries in the other boxes; only Box A is used for the purposes of this text.

13. Check your work for accuracy.

14. Save the changes.

15. Do not close the Patient List dialog box.

POLICY 2 TAB   The boxes in the Policy 2 tab are the same as those in the Policy 1 tab, with a few exceptions. The Copayment Amount, Capitated Plan, and Annual Deductible boxes appear only in the Policy 1 tab. Only the Policy 2 tab has a Crossover Claim box for supplemental insurance.

POLICY 3 TAB The Policy 3 tab does not contain the Copayment Amount, Capitated Plan, Annual Deductible, and Crossover Claim boxes. Otherwise, the boxes are the same as those in the Policy 1 and Policy 2 tabs.

MEDICAID AND MEDICAL TAB The Medicaid and Medical tab has two sections. The Medicaid section is used to enter additional information for patients covered by Medicaid. The Medical section stores information about the patient's medical condition and symptoms, disability, and hospitalization (see Figure 6-19).

Medicaid

Information in this section is entered when a patient is covered by the Medicaid program.

EPSDT stands for "Early and Periodic Screening, Diagnosis, and Treatment." This is a Medicaid program for patients under the age of 21 who need screening and diagnostic services to determine physical or mental problems as well as treatment for conditions discovered. It also includes well-baby checkup examinations. A check mark in the EPSDT box indicates that a patient's visit is part of the EPSDT program.

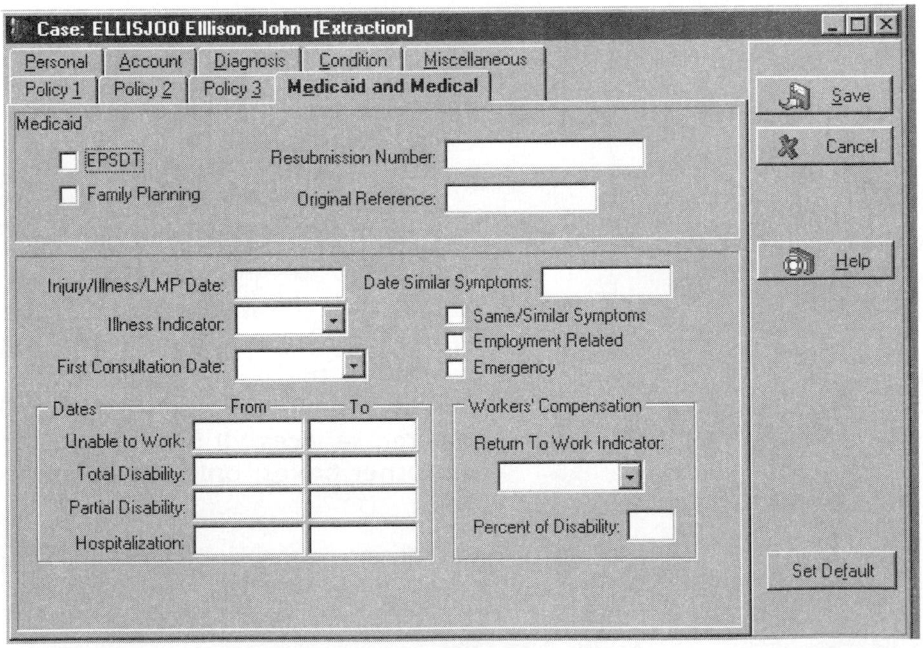

Figure 6-19   Medicaid and Medical tab.

Medical

Information in this section is entered when the dental treatment relates to emergencies or workers' compensation cases.

EDITING CASE INFORMATION ON AN ESTABLISHED PATIENT

Information in an existing case is modified by selecting the case to be edited and clicking the Edit Case button at the bottom of the Patient List dialog box. (The Case radio button must be clicked for the Edit Case button to be displayed.)

EXERCISE 6-6

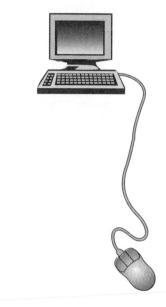

John Ellison, an established patient, has just remarried. Edit the information in his Case dialog box to reflect this change.

Date: October 1, 2007

1. Select John Ellison's case in the Patient List dialog box.

2. Click the Edit Case button to display his case information.

3. In the Personal tab, change the entry in the Marital Status box from Divorced to Married.

4. Check your work for accuracy.

5. Save the changes.

6. Close the Patient List dialog box.

7. Exit PractiSoft.

CHAPTER REVIEW

USING TERMINOLOGY

Match the terms on the left with the definitions on the right.

_____ 1. capitated plan

_____ 2. cases

_____ 3. chart

_____ 4. record of treatment and progress

_____ 5. referring provider

a. A folder that contains a patient's dental records.

b. A dentist's notes about a patient's condition and diagnosis.

c. A dentist who recommends that a patient make an appointment with a particular dentist.

d. A managed care insurance plan in which regular payments are made to primary care providers for patients, regardless of whether the patients visit the office during the time period covered by the payment.

e. Groupings of transactions organized around a patient's condition.

CHECKING YOUR UNDERSTANDING

Answer the questions below in the space provided.

6. Jimmy Barlow has no insurance of his own but is covered by his father's insurance policy. How would this be indicated in the Policy 1 tab for Jimmy?

_____

_____

7. Which tab in the Case dialog box contains information about a patient's allergies?

_____

8. Is it necessary to set up a new case when a patient changes insurance carriers? Why?

_____

_____

9. Which tab in the Case dialog box should you refer to if you need to determine when a patient first began orthodontic treatment?

_____

10. Which box in the Miscellaneous tab is used to enter the number that is preassigned by an insurance carrier to a plan of treatment?

_____

11. A patient has been seeing his dentist regularly for a series of fillings. Recently he has noticed bleeding in his gums. He has also changed his employment. Do you need to set up a new case for either of these situations? Explain.

_____

_____

_____

APPLYING KNOWLEDGE

Answer the questions below in the space provided.

12. While you are entering case information for a new patient, you realize that the patient's referring provider is not one of the choices in the Referring Provider box in the Account tab. What should you do?

_____

_____

13. One of the established patients has changed insurance carriers from BCBS of Florida to DeltaDental PPO. What specific boxes need to be changed in the Case dialog box?

_____

_____

AT THE COMPUTER

Answer the following questions at the computer:

14. Using the information contained in the Case dialog box, list Russell Klinger's primary insurance carrier. Does he have a secondary carrier?

15. Who is the guarantor for June Barlow's account?

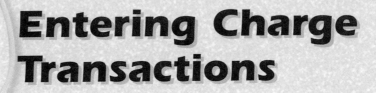

CHAPTER 7
Entering Charge Transactions

WHAT YOU NEED TO KNOW

To use this chapter, you need to know how to:

◆ Start PractiSoft, use menus, and enter and edit text.

◆ Edit information in an existing case.

◆ Work with chart and case numbers.

OBJECTIVES

When you finish this chapter, you will be able to:

1. **Record information about patients' visits, including procedure codes and charges.**
2. **Edit charge transactions.**
3. **Use PractiSoft's Search features to find specific transaction data.**

KEY TERMS

adjustments
charges
MultiLink codes
payments

TRANSACTION ENTRY OVERVIEW

charges the amounts a provider bills for services performed

payments monies received from patients and insurance carriers

adjustments changes to patients' accounts

Three types of transactions are recorded in PractiSoft: charges, payments, and adjustments. **Charges** are the amounts a provider bills for the services performed. **Payments** are monies received from patients and insurance carriers. **Adjustments** are changes to patients' accounts. Examples of adjustments include returned check fees, insurance write-offs, and changes in treatment. This chapter covers charge transactions. Chapter 8 covers payment and adjustment transactions.

The primary document needed to enter charge transactions in PractiSoft is a patient's encounter form (also called a charge ticket or superbill). Typically, the dentist circles or checks the appropriate procedure codes on the encounter form during or just after the patient visit. An insurance billing specialist enters charges and payments listed on the encounter form into the Transaction Entry dialog box in PractiSoft. After the information is entered, it is checked for accuracy. If all the information is correct, the transaction data are saved and a walkout receipt is printed for the patient. If it is incorrect, the data are edited and then saved.

THE TRANSACTION ENTRY DIALOG BOX

Transactions are entered in the Transaction Entry dialog box, which is accessed by clicking Enter Transactions on the Activities menu (see Figure 7-1 on page 116). The Transaction Entry dialog box lists existing transactions and provides options for editing existing transactions and creating new transactions. The following section provides an overview of the different areas of the Transaction Entry dialog box.

All transactions entered in PractiSoft begin with two critical pieces of information: a patient's chart number and the case number, which is related to the procedures performed. The chart number and case number must be selected in the Transaction Entry dialog box before a transaction can be entered. Boxes for entering these numbers are found at the top left of the dialog box.

Chart To begin entering a new transaction, a patient's chart number is selected on the drop-down list in the Chart box. Many practices have long lists of chart numbers in PractiSoft. The fastest way to enter a chart number is to key the first few letters of the patient's last name, which then displays that location in the drop-down list of chart numbers.

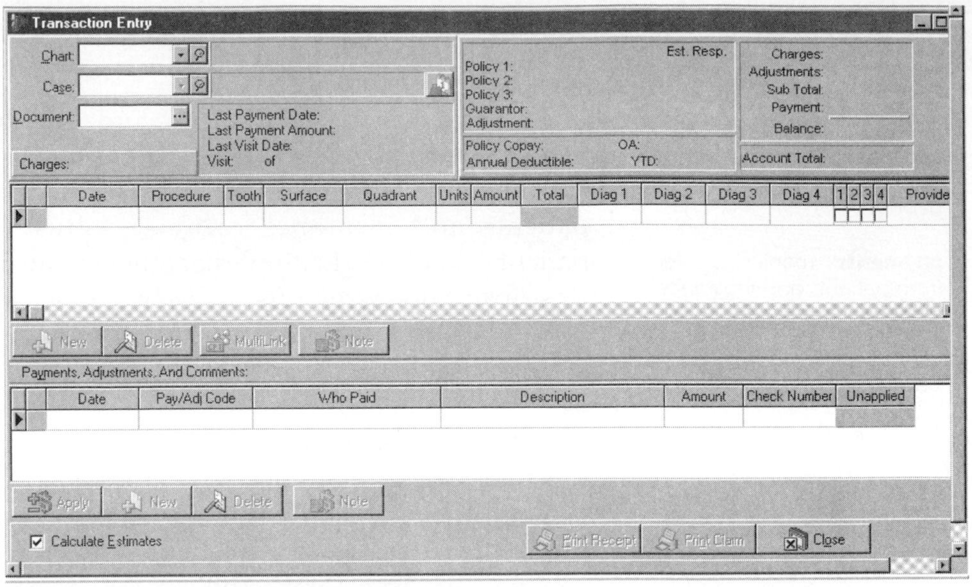

Figure 7-1 Transaction Entry dialog box.

Case After the chart number has been selected, the Case box displays a case number and description for a particular patient (see Figure 7-2). The patient's most recent case is displayed by default. If a patient has more than one active case, the drop-down list can be used to display the full list of cases. Only one case can be opened at a time. When transactions are listed at the bottom of the dialog box, they pertain to the particular case selected in the Case box. Transactions for other cases can be displayed by changing the selection in the Case box.

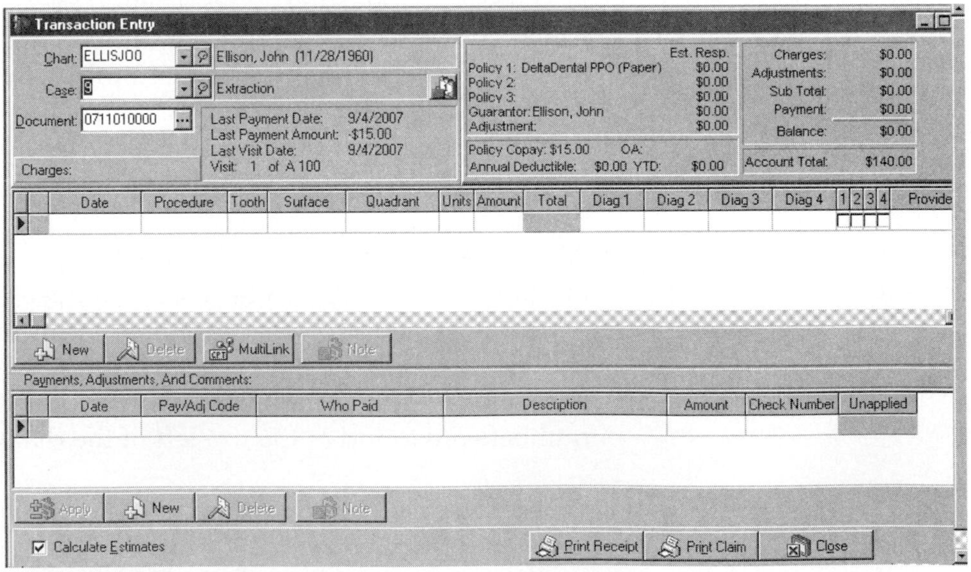

Figure 7-2 Transaction Entry dialog box with case data displayed.

After the chart and case numbers have been entered, a new transaction can be created or an existing transaction can be edited. Transactions already in the system for the patient whose chart number is active are listed in the two lower sections of the dialog box, the Charges section and the Payments, Adjustments, and Comments section, depending on the type of transaction. If the transaction was created prior to the current day, the Document box is clicked to open a Search box. A list of all document numbers and dates for the current case is displayed in the Search box. Click the appropriate document number or date to open the corresponding transaction data in the Transaction Data dialog box, where it can be edited.

The scroll bar at the bottom of the Transaction Entry dialog box may be used to display a full summary of the transactions for the lower section as well as part of the upper section (see Figure 7-3). To view the remaining information in the upper section, which is wider, use the scroll bar at the bottom of that section (see Figure 7-4).

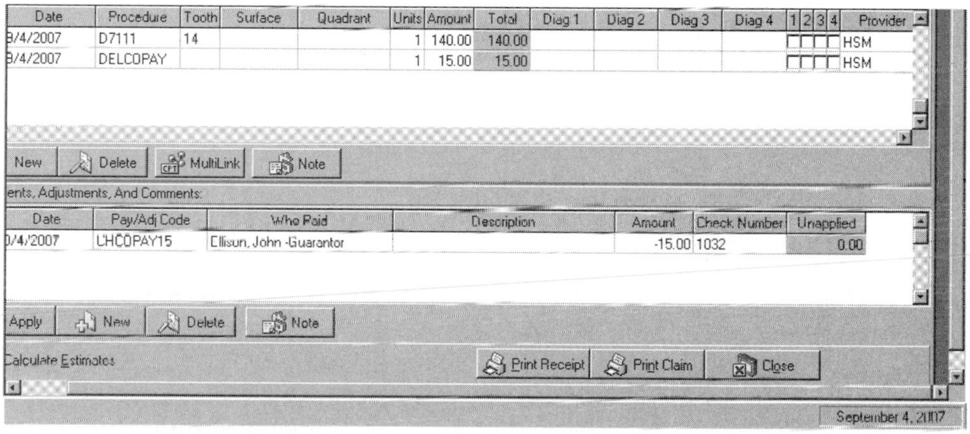

Figure 7-3 Information displayed when scrolling to the right in the lower section.

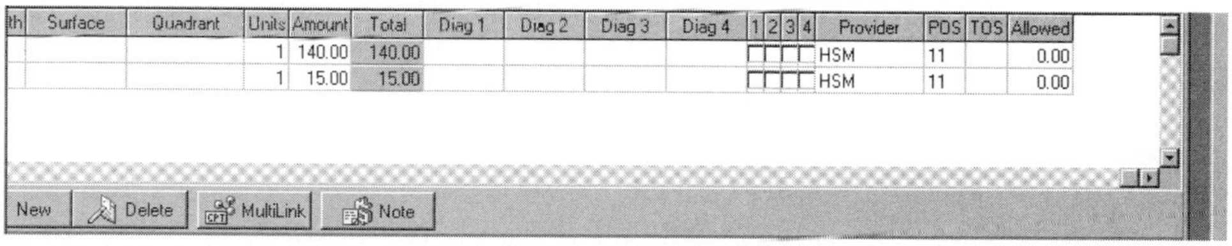

Figure 7-4 Information displayed when scrolling to the right in the upper section.

Charges for procedures are entered in the Charges section of the Transaction Entry dialog box (see Figure 7-5). The process of creating a new charge begins with clicking the New button (see Figure 7-6) in that section. (The steps for entering payment, adjustment, and comment transactions are described in Chapter 8.) The Charges section contains the following boxes:

Date When the New button is clicked in the Charges section, the pointer moves to the Date box. The asterisk to the left of the Date box indicates that a new charge is being created. In the Date box, the system automatically defaults to the current date, that is, the PractiSoft Program Date. If this is not the date on which the procedures were performed, the information in the Dates box needs to be changed to reflect the actual date of the procedures. Data can be changed by keying over the information that is already there or by selecting a date from the pop-up calendar that appears when the triangle button to the right of the box is clicked.

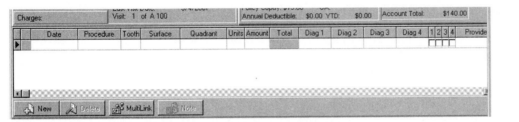

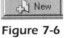

Figure 7-6
New button.

Figure 7-5 Charges section of the Transaction Entry dialog box.

If several transactions need to be entered for a date that is not the current date, the default date for the Date box can be changed. To change the default date for the Date box, close the Transaction Entry dialog box and change the PractiSoft program date using either the Set Program Date command on the File menu or the pop-up calendar on the PractiSoft status bar.

After the program date has been changed, the Transaction Entry dialog box is opened again and the appropriate selections are made in the Chart and Case boxes. When the New button is clicked for creating the new charge transaction, the correct date will be displayed in the Date box.

TIP . . . When entering a new transaction, if the Date box is changed without changing the PractiSoft program date, the Document number should also be changed. The Document box in the Transaction Entry dialog box, located directly below the Chart and Case boxes, displays a document number automatically whenever the Transaction Entry dialog box is opened; it is the current program date (listed in YYMMDD format instead of the usual MMDDYY format) followed by four zeros. The Document number is for reference only and is used in the Transaction Entry dialog box to help locate previous transactions for a particular patient.

In PractiSoft, a dental practice also has the option to use its own system of assigning document numbers. Up to 10 characters can be entered. If a practice uses numbered encounter forms, a common use of the Document box is to record the number found on each patient's encounter form. For the purposes of this book, the default document numbers based on the PractiSoft program date are used.

Procedure   The Procedure box is used to report the procedure code for the service that was performed. The procedure code is selected from the drop-down list of CDT codes already entered in the system. Only one procedure code can be selected for each transaction. If multiple procedures were performed for a patient, each must be entered as a separate transaction, or a MultiLink code, which is discussed in the next paragraph, must be used. After the code is selected from the drop-down list and the Tab key or Enter key is pressed, the charge for a procedure is displayed in the Amount box. If a CDT code is not listed, it will need to be added to the database by pressing the F8 key or by clicking Procedure/Payment/Adjustment Codes on the Lists menu. This can be done without exiting the Transaction Entry dialog box.

MULTILINK CODES

MultiLink codes   a time-saving feature for entering multiple procedure codes under a single code

PractiSoft provides a feature that saves time when entering multiple CDT codes that are related. **MultiLink codes** are groups of procedure code entries that relate to a single activity. Using MultiLink codes saves time by eliminating the need to enter related multiple procedure codes one at a time. For example, suppose a MultiLink code is created for the procedures used in evaluating a new patient. The MultiLink code NEWPTM is created. NEWPTM includes four procedures: D0150 Comprehensive Oral Evaluation, D0272 Bitewings—Two Films, D0330 Panoramic Film, and D1110 Prophylaxis—Adult.

When the MultiLink code NEWPTM is selected, all four procedure codes are entered automatically by the system, eliminating the need to make four different entries. The MultiLink feature saves time by reducing the number of procedure code entries, and it also reduces omission errors. When procedure codes are entered as a MultiLink, it is impossible to forget to enter a procedure, since all of the codes that are in the MultiLink group are entered automatically.

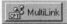

Figure 7-7
MultiLink button.

Clicking the MultiLink button (see Figure 7-7) at the bottom of the Charges section in the Transaction Entry dialog box displays the MultiLink dialog box. After a MultiLink code is selected from the MultiLink drop-down list, the Create Transactions button is clicked. The codes and charges for each procedure are automatically added to the list of transactions in the Charges section of the Transaction Entry dialog box.

Tooth   The number of the Tooth on which the procedure was performed is entered in the Tooth box. The drop-down list includes numbers 1 to 32 (representing the permanent, or second, set of teeth) and letters A to T (representing the primary, or first, set of teeth). On dental claims, teeth are numbered beginning with the person's upper right side. (See Figure 2-3 on page 23.)

Surface   The Surface box indicates which part of the tooth the procedure was performed on. Possible entries are displayed on the status bar as a guide when the Start box is clicked, for example, "L–Lingual" and "F–Facial." The lingual surface is the surface of the tooth directed toward the tongue; it is the opposite of the facial surface. The surface is indicated by the dentist on the encounter form when necessary, usually with restorative procedures.

Quadrant   The following options are available on the drop-down list in the Quadrant box: Full Mouth, Lower Left, Lower Right, Upper Left, Upper Right, indicating the general location in the mouth where the procedure was performed.

Units   The Units box indicates the quantity of the procedure. Normally, the number of units is one. In some cases, however, it may be more than one. For example, a patient may have three X rays done, in which case 3 would be entered in the Units box.

Amount   The Amount box lists the charge amount for a procedure. The amount is entered automatically by the system based on the CDT code and insurance carrier. Each CDT code stored in the system has a charge amount associated with it for each insurance carrier. The charge amount can be edited if necessary. To the right of the Amount box is the Total box. This area is used to display the total charges for the procedure(s) performed. To obtain a total, the number in the Units box is multiplied by the number in the Amount box. By default, PractiSoft does not calculate totals automatically. Only the amount of a single unit is displayed in the Total box. To enter a total for multiple units, key the total amount over the existing figure.

TIP . . . To change the default setting for totals, the Program Options dialog box can be accessed through the File menu. In the Data Entry tab, under Transactions, click the Multiply Units Times Amount check box.

Diag The Diag 1, 2, 3, and 4 boxes are used to report up to four different diagnosis codes associated with the procedure listed on the same line. Diagnosis codes are selected from the drop-down list of diagnosis codes already entered in the system. The four boxes to the right of the Diag 1,2,3, and 4 Diagnosis boxes are Diagnosis check boxes. A check mark appears in each Diagnosis check box for which a diagnosis was entered in the Diag 1, 2, 3, 4 boxes. This information is obtained from the Diagnosis tab of the Case folder.

Diagnosis codes are required only on dental claims that involve medical procedures, such as those performed by an oral surgeon. For this reason, no diagnosis codes have been used in the examples and exercises in this text, which focus on dental procedures only.

Provider The Provider box lists the code for a patient's assigned provider. If a patient sees a different provider for a visit, the Provider box can be changed to list that provider instead. The drop-down list inside the Provider box is used to select a new provider. The drop-down list contains the name and code of every provider in the database.

POS The POS, or Place of Service box, indicates where services were performed. The standard numerical codes used are:

11   **Provider's office**
21   **Inpatient hospital**
22   **Outpatient hospital**
23   **Hospital emergency room**

When PractiSoft is set up for use in a practice, an option is provided to set a default POS code. In addition, POS codes can be assigned to specific procedure codes when they are set up in the Procedure/Payment/Adjustment List. For purposes of this book, the default code has been set to 11 for Provider's office.

TOS TOS stands for "type of service." Dental offices may set up a list of codes to indicate the type of service performed. For example, 1 may indicate an examination, and 2 may indicate surgery. The TOS code is specified in the Procedure/Payment/Adjustment entry for each CDT code.

Allowed The Allowed box displays the allowed amount that the currently selected carrier will pay for the highlighted procedure code. This amount is recalculated each time an insurance carrier payment for a particular procedure code is entered into the database. The program uses the allowed amount to estimate a patient's portion of the charges for a procedure when it is entered in the Transaction Entry dialog box.

ENTERING ADDITIONAL CHARGES FOR THE SAME PATIENT

After information for the first charge transaction is entered, pressing the down arrow moves the pointer to a new line where information for a second charge can be entered. Clicking the New button accomplishes the same thing. The pointer moves to the Date box in the new row, where information for the next charge is entered.

ENTERING CHARGES FOR A DIFFERENT PATIENT OR CASE

After entering charge transactions for one patient, if other charges are to be entered for a different patient or case during the same session, the triangle button in the Chart and Case boxes is clicked, and the desired patient and case are selected. The New button is used to begin entering the charge information.

It is not necessary to close the Transaction Entry dialog box between charge transactions. Nor is it necessary to save any data that is entered in it. In the Transaction Entry dialog box, unlike in other dialog boxes in PractiSoft, information is saved automatically.

NOTE BUTTON

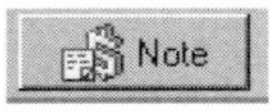

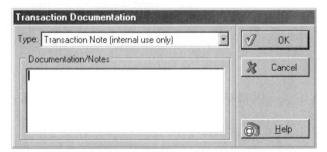

Figure 7-8
Note button.

When the Note button located at the bottom of the Charges section is clicked (see Figure 7-8), the Transaction Documentation dialog box is displayed (see Figure 7-9). This dialog box is used to store notes, which can be up to 255 characters long, about a particular transaction. The Transaction Documentation dialog box can also be accessed by clicking the right mouse button while in the Charges section of the Transaction Entry dialog box. A shortcut menu appears with the following options: New, Delete, MultiLink, and Note (the same options that are available on the four buttons at the bottom of the Charges section). Clicking Note opens the Transaction Documentation dialog box.

Figure 7-9   Transaction Documentation dialog box.

The Transaction Documentation dialog box is optional; it has to be completed only when there is additional information about a particular transaction that needs to be recorded on a claim. The note can be labeled as one of many types using the Type drop-down list. Examples of types on the drop-down list include Diagnostic Report, Prosthetics/Orthotic Certification, Statement Note, and Transaction Note (internal use only), which is the default setting. After information is entered in the Documentation/Notes box, it is saved by clicking the OK button. The information can be deleted by clicking the Cancel button. A Help button is also available within the Transaction Documentation dialog box.

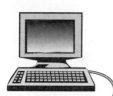

Using Source Document 4, enter the first procedure charge listed for Hannah Wilson's extraction case.

Date: October 1, 2007

1. Start PractiSoft and change the PractiSoft Program Date to October 1, 2007, if it is not already set to that date.

2. On the Activities menu, click Enter Transactions. The Transaction Entry dialog box is displayed.

3. Key *WI* in the Chart box and press Enter to select Hannah Wilson. Verify that the Extraction case is the active case in the Case box.

4. Click the New button in the Charge section. The pointer moves to the Date box in that section.

5. Verify that the entry in the Date box is 10/1/2007 and that the Document number is 0710010000 (for YYMMDD0000), reflecting the same date. (The Document box is located below the Chart and Case boxes.) Press Enter to move the pointer to the Procedure box.

6. Click the triangle button in the Procedure box to open the drop-down list of procedure codes. Select D7111 from the list to report the procedure code for the first service marked off on the encounter form. Press Enter to move to the next box.

TIP . . . To make a selection from the Procedure box drop-down list, the scroll bars can be used to scroll up or down the list until the desired entry is displayed, or, the first few letters of the desired entry can be keyed in the text box next to the drop-down list. When the first few characters of the procedure code are keyed, the system displays the entry in the list that most closely matches the characters keyed. The exact code can be selected by clicking it.

7. In the Tooth box, open the drop-down list and click the tooth number that corresponds to the first procedure marked off on the encounter form.

8. Leave the Surface box blank.

9. In the Quadrant box, select the appropriate quadrant from the drop-down list, as indicated on the encounter form. (See Figure 2-3 on page 23 for an illustration of how teeth are numbered and how the quadrants are labeled on dental insurance claims.)

10. Keep 1 in the Units box.

11. Accept the charge for the procedure that is displayed in the Amount box ($140.00) and Total box.

12. Press Tab or Enter eight times to leave the Diag 1–4 boxes and check boxes blank.

13. Accept the information displayed in the Provider box and the default entry of 11 in the POS box.

14. Press Enter to leave the TOS box blank.

15. When the pointer moves to the Allowed box, the amount is highlighted in blue. This is the end of the transaction line. Press Enter to accept the amount in the Allowed box (0.00).

16. After you press Enter in the Allowed box, an Information box should appear, reminding you that a $20 copayment is due for the office visit. Click the OK button to close the box.

17. To enter the charge for the $20 copayment, press the New button in the Charges section.

18. Press Tab to accept the default in the Date box, and then select the procedure code for the copayment (CIGCOPAY) and press Enter. PractiSoft enters 20 in the Amount and Total boxes automatically. The remaining boxes can be left as they are. (You will enter the $20 payment for the copay in Chapter 8, Entering Payments and Adjustments.)

Now complete the Charges section for the second procedure marked off on the encounter form by completing steps 19 through 30.

19. Press the New button in the Charges section.

20. Accept the default in the Date box.

21. Select the procedure code for the second service marked on the encounter form (D7140). Press Enter.

22. In the Tooth box, open the drop-down list and click the tooth number that corresponds with the second procedure.

23. Leave the Surface box blank.

24. In the Quadrant box, select the appropriate quadrant from the drop-down list.

25. Keep 1 in the Units box.

26. Accept the charge for the procedure that is displayed in the Amount box ($100.00) and Total box.

27. Leave the Diag 1–4 boxes and check boxes blank.

28. Accept the information displayed in the Provider box.

29. Accept the default entry of 11 in the POS box; leave the TOS box blank; and press Enter to accept the information in the Allowed box (0.00).

30. Check your entries for accuracy.

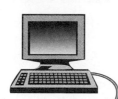

EXERCISE 7-2

Using Source Document 5, enter a charge transaction for Luz Vasquez's case.

Date: October 1, 2007

1. If necessary, change the PractiSoft program date to October 1, 2007, and open the Transaction Entry dialog box.

2. Key *V* in the Chart box and press Enter to select Luz Vasquez. Verify that the Preventive case is the active case in the Case box.

3. Click the New button in the Charge section. The pointer moves to the Date box in that section.

4. Verify that the entry in the Date box is 10/1/2007 and that the Document number is 0710010000 (for YYMMDD0000), reflecting the same date. Press Enter to move the pointer to the Procedure box.

5. Key *D29* in the Procedure box to locate procedure code D2920 from the drop-down list of codes. Once code D2920 is selected, press Enter.

6. In the Tooth box, open the drop-down list and click the tooth number as recorded on the encounter form.

7. Leave the Surface and Quadrant boxes blank, according to the encounter form.

8. Keep 1 in the Units box.

9. Accept the charge for the procedure that is displayed in the Amount box ($60.00) and Total box.

10. Press Enter eight times to leave the Diag 1-4 boxes and check boxes blank.

11. Accept the information displayed in the Provider box.

12. Accept the default entry of 11 in the POS box.

13. Leave the TOS box blank, and press Enter to accept the information in the Allowed box (0.00).

14. Use the left scroll arrow at the bottom of the Charges section to scroll back and check your entries for accuracy.

Note: Notice that no copayment charge was entered for Luz Vasquez. This is because his insurance, BCBS of Florida, as displayed in the top panel of the Transaction Entry dialog box, does not require a copay.

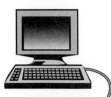

EXERCISE 7-3

Using Source Document 6, enter the first procedure charge listed for John Ellison's extraction case.

Date: October 1, 2007

1. If necessary, change the PractiSoft program date to October 1, 2007, and open the Transaction Entry dialog box.

2. In the Chart box, key *E*. Notice that the chart number for John Ellison is highlighted on the drop-down list. Press the Enter key. Verify that Extraction is the active case in the Case box.

3. Click the New button in the Charge section. The pointer moves to the Date box in that section.

4. Verify that the entry in the Date box is 10/1/2007 and that the Document number is 0710010000 (for YYMMDD0000), reflecting the same date. Press Enter to move the pointer to the Procedure box.

5. Click the triangle button in the Procedure box to open the drop-down list of procedure codes. Select the procedure code for the first procedure marked off on the encounter form *(D5211)*. Press Enter.

6. Leave the Tooth, Surface, and Quadrant boxes blank.

7. Keep 1 in the Units box.

8. Accept the charge for the procedure that is displayed in the Amount box ($720.00) and Total box.

9. Press Enter eight times to leave the Diag 1–4 boxes and check boxes blank.

10. Accept the information displayed in the Provider box and the default entry of 11 in the POS box.

11. Leave the TOS box blank, and press Enter twice to accept the amount in the Allowed box (0.00).

12. After you press Enter in the Allowed box, an Information box is displayed, stating that a $15 copayment is due for the office visit. Click the OK button.

13. To enter the charge for the $15 copayment, press the New button in the Charges section.

14. Press Tab to accept the default in the Date box, and then select the procedure code for the copayment (DELCOPAY) and press Enter. PractiSoft enters 15 in the Amount and Total boxes automatically. (You will enter the $15 payment for the copay in Chapter 8.)

Now complete the Charge section for the second procedure marked off on the encounter form by completing steps 15 through 25.

15. Press the New button in the Charge section.

16. Accept the default in the Date box.

17. Select the procedure code for the second service marked on the encounter form (D5212). Press Enter.

18. Leave the Tooth, Surface, and Quadrant boxes blank.

19. Keep 1 in the Units box.

20. Accept the charge for the procedure that is displayed in the Amount box ($720) and Total box.

21. Leave the Diag 1–4 boxes and check boxes blank.

22. Accept the information displayed in the Provider box.

23. Accept the default entry of 11 in the POS box; leave the TOS box blank; and press Enter to accept the information in the Allowed box (0.00).

24. Check your entries for accuracy.

25. Close the Transaction Entry dialog box.

EDITING AND DELETING TRANSACTIONS

All transactions entered in PractiSoft can be edited within the Transaction Entry dialog box. To edit a transaction, click in the field to be edited and make the change. Changes will be saved automatically.

Transactions can also be deleted from the Transaction Entry dialog box. To delete a charge transaction, click anywhere in the transaction line, and then click the Delete button at the bottom of the Charges section. Alternatively, position the pointer in the transaction line, click the right mouse button to display the shortcut menu, and select Delete. Selecting Delete causes a Confirm dialog box to be displayed, asking "Are you sure you want to delete this charge?" Clicking the Yes button deletes the transaction; clicking the No button cancels the action.

PRETREATMENT PLAN/ESTIMATE

Some insurance carriers require the patient to submit a pretreatment estimate, an estimate of the scope and cost of proposed dental work prepared by a dentist before treating a patient. The purpose of submitting the pretreatment estimate is to protect the patient from unexpected costs incurred for procedures or materials that are not covered by the patient's insurance plan. The insurance carrier reviews the pretreatment plan and associated costs and either approves it or suggests changes. After receiving the insurance carrier's response, the patient and dentist decide on a final plan of treatment based on what the insurance will cover.

PractiSoft's Pretreatment Plan/Estimate feature is designed to create claim forms marked "Pretreatment" that serve as pretreatent estimates for insurance carriers. There are two steps to creating pretreatment estimates. First, the proposed transactions are entered in the Pretreatment Plan/Estimate dialog box. Then the estimate is created and printed using the Claim Management—Pretreatment Plan/Estimate dialog box.

ENTERING PRETREATMENT TRANSACTIONS

Charges for pretreatment plans are entered in the Pretreatment Plan/Estimate dialog box (see Figure 7-10). The same method is used for entering an estimate that is used for entering charges in the Transaction Entry dialog box. In fact, the Pretreatment Plan/Estimate dialog box looks the same as the Transaction Entry dialog box, except that it has a different name, and the lower section, Payments, Adjustments, and Comments, is not included. Because the information entered in the Pretreatment Plan/Estimate dialog box serves a different purpose than that entered in the Transaction Entry dialog box, it is stored in a separate file in the PractiSoft database. Pretreatment data is used to create estimates for insurance carriers, while transaction entry data are used to create actual claims.

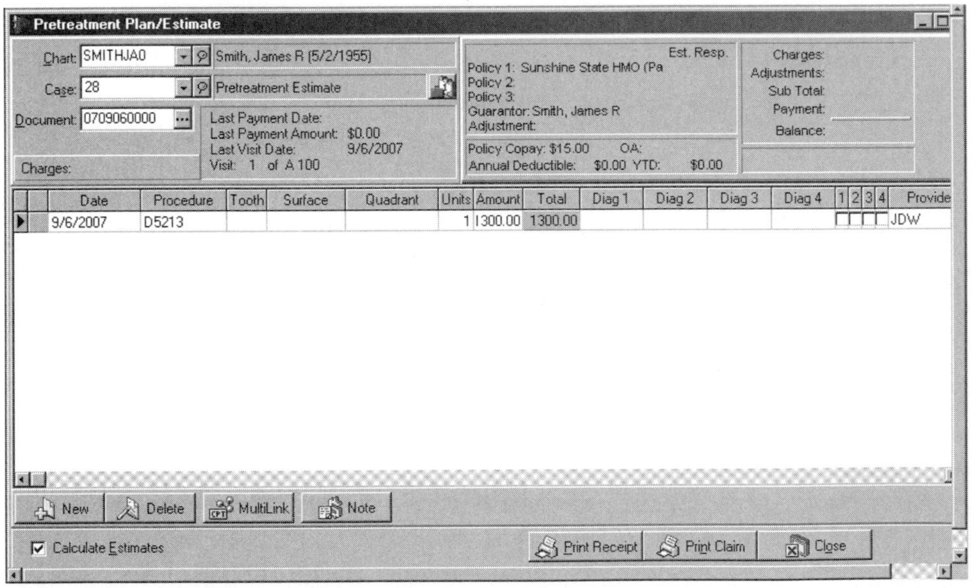

Figure 7-10   Pretreatment Plan/Estimate dialog box.

Figure 7-11
Pretreatment
Transaction Entry
toolbar button.

The Pretreatment Plan/Estimate dialog box is accessed by clicking Enter Pretreatment Estimates on the Activities menu or by clicking the Pretreatment Transaction Entry button on the toolbar (see Figure 7-11). As in the Transaction Entry dialog box, the patient's chart number and case number must be selected before a transaction can be entered. After the proposed transactions are entered in the Pretreatment Plan/Estimate dialog box, the Claim Management—Pretreatment Plan/Estimate dialog box is accessed to create and print the pretreatment estimate for submission to the insurance carrier. This procedure is covered in Chapter 10.

LOCATING TRANSACTION INFORMATION

Sometimes it is necessary to locate certain patients or cases before editing a transaction. PractiSoft provides two features within the Transaction Entry dialog box that make it easy to locate transaction information: the Search button and the Briefcase button.

SEARCH BUTTON   The Search button, indicated by a magnifying glass, appears in many PractiSoft dialog boxes that contain drop-down lists. In the Transaction Entry dialog box, there is a Search button located next to the Chart box for locating a particular patient and next to the Case box for locating a particular case. When the Search button next to the Chart box is clicked, the Patient Search Window dialog box appears (see Figure 7-12). Patients are listed in alphabetical order by chart number. (If the chart numbers begin with numbers, PractiSoft sorts them numerically.) The patient list can be viewed in a different order by clicking the Field drop-down list and selecting a different sorting field. The Field drop-down list includes the following options:

- Chart Number (the default setting)
- Assigned Provider
- Last Name, First Name
- Patient ID #2 (an optional field used to classify patients according to a criterion set by the practice)
- Last Name, First Name, Middle initial, Chart Number
- Social Security Number

The Locate buttons within the Patient Search Window dialog box can be used to perform searches for specific information, such as an assigned provider, employer, date of birth, last payment amount, and so forth. There are two Locate buttons—Locate and Locate

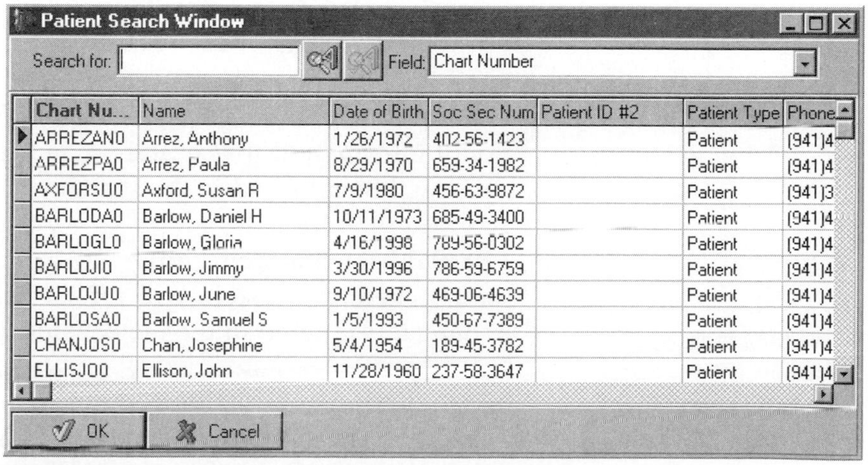

Figure 7-12   Patient Search Window dialog box.

Next—indicated by two magnifying glasses to the right of the Search For box (see Figure 7-13). When the Locate button is clicked, the Locate Patient dialog box appears (see Figure 7-14).

Figure 7-13
Locate and Locate Next buttons.

Figure 7-14
Locate Patient dialog box.

The Locate Patient dialog box contains the following boxes:

Field Value   In the Field Value box, the specific characters that match or come close to matching the sought-after information are entered. For example, if someone were searching for a patient with the last name of Silverman, *Silverman* would be entered in the Field Value box. If a search were being conducted for patients of Dr. Singh, *Singh* would be entered.

Search Type   The boxes in the Search Type area of the Locate dialog box provide options that limit the parameters of the search.

Case Sensitive   A check mark in the Case Sensitive box indicates that the items found in the search must match the case of the characters entered in the Field Value box. If this box were checked, a search for "singh" would not return any matches, since the provider's name is in the database as "Singh," with an uppercase *S*.

Exact Match   A check mark in the Exact Match box signifies that only information that exactly matches the entry in the Field Value box will be returned in the search.

Partial Match at Beginning   If the Partial Match at Beginning box is checked, the system will return items that match the beginning characters entered in the Field Value box.

Partial Match Anywhere   If the Partial Match Anywhere box is checked, the system will return items that match the characters entered in the Field Value box if they appear anywhere in the item. For example, if "son" were entered in the Field Value box, the system would return entries such as "Masterson," "Sonya," and "Wilson's Hardware."

Fields   Searches can be conducted on a variety of different fields of information. In PractiSoft, the choices in the Fields drop-down list vary depending on which dialog box the search is initiated from. In the Locate Patient dialog box, there are 35 choices of fields, including assigned provider, chart number, last name, phone number (1 and 2), Social Security number, and zip code.

First   When the First button is clicked, the system locates the first patient that matches the search criterion and displays that patient's Transaction Entry dialog box. For example, if a search were conducted from the Chart box for patients whose primary phone number begins with (908)508, clicking the First button would display, in the Patient Search Window dialog box, the first patient (in order of last name) whose phone number begins with (908)508. Clicking OK would display the Transaction Entry dialog box for that patient.

Next   When the Next button is clicked, the system locates the next patient who matches the criterion and displays the name in the Patient Search Window dialog box. Clicking OK displays his or her Transaction Entry dialog box.

Cancel   When the Cancel button is clicked, the search is terminated, the Locate Patient dialog box is closed, and the Patient Search Window dialog box is redisplayed.

The Search and Locate features work the same way in all PractiSoft drop-down list boxes.

EXERCISE 7-4

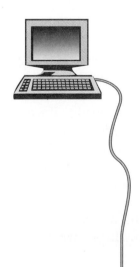

Use the Search feature to locate transactions for an unknown patient based on the patient's Social Security number.

Date: October 1, 2007

1. Open the Transaction Entry dialog box if it is not already open.

2. Suppose you need to locate a procedure charge that was entered last month. Although you do not have the patient's name, you have a Social Security number. Click the Search button next to the Chart box. The Patient Search Window dialog box is displayed.

3. Change the Field box to Social Security Number.

4. Click in the Search For box to make it active. Key the first three digits of Social Security number *456-63-9872*, and watch what happens.

5. After the third digit is keyed, Susan Axford's information is sin-
gled out. Check to see that the rest of the number is correct.

6. Click Susan Axford's chart number to highlight it, and then
click the OK button.

7. The Patient Search Window dialog box closes, and the
Transaction Entry dialog box reappears with Susan Axford's
chart number displayed. Click the triangle button in the Case
box to list any cases she may have; then click the one case
listed.

8. Click the small ellipses to the right of the document number
to display a list of document numbers and dates associated
with that case.

9. There is only one document number listed. Notice that the
transaction date is from last month (9/3/2007). Click the OK
button to select the transaction.

10. Susan Axford's transaction data for September 3, 2007, are
displayed in the Transaction Entry dialog box, including a
charge for procedure D2150. The search is successful.

11. Close the Transaction Entry dialog box.

12. Open the Patient List dialog box. Notice the option in the
Field box is now Social Security Number because of the
recent search. For future use, change the Field setting in the
Patient List dialog box back to Chart Number. Then close the
Patient List dialog box.

BRIEFCASE BUTTON

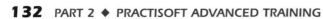

Figure 7-15
Briefcase
button.

The Briefcase button (see Figure 7-15) in the Transaction Entry
dialog box provides the opportunity to select cases for a particular
patient by transaction date, procedure code, and/or amount. This
action is accomplished in the Select Case by Transaction Date dialog
box (see Figure 7-16), which appears when the Briefcase button is
clicked. The right side of this dialog box lists all transactions in the
system for a particular patient. The left side contains several boxes
that can be used to locate transactions that match certain criteria.
These boxes are Date From, (Procedure) Code, and Amount. Any
combination of the procedure dates, codes, and/or transaction
amounts can be entered in their respective boxes.

For example, suppose a billing clerk needs to locate all transactions
for procedures performed on a particular patient on May 24, 2007.
To search for that information, the patient's chart number would be
selected in the Chart box, and then the Briefcase button would be
clicked. In the Select Case by Transaction Date dialog box, 05242007
would be entered in the Date From box, and then the Apply Filter
button would be clicked. Instead of listing all transactions for the
patient, the right side of the dialog box now lists only those transactions performed on May 24, 2007.

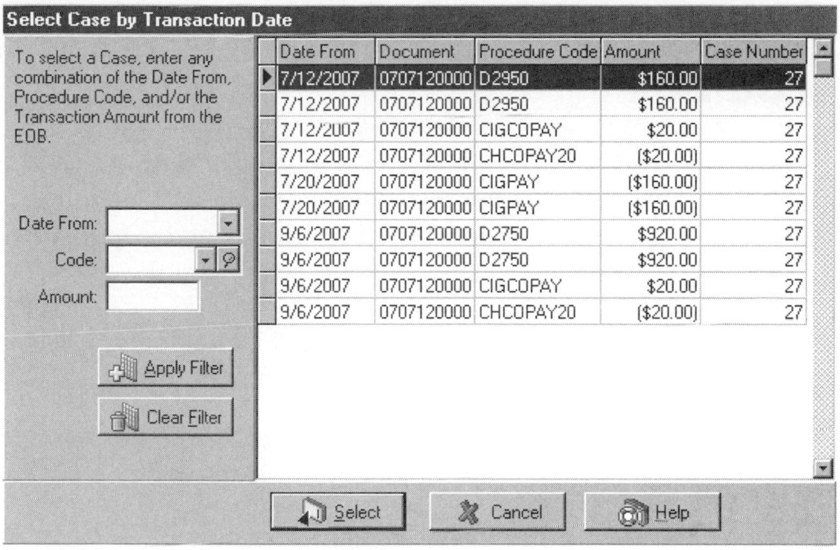

Select Case by Transaction Date

To select a Case, enter any combination of the Date From, Procedure Code, and/or the Transaction Amount from the EOB.

Date From: [_____ ▼]

Code: [_____ ▼ 🔍]

Amount: [_____]

[🗂 Apply Filter]

[🗂 Clear Filter]

Date From	Document	Procedure Code	Amount	Case Number
▶ 7/12/2007	0707120000	D2950	$160.00	27
7/12/2007	0707120000	D2950	$160.00	27
7/12/2007	0707120000	CIGCOPAY	$20.00	27
7/12/2007	0707120000	CHCOPAY20	($20.00)	27
7/20/2007	0707120000	CIGPAY	($160.00)	27
7/20/2007	0707120000	CIGPAY	($160.00)	27
9/6/2007	0707120000	D2750	$920.00	27
9/6/2007	0707120000	D2750	$920.00	27
9/6/2007	0707120000	CIGCOPAY	$20.00	27
9/6/2007	0707120000	CHCOPAY20	($20.00)	27

[🗂 Select] [✗ Cancel] [🗂 Help]

Figure 7-16 Select Case by Transaction Date dialog box.

Similarly, a search can be conducted by procedure code or amount. Searches can be conducted using just one of the criteria, or they may include two or three criteria. When the Clear Filter button is clicked, the full list of transactions is displayed again on the right side of the dialog box. Clicking the Select button selects the particular transaction to which the arrow is pointing. The Cancel button closes the dialog box without making any selection.

EXERCISE 7-5

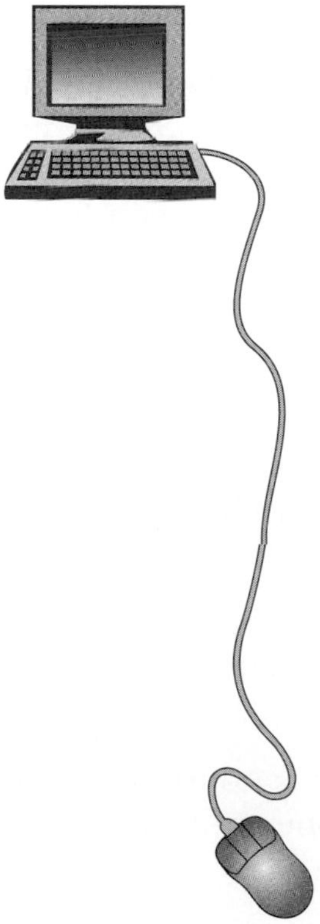

Using the Briefcase button, locate all copayment charges for Sally Smith, indicated by code CIGCOPAY.

Date: October 1, 2007

1. Open the Transaction Entry dialog box.
2. Key *SMITHS* in the Chart box to select Sally Smith. Press the Enter key.
3. Click the Briefcase button. The Select Case by Transaction Date dialog box is displayed. Notice that there are several transactions listed for Sally Smith.
4. In the Code box, click CIGCOPAY (for CIGNA copayment).
5. Click the Apply Filter button to execute the search. All transactions that do not match the search criteria are hidden from view; only the two transactions that match code CIGCOPAY remain visible.
6. Highlight the first transaction, dated 7/12/2007.
7. Press the Select button. The transaction data associated with the 7/12/2007 CIGCOPAY transaction appear in the Transaction Entry dialog box.
8. Close the Transaction Entry dialog box.
9. Exit PractiSoft.

ADDITIONAL INFORMATION IN THE TRANSACTION ENTRY DIALOG BOX

The Transaction Entry dialog box also includes other useful information. These data cannot be edited but provide valuable information about a patient and a patient's account. This information is listed in three sections in the Transaction Entry dialog box.

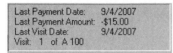

Figure 7-17   Last payment and last visit area of Transaction Entry dialog box.

The left section of the dialog box lists information about the patient's most recent payment and most recent visit (see Figure 7-17).

Last Payment Date   The Last Payment Date line lists the date of the last payment received on a patient's account.

Last Payment Amount   The Last Payment Amount line lists the amount of the last payment received on a patient's account.

Last Visit Date   This line lists the date of a patient's most recent visit to a particular provider.

Visit   The Visit line lists the visit series information as entered in the Account tab of the Case dialog box. The Visit line can be edited from within the Transaction Entry dialog box.

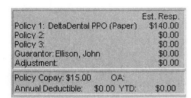

Figure 7-18   Financial responsibilities area of Transaction Entry dialog box.

The center section of the dialog box displays information about the financial responsibilities of the guarantor and the insurance carrier. An estimate of the portion of a bill that will be paid by the insurance carrier(s) is listed, followed by the amount the guarantor is responsible for paying (see Figure 7-18).

Policy 1, Policy 2, Policy 3   A patient's insurance carriers are listed in the Policy 1, Policy 2, and Policy 3 lines. To the right of the insurance policy is a column labeled "Est. Resp." This is the dollar amount of the estimated responsibility for each insurance carrier for the transaction currently selected in the Transaction Entry dialog box. The Calculate Estimates check box at the bottom left of the Transaction Entry dialog box must be checked first before the figures in the Est. Resp. column (as well as in the subtotals column to the far right) are displayed.

Guarantor   The system automatically calculates the dollar amount that the guarantor is responsible for paying, after deducting the estimated amount paid by the insurance carrier. This amount is listed in the Guarantor line after the guarantor's last name and first name.

Policy Copay   The Policy Copay box lists the amount of a patient's copayment, if applicable.

Adjustment   If an adjustment, such as a courtesy discount, has been made to a transaction charge, the amount of the adjustment is listed in the Adjustment line.

OA The Other Arrangements box indicates whether special conditions have been set up for a patient's billing. The system automatically enters information recorded in the Other Arrangements box in the Account tab of the Case dialog box.

Annual Deductible The Annual Deductible box lists the amount of the patient's annual insurance deductible, if one exists. The YTD (Year-to-Date) box indicates how much of the annual deductible has been meet so far in the current year.

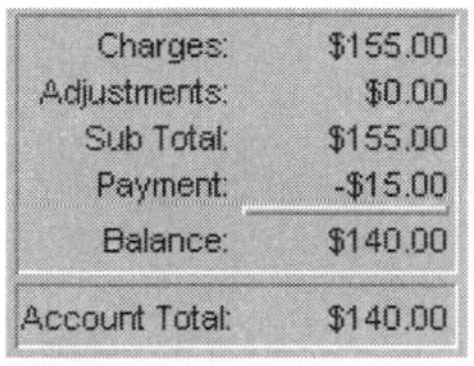

The right side of the dialog box contains a summary of a patient's account, including charges, adjustments, and payments, for an active case (see Figure 7-19).

Charges The Charges line lists the total of the charges for a particular case.

Adjustments The Adjustments line lists the total of the adjustments for this case.

Sub Total The Sub Total line lists a subtotal of the amounts shown in the Charges and Adjustments boxes. If the amount in the Adjustments box is preceded by a minus sign, that amount is subtracted from the amount in the Charges box.

Payment The Payment line lists the total payments received to date for this case.

Balance The Balance line lists the amount owed for this case.

Account Total The Account Total line lists the amount owed for a particular patient for all cases, not just the case currently displayed in the Transaction Entry dialog box.

The last two sections described make up the Estimates tab in the top right portion of the Transaction Entry dialog box. A second tab, the Charge tab, is also available. When the Charge tab is opened, as illustrated in Figure 7-20, charge information for the currently active transaction is displayed in place of estimate information. The Charge tab details who the responsible parties are for the charge in the current transaction (indicated by the pointer), who has been billed for the charge, and how much each responsible party has paid to date.

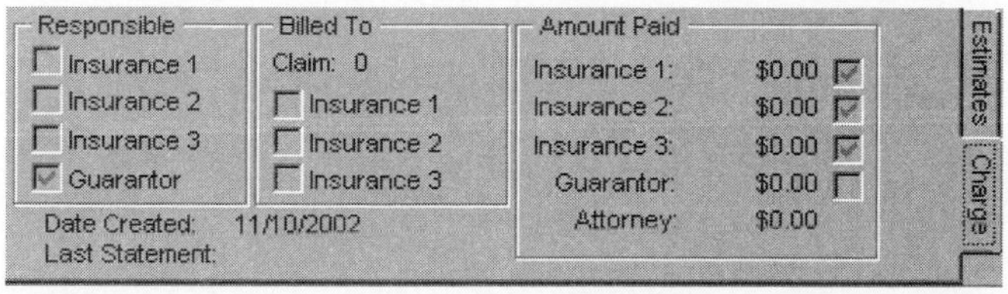

Charges:	$155.00
Adjustments:	$0.00
Sub Total:	$155.00
Payment:	-$15.00
Balance:	$140.00
Account Total:	$140.00

Figure 7-19
Account area of Transaction Entry dialog box.

Figure 7-20 Charge tab in the Transaction Entry dialog box.

CHAPTER REVIEW

USING TERMINOLOGY

Match the terms on the left with the definitions on the right.

_____ 1. payments

_____ 2. charges

_____ 3. MultiLink codes

_____ 4. adjustments

a. Changes to patients' accounts.

b. The amounts billed by a provider for particular services.

c. Monies paid to a dental practice by patients and insurance carriers.

d. A time-saving feature for entering several procedure codes under a single code.

CHECKING YOUR UNDERSTANDING

Answer the questions below in the space provided.

5. What are the two key pieces of information you must have before entering a procedure charge?

_____

_____

6. List two advantages of using MultiLink codes.

_____

_____

7. On a dental claim, what number and quadrant would be used to describe a person's two front teeth in the top portion of the mouth?

_____

_____

8. In the Transaction Entry dialog box, what is the difference between the Search button and the Briefcase button?

_____

_____

9. What is the Transaction Documentation feature used for?

_____

_____

10. An established patient of Dr. Miller comes in for an emergency visit but cannot get an appointment with him. Instead, she sees Dr. Josephine Wu. When entering the charge for the visit, how would you indicate that the patient saw Dr. Wu, not Dr. Miller, for that particular office visit?

_____

_____

APPLYING KNOWLEDGE

Answer the questions below in the space provided.

11. After you have entered a charge for procedure code D3310 (Root canal 1, $400), you realize it should have been D3110 (Pulp cap, $60). What should you do?

_____

_____

_____

12. The receptionist working at the front desk phones to tell you that Herb Fonagy has just seen the dentist and would like to know before he leaves the office what the charges were for his September 4, 2007, office visit. You are in the middle of entering charges from an encounter form for another patient. What should you do first? What is your reasoning?

_____

_____

_____

AT THE COMPUTER

Answer the following questions at the computer.

13. Use the Briefcase button to conduct a search for charge transactions for Russell Klinger that occurred on September 4, 2007. What are the procedure codes and charges for those transactions?

14. What is the amount of the procedure charge entered on September 7, 2007, for patient Rosina Vasquez?

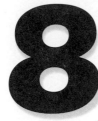

CHAPTER

8

Entering Payments and Adjustments

WHAT YOU NEED TO KNOW

To use this chapter, you need to know how to:

◆ Start PractiSoft, use menus, and enter and edit text.
◆ Edit information in an existing case.
◆ Work with chart and case numbers.
◆ Select patients and cases for transaction entry.

OBJECTIVES

In this chapter, you will learn how to:

1. Record and apply payments received from patients.
2. Print walkout receipts.
3. Record and apply payments received from insurance carriers.

KEY TERMS

capitation payments
insurance payments
patient payments

ENTERING PAYMENTS IN PRACTISOFT

Payments are entered in two different areas of the PractiSoft program: the Transaction Entry dialog box, which was introduced in Chapter 7, and the Deposit List dialog box, which will be discussed shortly. Practices may have different preferences for how payments are entered, depending on their billing procedures. In this book, you will be introduced to both methods of payment entry. **Patient payments**—payments to the practice made directly by the patient or guarantor—will be entered in the Transaction Entry dialog box. This method is convenient for entering patient copayments that are made at the conclusion of an office visit. **Insurance payments**—payments made to the practice on behalf of a patient by an insurance carrier—will be entered in the Deposit List dialog box. The Deposit List feature is more efficient for entering large insurance payments that must be split up and applied to a number of different patients.

patient payments payments made to the practice from a patient or guarantor

insurance payments payments made to the practice on behalf of a patient by an insurance carrier

ENTERING PATIENT PAYMENTS

Patient payments are entered in the Payments, Adjustments, and Comments section of the Transaction Entry dialog box (see Figure 8-1). The payment area, located at the bottom of the Transaction Entry dialog box, contains the following fields:

Date   In the Date box, the date when the payment was received is entered. The value in this box defaults to the current date (PractiSoft Program Date).

Pay/Adj Code   From the drop-down list in the Pay/Adj Code box, the type of payment is selected, such as patient payment, cash; patient payment, check; and various copayment selections.

Who Paid   From the drop-down list in the Who Paid box, the party that made the payment is selected. The choices include the patient (or the patient's guarantor) and the patient's insurance carrier(s).

Description   If a payment is not made by check, the Description box can be used to record other information about the payment. Otherwise this box can be left blank.

Amount   The amount of a payment is entered in the Amount box.

Check Number   If a payment is made by check, the check number is entered in the Check Number box.

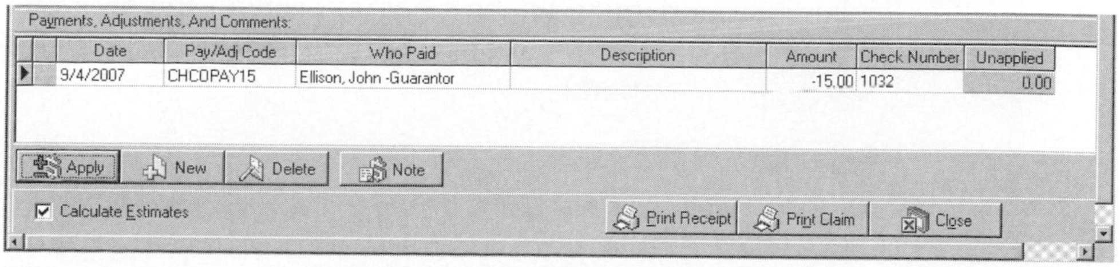

Date	Pay/Adj Code	Who Paid	Description	Amount	Check Number	Unapplied
9/4/2007	CHCOPAY15	Ellison, John -Guarantor		-15.00	1032	0.00

Figure 8-1 Payment section of the Transaction Entry dialog box.

APPLYING PATIENT PAYMENTS

After the payment section's fields have been completed and checked for accuracy, the payment must be applied to charges. This is accomplished by clicking the Apply button. The Apply Payment to Charges dialog box is then displayed (see Figure 8-2). The dialog box lists information about all unpaid charges for a patient, including the date of the procedure, the document number, the procedure code, the charge, the balance, and the payor total. In the top right corner of the dialog box, the amount of payment that has not yet been applied to charges is listed in the Unapplied box. The cursor appears in the first box of the column labeled "This Payment." Clicking on the zeros in the This Payment box moves the zeros to the top left corner of the box. This indicates that the box is active and ready for entry. The amount of a payment that is to be applied to a charge is entered with or without a decimal point.

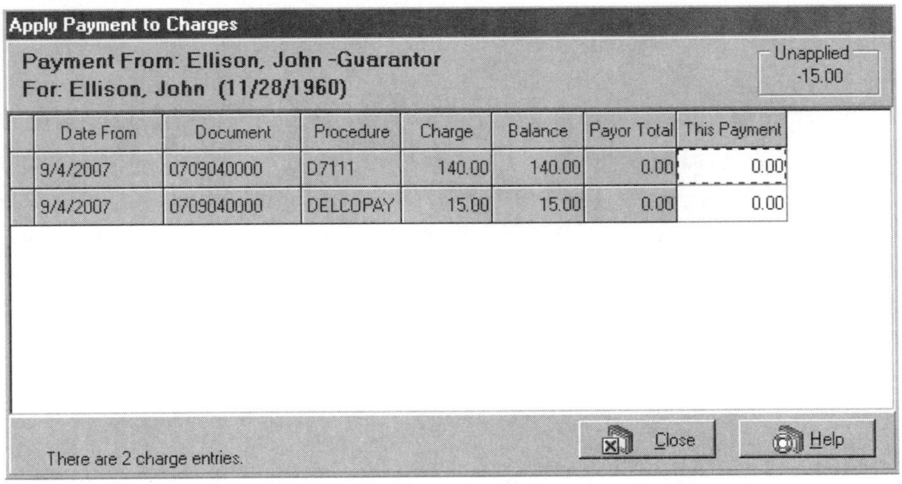

Apply Payment to Charges

Payment From: Ellison, John -Guarantor
For: Ellison, John (11/28/1960)

Unapplied
-15.00

Date From	Document	Procedure	Charge	Balance	Payor Total	This Payment
9/4/2007	0709040000	D7111	140.00	140.00	0.00	0.00
9/4/2007	0709040000	DELCOPAY	15.00	15.00	0.00	0.00

There are 2 charge entries.

Close   Help

Figure 8-2   Apply Payment to Charges dialog box.

Payments can be applied to more than one charge. For example, suppose that the amount in the Unapplied box is $200 and there are three charges that have not been paid. The $200 payment can be applied to one of the charges or two of the charges, or it can be distributed among the three charges. It is not even necessary to apply the entire payment amount. A balance can remain in the Unapplied box, or the balance can be used to reduce the amount due on another charge. Clicking the Close button exits the Apply Payment to Charges dialog box, and the Transaction Entry dialog box is again displayed.

The Transaction Documentation feature is also available in the payment area by clicking the payment for which a note is to be entered and then clicking the Note button at the bottom of the section. (Unlike in the Charges section, the shortcut menu displayed with the right mouse button in this section does not include a Note option.)

ENTERING AND APPLYING CREDIT CARD PAYMENTS

Credit cards payments can also be entered and applied in the Transaction Entry dialog box. However, for a dental office to use this option, enrollment in a credit card processing program known as Global Payments is required. Enrollment is done through MediSoft. As part of the enrollment process, MediSoft sends enrollment forms, an instructional video, and a magnetic stripe reader for swiping credit cards. When approved for credit card processing, the practice is assigned a Transaction ID number and a Merchant ID. The first time a credit card transaction is attempted, a Receiver Settings dialog box is displayed requesting the assigned information. After successfully transmitting the information electronically, credit card processing becomes available.

Entering credit card transactions in PractiSoft is a two-part process. The first step is to create the credit card transaction in the Transaction Entry dialog box. Credit card transactions are created the same way as other transactions. In the Pay/Adj Code box, however, a credit card payment or credit card adjustment code must be entered. (Credit card codes are set up in the Procedure/Payment/ Adjustment Code dialog box.) Any time a credit card code is entered in the Pay/Adj Code box, an Authorize button appears at the bottom of the Payments, Adjustments, and Comments section. The Authorize button is clicked to obtain electronic approval from Global Payments. Funding is then authorized, and the payment is applied to the transaction in the Transaction Entry dialog box.

The second step in the two-part process is to balance all credit card transactions created during the day in the Credit Card Management dialog box, accessed through the Activities menu. Balancing is usually done at the end of the day to make sure all credit card transactions have been properly processed and to spot and correct any obvious errors.

ENTERING COMMENTS

In addition to entering payments and adjustments, the payment section of the Transaction Entry dialog box can be used to enter comments. To enter a comment, the New button is clicked and a comment code is selected from the Pay/Adj Code box. The comment is keyed in the Description box in the same transaction line.

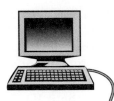

EXERCISE 8-1

Using Source Document 4, enter the copayment made by Hannah Wilson for her October 1, 2007, office visit.

Date: October 1, 2007

1. If necessary, start PractiSoft and change the PractiSoft Program Date to October 1, 2007.

2. Open the Transaction Entry dialog box.

3. In the Chart box, key *WI* and press Enter to select Hannah Wilson. Verify that Extraction is the active case in the Case box and that the Document number displayed reflects today's date (0710010000).

4. In the Payments, Adjustments, and Comments section, click the New button. The pointer moves to the Date box in that section.

5. Press Enter to accept the default entry of 10/1/07 in the Date box.

6. In the Pay/Adj Code drop-down list, click CHCOPAY20 (the copayment amount required by CIGNA PPO) and press Enter.

7. On the Who Paid drop-down list, click Wilson, Hannah - Guarantor, if she is not already selected.

8. Leave the Description box blank.

9. Accept the amount displayed in the Amount box (-20.00).

10. Key *123* in the Check Number box and press Enter.

11. The amount of the payment (-20.00) is displayed in the Unapplied box at the end of the transaction line. To apply the payment, click the Apply button at the bottom of the Payment section.

12. The Apply Payment to Charges dialog box is displayed. Notice that the amount of this payment (-20.00) is listed in the Unapplied box at the top right of the dialog box.

13. Click the zeros in the This Payment box located on the same line as the CIGCOPAY charge.

14. Key *20* in the This Payment box. Press Enter. Notice that the system inserts a decimal point automatically and the Unapplied box at the top right now displays 0.00.

15. Click the Close button. The Transaction Entry dialog box is displayed again. Now the Unapplied box in the Transaction Entry dialog box also displays 0.00.

16. Check your entries for accuracy. Do not close the Transaction Entry dialog box.

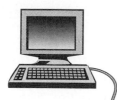

EXERCISE 8-2

Using Source Document 6, enter the copayment made by John Ellison for his October 1, 2007, office visit.

Date: October 1, 2007

1. Make sure the Transaction Entry dialog box is open.

2. In the Chart box, key *E* and press Enter to select John Ellison. Verify that Extraction is the active case in the Case box and that the Document number displayed reflects today's date (0710010000).

3. Click the New button in the Payments, Adjustments, and Comments section. The pointer moves to the Date box in that section.

4. Press Enter to accept the default entry of 10/1/2007.

5. In the Pay/Adj Code drop-down list, click the code for Check Copayment $15 (the copayment amount required by DeltaDental PPO).

6. On the Who Paid drop-down list, click Ellison, John - Guarantor, if he is not already selected.

7. Leave the Description box blank.

8. Accept the amount displayed in the Amount box (-15.00).

9. Key *456* in the Check Number box and press Enter.

10. The amount of the payment (-15.00) is displayed in the Unapplied box at the end of the transaction line. To apply the payment, click the Apply button at the bottom of the Payment section.

11. The Apply Payment to Charges dialog box is displayed. Click the zeros in the This Payment box located on the same line as the DELCOPAY charge.

12. Key *15* in the This Payment box. Press Enter. The system inserts a decimal point automatically, and the Unapplied box at the top right now displays 0.00.

13. Click the Close button. The Transaction Entry dialog box is displayed again, with the Unapplied box now displaying 0.00.

14. Check your entries for accuracy. Do not close the Transaction Entry dialog box.

PRINTING WALKOUT RECEIPTS

A walkout receipt includes information on the procedures and charges for a visit. If required, a patient can attach the receipt to an insurance form and submit it directly to his or her carrier. If there is a balance due, the receipt serves as a reminder of the amount owed.

After a patient payment has been entered in the Transaction Entry dialog box, a walkout receipt is printed and given to the patient before the patient leaves the office. In the Transaction Entry dialog box, a walkout receipt is printed by clicking the Print Receipt button. The Open Report dialog box is displayed, and the available reports are listed under the Report Title heading (see Figure 8-3). The report options include a walkout receipt that prints all transactions, one that prints charges only, and one that records a credit card transaction. Click the desired option to select the report title, and then click the OK button. PractiSoft then asks whether the report is to be previewed on the screen, sent directly to the printer, or exported to a file. If the report is to be previewed on screen, it can subsequently be printed directly from the Preview Report window. After the preview/print/export choice has been made, the Data Selection Questions dialog box is displayed that confirms the date of the transaction. The system automatically enters default data based on the transaction that is active. Clicking the OK button accepts the default data and sends the report to the printer.

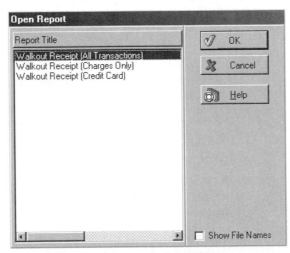

Figure 8-3   Open Report dialog box.

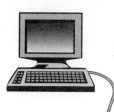

EXERCISE 8-3

Create a walkout receipt for John Ellison.

Date: October 1, 2007

1. With the Transaction Entry dialog box open to John Ellison's extraction case, click the Print Receipt button. The Open Report dialog box is displayed.

2. Verify that Walkout Receipt (All Transactions) is highlighted, and then click the OK button.

3. In the Print Report Where? dialog box, accept the default selection to preview the report on the screen. Click the Start button.

4. The Data Selection Questions dialog box is displayed. Accept the default entries in the Date From Range boxes and click the OK button. The Preview Report window opens, displaying the walkout receipt.

5. Review the charge and payment entries listed in the top half of the receipt.

6. Scroll down and review the total charges, payments, and adjustments listed at the lower right area of the receipt.

7. Click the Close button at the top of the window to exit the Preview Report window.

8. Close the Transaction Entry dialog box.

ENTERING INSURANCE CARRIER PAYMENTS

Information about payments from insurance carriers is mailed or electronically transmitted to a provider through an electronic remittance advice (RA). A remittance advice lists patients, dates of service, charges, and the amount paid or denied by the insurance carrier. Most RAs also provide an explanation of unpaid charges. Sometimes a paper check is attached to the RA; in other cases the payment is deposited directly in the practice's bank account.

Payment information located on the RA is entered in the Deposit List dialog box. This dialog box is opened by clicking Enter Deposits/ Payments on the Activities menu. The Deposit List dialog box displays a list of all deposits already entered in the program (see Figure 8-4 on page 146). It contains the following information:

Deposit Date The computer's system data is displayed as the default. The date can be changed by keying over the default date or by activating the pop-up calendar to the right of the Deposit Date box and selecting a date.

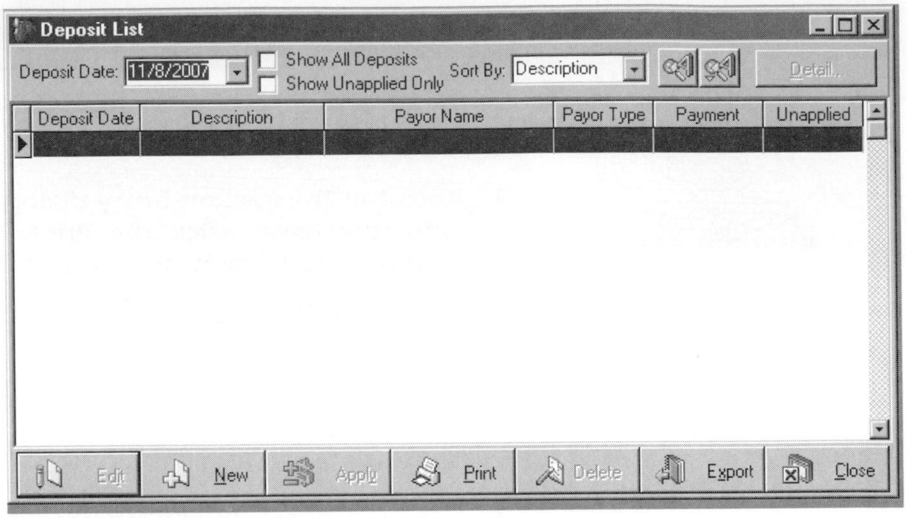

Figure 8-4   Deposit List dialog box.

Show All Deposits   If this box is checked, all payments are displayed—those entered in the Transaction Entry dialog box and those entered in the Deposit List dialog box. If this box is not checked, only payments that were entered in the Deposit List box are visible.

Show Unapplied Only   If the Show Unapplied Only box is checked, only payments that have not been fully applied to charge transactions are displayed. If the box is not checked, all payments—both applied and unapplied—are listed.

Sort By   The Sort By drop-down list offers two choices for how payment information is listed: the default is sorting payments by description. Payments can also be sorted by the payor name.

Detail   To view detail about a specific deposit, highlight the deposit and click the Detail button.

In the middle section of the Deposit List window, information is listed for each deposit/payment, including:

Deposit Date lists the date of the deposit or payment.

Description displays whatever was entered in the Description or Bank Number box in the Deposit dialog box. The Deposit dialog box is where new payments and deposits are recorded (see Figure 8-5). It is accessed by clicking the New button in the Deposit List dialog box.

Payor Name lists the name of the insurance carrier or individual who made the payment.

Payor Type is a classification column; it lists whether the payment is an insurance payment, a patient payment, or a capitation payment.

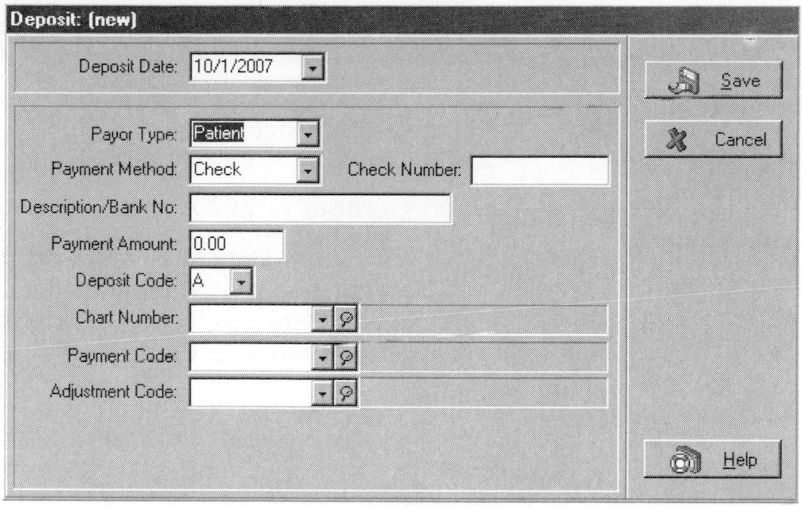

Figure 8-5 Deposit (new) dialog box.

capitation payments
payments made on a regular basis from an insurance carrier to a provider for providing services to plan members

Capitation payments are payments made to providers on a regular basis (such as monthly) for providing services to patients in a managed care insurance plan. In traditional insurance plans, dentists are paid based on the specific procedure they perform and the number of times the procedure is performed. Under a capitated plan, a flat fee is paid to the dentist no matter how many times a patient receives treatment. For example, a dentist who is the primary dental care provider for 50 patients may receive a payment of $2,500 per month to provide care for those patients, regardless of whether they have been seen by the dentist during that month.

Payment lists the amount of the payment.

Unapplied displays the amount of the payment that has not yet been applied to charges.

At the bottom of the Deposit List dialog box are buttons that perform the following actions:

Edit Opens the highlighted payment/deposit for editing.

New Opens the Deposit dialog box, where new payments and deposits are recorded.

Apply Applies payments to specific charge transactions.

Print Sends a command to print the deposit list.

Delete Deletes the highlighted transaction.

Export Exports the deposit list to a file.

Close Exits the Deposit List dialog box.

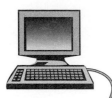

EXERCISE 8-4

Using Source Document 7, enter the payment received from John Ellison's insurance carrier for services provided on September 4, 2007.

Date: October 1, 2007

1. Click Enter Deposits/Payments on the Activities menu. The Deposit List dialog box is displayed. Key *10012007* in the Deposit Date box, and press the Tab key. Notice that the copayments entered in Exercise 8-1 and 8-2 appear on the deposit list.

2. Click the New button. The Deposit (new) dialog box is displayed.

3. Verify that the entry in the Deposit Date box is 10/01/2007.

4. Since this is a payment from an insurance carrier, change the selection in the Payor Type box to Insurance.

5. Accept the default entry (Check) in the Payment Method box.

6. Key *412877429* in the Check Number box.

7. The Description/Bank No. field can be left blank.

8. Key *140* in the Payment Amount box.

9. Accept the default entry (A) in the Deposit Code box.

10. Select DeltaDental PPO from the Insurance drop-down list. When an insurance carrier is selected in the Insurance box, PractiSoft automatically enters the corresponding Payment, Adjustment, Withhold, and Deductible codes for DeltaDental PPO. You will apply the payment from DeltaDental using one of these codes in the Apply Payment/Adjustments to Charges dialog box that follows.

11. Click the Save button to save the entries and close the Deposit dialog box.

12. The Deposit List box reappears. The insurance payment appears in the list of deposits. Now the payment must be applied to the specific procedure charge to which it is related.

13. With the DeltaDental PPO payment entry highlighted, click the Apply button. The Apply Payment/Adjustments to Charges dialog box appears (see Figure 8-6). Notice the three check boxes and corresponding options that appear at the bottom of the dialog box. For the purposes of this exercise, make sure all three boxes are checked, which is the default setting.

14. Key *E* in the For box and press Enter to select John Ellison, since this payment was for his account. All the charge entries for John Ellison that have not been paid in full are listed.

Figure 8-6 Apply Payment/Adjustments to Charges dialog box.

15. Since this payment is for the D7111 procedure completed on 09/04/2007, that is the line in which the payment will be applied. Notice that the Payment box is highlighted by default. Depending on the type of payment being applied, the Deductible, Withhold, or Adjustment boxes could also be used. In this case, the appropriate box is Payment.

16. Key *140* in the Payment box and press Enter. PractiSoft automatically places a minus sign before the amount. Notice that once the payment is applied, the Complete box to the right of the dialog box is checked. This indicates that the transaction is complete.

17. Click the Save Payments/Adjustments button to save your entry.

18. If an Information box displays, alerting you that the claim for the primary insurance has been done, click OK. (This appears whenever the Alert When Claims Are Done checkbox is checked at the bottom of the Apply Payment/Adjustments to Charges dialog box.)

19. The Open Report dialog box displays, giving you the option to print a patient statement at this point. (This option appears whenever the Print Statement checkbox at the bottom of the dialog box is checked.) For now, Click Cancel.

20. The Apply Payment/Adjustments to Charges dialog box is cleared of the current transactions and is ready for a new transaction.

21. Click the Close button to exit the Apply Payment/Adjustments to Charges dialog box. The Unapplied box for the DeltaDental PPO payment on 10/1/2007 is now 0.00.

22. Without closing the Deposit List dialog box, open the Transaction Entry dialog box, select John Ellison, and click the ellipses in the Document box.

23. In the Search box that appears, double click document number 0709040000 to display the transaction data for the September 4, 2007, visit to which the DeltaDental PPO payment was made. Verify that an insurance carrier payment appears in the list of transactions. Payments entered in the Deposit List dialog box also appear in the Transaction Entry dialog box.

24. Close the Transaction Entry dialog box.

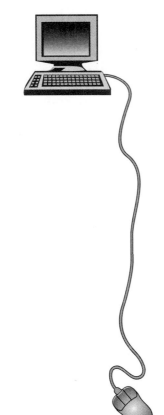

EXERCISE 8-5

Using Source Document 8, enter a capitation payment from Sunshine State HMO for the month of September 2007.

Date: October 1, 2007

1. Click the New button in the Deposit List dialog box.

2. Verify that the entry in the Deposit Date box is 10/01/2007.

3. In the Payor Type box, select Capitation.

4. Accept the default entry of Check in the Payment Method box.

5. Key *98721043* in the Check Number box.

6. Leave the Description/Bank No. box blank.

7. Key *2500* in the Payment Amount box and press Enter.

8. Accept the default entry of A in the Deposit Code box.

9. Click Sunshine State HMO in the Insurance drop-down list.

10. Click the Save button. The Deposit List window reappears, displaying the payment just entered. Notice that, for this payment, the Unapplied box in the right-most column of the dialog box is blank. This is because capitated payments do not need to be applied to individual patients and procedures.

ENTERING INSURANCE PAYMENTS WITH ADJUSTMENTS

Many times insurance carriers do not pay claims in full. Payment may be 80 percent or 50 percent of the charges, or some other amount. Sometimes a change, or an adjustment, needs to be made to a patient's account. When a dental office receives an RA with payments for less than the amount billed, an adjustment transaction must be entered to offset the unpaid charges.

When a payment amount from an insurance carrier is less than the charge amount, PractiSoft calculates an estimated adjustment based on data previously entered for that procedure code and insurance carrier. For example, if the charge amount is $60.00 and the insurance carrier paid $48.00 the last time a payment was entered, the program will estimate the adjustment amount to be $12.00 the next time a payment for that procedure code is entered.

EXERCISE 8-6

The dental office has just received an RA from Aetna (see Source Document 9). The total amount of the check is $1,388.00. This amount includes payments for a number of patients. Enter the insurance carrier payment for each patient.

Date: November 15, 2007

1. Change the entry in the Deposit Date box to 11/15/2007 and press the Tab key.

2. Click the New button in the Deposit List dialog box.

3. Select Insurance in the Payor Type box.

4. Key *1098* in the Check Number box.

5. Key the RA number, *100432*, in the Description/Bank No. box.

6. Key *1388.00* in the Payment Amount box.

7. Accept the default entry in the Deposit Code box.

8. Select Aetna in the Insurance box. PractiSoft automatically completes the Payment, Adjustment, Withhold, and Deductible code boxes for Aetna.

9. Click the Save button.

10. The payment entry appears in the Deposit List dialog box. Notice the amount of $1,388.00 listed in the Unapplied column for this payment.

Now apply the payment to the specific transaction charges.

11. With the Aetna line highlighted, click the Apply button. The Apply Payment/Adjustments to Charges dialog box is displayed.

12. Key *FONC* in the For box to select Georgette Foncet, and press Enter.

13. Locate the charge for procedure code D2740 on 10/30/2007. Key the amount of the payment, *840.00* in the Payment box and press Enter. PractiSoft automatically checks the Complete box, since Foncet only has one insurance carrier (no payment is forthcoming from any other carrier, so the charge is complete).

14. Now enter the payment for the next procedure listed on the RA. Notice that when you click in the Payment box for the second payment entry, PractiSoft calculates the amount still owed on the first procedure charge—the remainder—and displays it in the Remainder column for that charge. In this instance, the remainder is $210.00. Continue entering payments for Foncet's other procedures.

15. Click the Save Payments/Adjustments button.

16. Click OK in the Information box that displays, alerting you that the claim for the primary insurance has been done.

17. In the Open Reports dialog box that displays, click the Cancel button. The information for Georgette Foncet that was visible in the Apply Payment/Adjustments to Charges dialog box is cleared, and the dialog box is ready for the next payment or adjustment. Notice also that the amount listed in the Unapplied column for Aetna has been reduced by the amount applied. The unapplied amount is now $360.00.

Now enter the payments for the next patient listed on the RA, Juliet Schubert-Seku.

18. Key *SC* in the For box and press Enter to select Juliet Schubert-Seku.

19. Enter the payment of *180.00* in the Payment box for the D4341-LR charge on 10/30/2007. Press Enter.

20. Enter the other payment for Juliet Schubert-Seku.

21. Click the Save Payments/Adjustments button. Click the OK button in the Information dialog box. Elect not to print a statement at this time.

22. Notice that the amount listed in the Unapplied area of the Apply Payment/ Adjustments to Charges dialog box is now 0.00, indicating that the entire payment has been entered.

23. Close the Apply Payment/Adjustments to Charges dialog box.

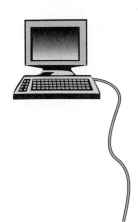

EXERCISE 8-7

The dental office has just received an RA from CIGNA PPO (see Source Document 10). The total amount of the check is $400.00. This amount includes payments for a number of patients. Enter the insurance carrier payments for each patient.

Date: October 1, 2007

1. Change the entry in the Deposit Date box to 10/01/2007 and press the Tab key.

2. Click the New button in the Deposit List dialog box.

3. Select Insurance in the Payor Type box.

4. Key *6549870* in the Check Number box.

5. Key the RA number, *010101*, in the Description/Bank No. box.

6. Key *400.00* in the Payment Amount box and press Tab.

7. Accept the default entry in the Deposit Code box.

8. Select CIGNA PPO in the Insurance box. PractiSoft automatically completes the Payment, Adjustment, Withhold, and Deductible code boxes with the corresponding codes for CIGNA PPO.

9. Click the Save button.

10. The payment entry appears in the Deposit List dialog box. Notice the amount of $400.00 listed in the Unapplied column for this payment.

Now apply the payment to the specific transaction charges.

11. With the CIGNA PPO line highlighted, click the Apply button. The Apply Payment/Adjustments to Charges dialog box is displayed.

12. For now, uncheck the Alert When Claims Are Done and the Print Statement Now check boxes at the bottom of the Apply Payment/Adjustments to Charges dialog box.

13. Key *AX* in the For box and press Enter to select Susan Axford.

14. Locate the charge for procedure code D2150 on 09/03/2007. Key the amount of the payment, *120.00*, in the Payment box and press Enter. Notice that PractiSoft automatically checks the Complete box, since Susan Axford has only one insurance carrier (there is no payment forthcoming from any other carrier, so the charge is complete).

15. Click the Save Payments/Adjustments button. The information for Susan Axford that was visible in the Apply Payment/Adjustments to Charges dialog box is cleared, and the dialog box is ready for the next payment or adjustment. Notice also that the amount listed in the Unapplied column for CIGNA PPO has been reduced by the amount applied. The unapplied amount is now $280.00.

Now enter the payment for the next patient listed on the RA, Daniel Barlow.

16. Key *B* in the For box and press Enter to select Daniel Barlow.

17. Enter the payment of *60.00* in the Payment box for the D1110 procedure on 09/03/2007. Press Enter.

18. Click the Save Payments/Adjustments button.

Apply the insurance carrier payment to June Barlow's D0120 and D1110 procedures for September 3, 2007.

19. Click June Barlow's name in the For box to display her charges.

20. Enter the payment of *25.00* in the Payment box for the D0120 charge on 09/03/2007. Press Enter.

21. Enter the payment of *60.00* in the Payment box for the D1110 charge on 09/03/2007. Press Enter.

22. Click the Save Payments/Adjustments button.

23. Continue to apply the insurance payments for Jimmy Barlow, Samuel Barlow, and Gloria Barlow in the same way, using the information on Source Document 10. When you have applied all the payments, the amount in the Unapplied box for the CIGNA PPO payment should be 0.00.

24. Close the Apply Payment/Adjustments to Charges dialog box.

25. Close the Deposit List dialog box.

26. Exit PractiSoft.

As you can see, the Deposit List feature makes it possible to enter a number of payment transactions in a short period of time.

USING TERMINOLOGY

Match the terms on the left with the definitions on the right.

_____ **1.** capitation payments

_____ **2.** insurance payments

_____ **3.** patient payments

a. Monies paid to the practice by an insurance carrier for procedure charges.

b. Monies paid to the practice by an insurance carrier for providing treatment to a certain number of patients for a specified period of time.

c. Monies paid to a dental practice by patients in exchange for services.

CHECKING YOUR UNDERSTANDING

Answer the questions below in the space provided.

4. When is it appropriate to print a walkout receipt?

_____

_____

5. Why is it easier to enter large insurance payments in the Deposit List dialog box than in the Transaction Entry dialog box?

_____

_____

6. When all payments on a remittance advice have been successfully entered and applied to charges, what should appear in the Unapplied box in the upper right corner of the Deposit List dialog box?

_____

7. What information does PractiSoft use to calculate an estimated adjustment amount?

_____

_____

APPLYING KNOWLEDGE

Answer the questions below in the space provided.

8. After you have entered a payment for $30, you realize it should have been $300. What should you do?

_____

_____

_____

9. The phone rings and it is Russell Klinger. He would like to know whether Sunshine State HMO has paid any of his charges for his September office visit. How would you look up this information in PractiSoft?

_____

_____

_____

AT THE COMPUTER

Answer the following questions at the computer.

10. What is the total amount that John Ellison paid in copayments in September 2007? (*Hint*: Include his daughter Ruby in the calculation.)

11. Today is November 12, 2007. A check for $56.00 arrives from BCBC of Florida as payment for Fran Mitchell-Dean's prophylaxis performed on October 30, 2007. What is the remaining amount of the charge that is Fran's responsibility to pay? (Do not actually enter the payment in the computer; use PractiSoft to look up the information required to calculate the remaining amount.)

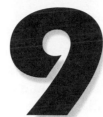

Scheduling

WHAT YOU NEED TO KNOW

To use this chapter, you need to know how to:

◆ Start PractiSoft, use menus, and enter and edit text.

◆ Work with chart numbers and codes.

OBJECTIVES

When you finish this chapter, you will be able to:

1. Start Office Hours.
2. View the appointment schedule.
3. Enter an appointment.
4. Search for available appointment time.
5. Change or delete an appointment.
6. Create a recall list.
7. Enter a break in a provider's schedule.
8. Preview and print providers' schedules.

KEY TERMS

Office Hours break
Office Hours schedule

INTRODUCTION TO OFFICE HOURS

Appointment scheduling is one of the most important tasks in a dental office. Different procedures take different lengths of time, and each appointment must be the right length. On the one hand, dentists want to be able to go from one appointment to another without unnecessary breaks. On the other hand, patients should not be kept waiting more than a few minutes for a dentist. Managing and juggling the schedule is usually the job of a dental office assistant working at the front desk. PractiSoft provides a special program called Office Hours to handle appointment scheduling.

OVERVIEW OF THE OFFICE HOURS WINDOW

The Office Hours program has its own window (see Figure 9-1) with a menu bar and toolbar. The Office Hours menu bar lists the menus available: File, Edit, View, Lists, Reports, Tools, and Help (see Figure 9-2). Below the menu bar is a toolbar with shortcut buttons. The functions of Office Hours are accessed by selecting a choice from one of the menus or by clicking a button on the toolbar.

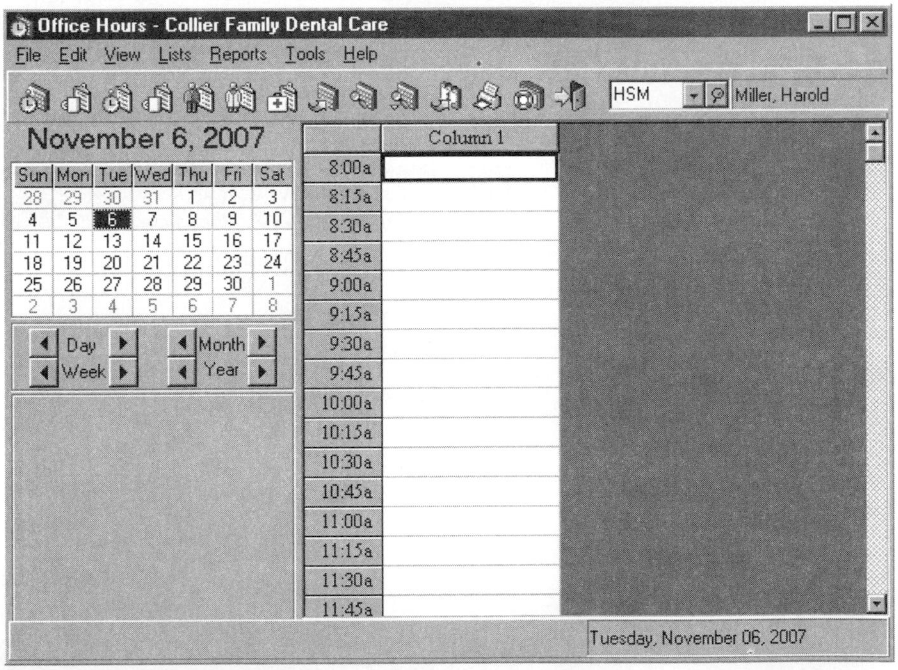

Figure 9-1   The Office Hours window.

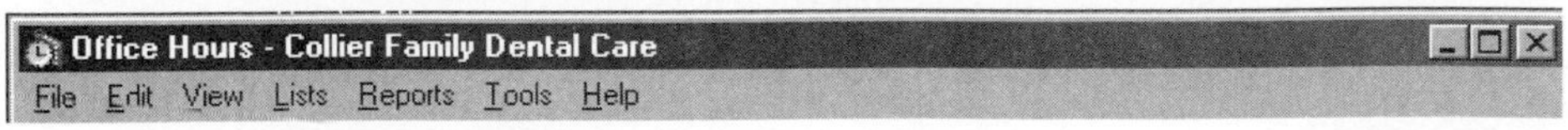

Figure 9-2   The Office Hours menu bar.

Located just below the menu bar, the toolbar contains a series of buttons that represent the most common activities performed in Office Hours. These buttons are shortcuts for frequently used menu commands. The toolbar displays 14 buttons (see Figure 9-3 and Table 9-1).

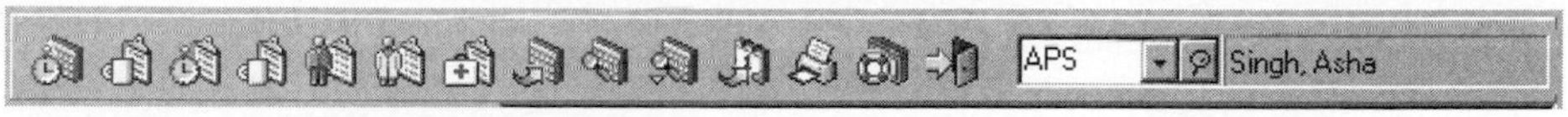

Figure 9-3   The Office Hours toolbar.

Table 9-1   Office Hours Toolbar Buttons

BUTTON	BUTTON NAME	ASSOCIATED FUNCTION	ACTIVITY
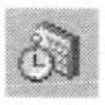	Appointment Entry	New Appointment Entry dialog box	Enter appointments.
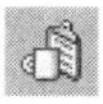	Break Entry	New Break Entry dialog box	Enter break.
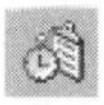	Appointment List	Appointment List dialog box	Display list of appointments.
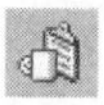	Break List	Break List dialog box	Display list of breaks.
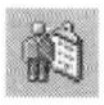	Patient List	Patient List dialog box	Display list of patients.
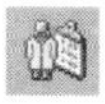	Provider List	Provider List dialog box	Display list of providers.
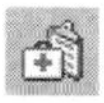	Resource List	Resource List dialog box	Display list of resources.
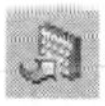	Go to a Date	Go to Date dialog box	Change calendar to a different date.
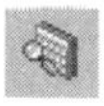	Search for Open Time Slot	Find Open Time dialog box	Locate first available time slot.
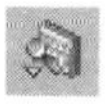	Search Again	Find Open Time dialog box	Locate next available time slot.
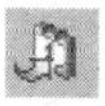	Go to Today		Return calendar to current date.
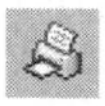	Print Appointment List		Print appointment list.
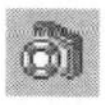	Help	Office Hours Help	Display Office Hours Help contents.
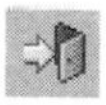	Exit		Exit the Office Hours program.

The left half of the Office Hours screen displays the current date and a calendar of the current month (see Figure 9-4). The current date is highlighted on the calendar. When a different date is clicked on the calendar, the calendar switches to the new date.

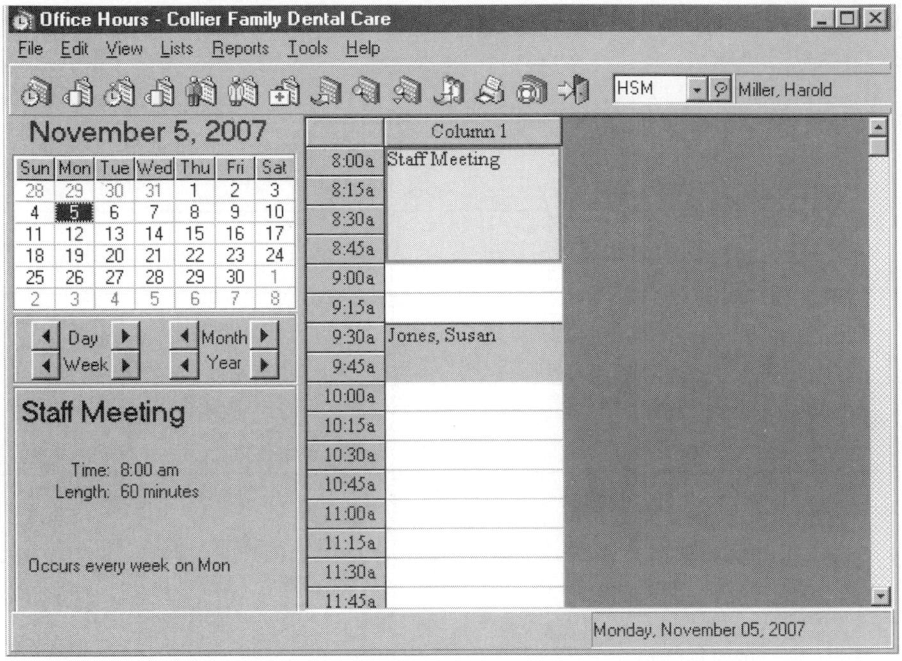

Figure 9-4 *The left side of the Office Hours window displays the current date and a monthly calendar. The right side of the window contains the selected provider's schedule for the current day.*

Office Hours schedule *a listing of time slots for a particular day for a specific provider*

The **Office Hours schedule**, shown in the right half of the screen, is a listing of time slots for a particular day for a specific provider. The provider's name and code is displayed at the top to the right of the shortcut buttons. The provider can be easily changed by clicking the triangle button in the Provider box.

PROGRAM OPTIONS

When Office Hours is installed in a dental practice, it is set up to reflect the needs of that particular practice. Most offices that use PractiSoft already have Office Hours set up and running. However, if PractiSoft is just being installed, options for setting up the program, such as the option for defining the practice's start time and end time, can be found in the Program Options dialog box, which is accessed by clicking Program Options on the Office Hours File menu.

ENTERING AND EXITING OFFICE HOURS

Office Hours can be started from within PractiSoft or directly from Windows. To access Office Hours from within PractiSoft, Appointment Book is clicked on the Activities menu. Office Hours can also be started by clicking the corresponding shortcut button on the toolbar.

To start Office Hours without entering PractiSoft first:

1. **Click the Start button on the Windows task bar.**

2. **Click PractiSoft on the Programs submenu.**

3. **Click Office Hours on the PractiSoft submenu.**

The Office Hours program is closed by clicking Exit on the Office Hours File menu, or by clicking the Exit button on its toolbar. If Office Hours was started from within PractiSoft, exiting will return you to PractiSoft. If Office Hours was started directly from Windows, clicking Exit will return you to the Windows desktop.

ENTERING APPOINTMENTS

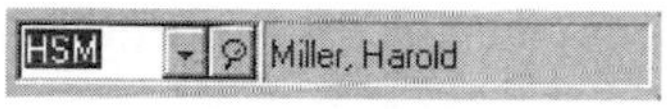

Figure 9-5   Provider box.

Entering an appointment begins with selecting the provider for whom the appointment is being scheduled. The current provider is listed in the Provider box at the top right of the screen (see Figure 9-5). Clicking the triangle button displays a drop-down list of providers in the system. To choose a different provider, click the name of the provider on the drop-down list.

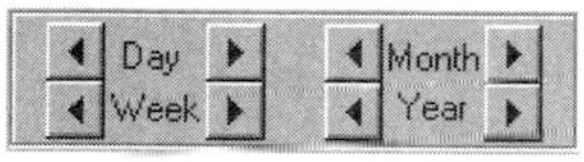

**Figure 9-6
Day, Week, Month, and
Year triangle buttons**

After the provider is selected, the date of the desired appointment must be chosen. Dates are changed by clicking the Day, Week, Month, and Year right and left triangle buttons located under the calendar (see Figure 9-6). After the provider and date have been selected, patient appointments can be entered.

Appointments are entered by clicking the Appointment Entry shortcut button or by double-clicking in a time slot on the schedule. When either of those actions is taken, the New Appointment Entry dialog box is displayed (see Figure 9-7). The dialog box contains the following fields:

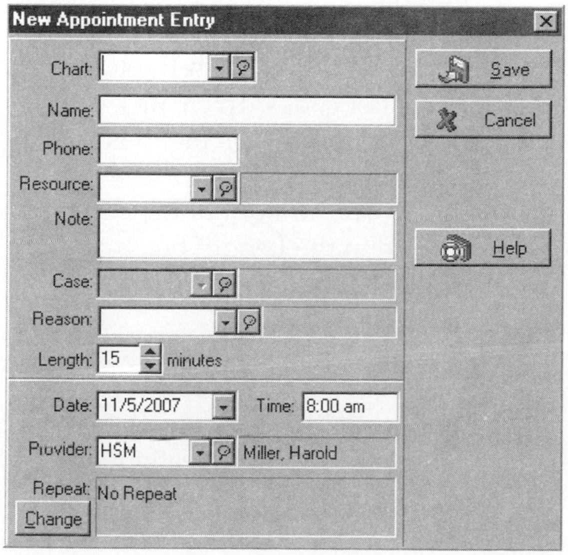

Figure 9-7   New Appointment Entry dialog box.

Chart A patient's chart number is chosen from the Chart drop-down list. To select the desired patient, click on the name and press Enter. After pressing Enter, PractiSoft automatically displays information on the patient in several other fields. If you are setting up an appointment for a new patient who has not been assigned a chart number, skip this box and key the patient's name in the Name box.

Name Once a patient's chart number is selected from the Chart drop-down list and the Enter key is pressed, PractiSoft displays the patient's name in the Name box. If a patient does not have a chart number, key the patient's name in this box.

Phone After selecting a patient's chart number and pressing Enter, that patient's phone number is automatically entered in the Phone box.

Resource This box is used if the practice assigns codes to resources, such as exam rooms or equipment.

Note Any special information about an appointment is entered in the Note box.

Case The case that pertains to the appointment is selected from the drop-down list of cases.

Reason This box is used if the practice assigns reason codes for patients' appointments. In the Collier Family Dental Care database used in the exercises in this text, no reason codes are used. However, a practice might assign reason codes such as the code NEWPAT00 for new patients or URGENT00 for urgent visits. Providers can designate time slots for handling particular types of appointments each day, as well as a default length of time for an appointment. When setting up a new appointment, if the reason code selected in the Reason box does not match the requirements set up for that type of appointment, Office Hours will display a warning message. The appointment can then be scheduled or not, as desired. A reason code can be keyed directly in the Reason box or selected from the drop-down list of codes. To create a reason list, the Reason List option on the Office Hours Lists menu is used.

Length The amount of time an appointment will take (in minutes) is entered in the Length box by keying the number of minutes or by using the up and down arrows.

Date The Date box displays the date that is currently displayed on the calendar. If this is not the desired date, it may be changed by keying in a different date or by clicking the triangle button to the right of the box and selecting a date from the pop-up calendar that appears.

Time   The Time box displays the appointment time that is currently selected on the schedule. If this is not the desired time, it may be changed by keying in a different time.

Provider   The provider who will be treating the patient during this appointment is selected from the drop-down list of providers.

Repeat   The Repeat box is used to enter appointments that recur on a regular basis.

After the boxes in the New Appointment Entry dialog box have been completed, clicking the Save button enters the information on the schedule. The patient's name appears in the time slot corresponding to the appointment time. In addition, information about the appointment appears in the lower left corner of the Office Hours window.

LOOKING FOR A FUTURE DATE

Often a patient will need a follow-up appointment at a certain time in the future. For example, suppose a dentist has seen a certain patient on a particular day and would like a checkup appointment in three weeks. The most efficient way to search for a future appointment in Office Hours is to use the Go to a Date shortcut button on the toolbar. (This feature can also be accessed on the Edit menu.)

Clicking the Go to a Date shortcut button displays the Go To Date dialog box (see Figure 9-8). Within the dialog box, five boxes offer options for choosing a future date.

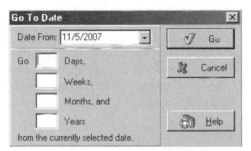

Figure 9-8   Go To Date dialog box.

Date From   This box indicates the current date in the appointment search.

Go __ Days   This box is used to locate a date a specific number of days in the future. For example, if a patient needs an appointment ten days from the current day, 10 would be entered in this box.

Go __ Weeks   This box is used when a patient needs an appointment a specific number of weeks in the future, such as six weeks from the current day.

Go __ Months This box is used when a patient needs an appointment a specific number of months in the future, such as three months from the current day.

Go __ Years Similar to the weeks and months options, this box is used when an appointment is needed one or several years in the future.

After a future date option has been selected, clicking the Go button closes the dialog box and begins the search. The system locates the future date and displays the calendar schedule for that date.

EXERCISE 9-1

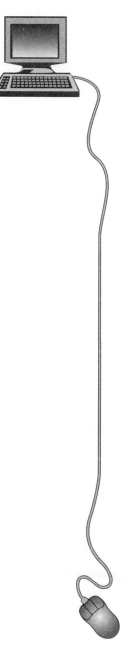

Enter an appointment for Daniel Barlow at 2:30 p.m. on Monday, November 12, 2007. The appointment is 60 minutes in length and is with Dr. Harold Miller.

1. Start PractiSoft. Start Office Hours by clicking the Appointment Book shortcut button on the toolbar.

2. Click HSM – Miller, Harold on the drop-down list in the Provider box to select Harold Miller if he is not already selected.

3. Change the date on the calendar to Monday, November 12, 2007. Use the forward or backward arrow keys to change the month and year, then click the day in the calendar itself.

4. In the schedule, double-click the 2:30 p.m. time slot. (You will need to use the scroll bar to view 2:30 p.m.) The New Appointment Entry dialog box is displayed.

5. Click Daniel Barlow from the list of names on the drop-down list in the Chart box and press Enter. The system automatically fills in a number of boxes in the dialog box, such as the patient's name and phone number.

6. Leave the Resource and Note boxes blank.

7. Accept the default entry in the Case box, and leave the Reason box blank.

8. Notice that the Length box already contains an entry of 15 minutes. This is the default appointment length set up in PractiSoft. In this instance, because Daniel Barlow's appointment is for periodontal work that is expected to take an hour, this entry must be changed. Key *60* in the Length box or use the up arrow next to the length box to change the appointment length to 60 minutes.

9. Verify the entries in the Date, Time, and Provider boxes, and click the Save button. PractiSoft saves the appointment, closes the dialog box, and displays the appointment on the schedule, as well as in the lower left corner of the Office Hours window. Daniel Barlow's name is displayed in the 2:30 p.m. time slot on the schedule.

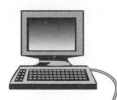

EXERCISE 9-2

Enter the following appointments with Dr. Harold Miller.

1. The first appointment is Monday (November 12, 2007) at 3:30 p.m. for John Ellison, 30 minutes in length. Verify that HSM – Miller, Harold is displayed in the Provider box.

2. In the schedule, double-click the 3:30 p.m. time slot.

3. Select John Ellison on the Chart drop-down list.

4. Press the Enter key. The program automatically completes several boxes in the dialog box.

5. Press the Tab key until the entry in the Length box is highlighted.

6. Key *30* in the Length box or click the up arrow once to change the length to 30 minutes.

7. Click the Save button. Verify that the appointment for John Ellison appears on the schedule for November 12, 2007, at 3:30 p.m. for a length of 30 minutes.

8. Enter an appointment on Monday, November 12, 2007, at 4:00 p.m. for Sheila Rossi, 15 minutes in length.

9. Enter an appointment on Tuesday, November 13, 2007, at 12:15 p.m. for Sally Smith, 30 minutes in length. In the case box, select Preventive.

10. To schedule an appointment two weeks after November 13, 2007, for Sally Smith at 12:15 p.m., 15 minutes in length, click the Go To a Date shortcut button.

11. Key 2 in the Go _____ Weeks box. Click the Go button. The program closes the Go To a Date box and displays the appointment schedule for November 27, 2007.

12. Enter Sally Smith's appointment. Again, select the Preventive case.

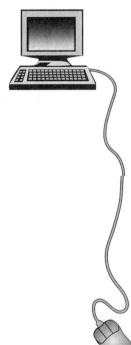

EXERCISE 9-3

Enter the following three appointments with Collier Family Dental Care's oral hygienist, Asha Singh.

1. Select Asha Singh from the drop-down list in the Provider box.

2. Enter an appointment for Friday, November 16, 2007, at 2:00 p.m. for June Barlow, 30 minutes in length.

3. Use Office Hours' Go To Date feature to schedule an appointment three weeks from November 16, 2007, at 1:15 p.m. for Jimmy Barlow, 15 minutes in length.

4. Schedule an appointment for Ruby Ellison one week from November 16, 2007, at 9:00 a.m., 30 minutes in length.

5. Temporarily leave Office Hours by clicking the minimize button in the upper right corner of the window.

EXERCISE 9-4

Enter an appointment on Thursday, November 8, 2007, at 9:00 a.m. for Herb Fonagy, 30 minutes in length. You do not know his provider, so this information must be looked up in PractiSoft before you enter the appointment.

1. In PractiSoft, click Patients/Guarantors and Cases on the Lists menu.

2. In the Patient List dialog box that appears, select Herb Fonagy as the patient. Click the Edit Patient button.

3. Click the Other Information tab to find his assigned provider.

4. Click the Office Hours button on the Windows task bar (bottom of screen). Notice that the Patient List dialog box is still partially visible beneath the Office Hours window.

5. Select Fonagy's provider in the Provider box in Office Hours.

6. Enter the appointment.

7. Minimize Office Hours.

8. In PractiSoft, close the open dialog boxes.

SEARCHING FOR AVAILABLE APPOINTMENT TIME

Often it is necessary to search for available appointment space on a particular day of the week and at a specific time. For example, a patient needs a 30-minute appointment and would like it to be during his lunch hour, which is from 12:00 p.m. to 1:00 p.m. He can get away from the office only on Mondays and Fridays. Office Hours makes it easy to locate an appointment slot that meets these requirements with the Search for Open Time Slot shortcut button. This shortcut button (or the Find Open Time option on the Edit menu) displays the Find Open Time dialog box.

Before accessing the Find Open Time dialog box, the required dentist is selected in the Provider box. After the dialog box opens, the length of the appointment and the start and end times are indicated. The days the patient is available are also indicated. When the Search button is clicked, PractiSoft locates the first available time that meets the criteria.

EXERCISE 9-5

Search for the next available appointment slot beginning November 8, 2007, with Dr. Miller, on a Monday or Wednesday, between the hours of 11:00 a.m. and 2:00 p.m.

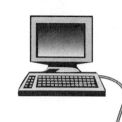

1. Click the Office Hours button on the Windows taskbar. Select Dr. Miller in the Provider box.

2. On the Edit menu, click Find Open Time, or click the Search for Open Time Slot shortcut button. The Find Open Time dialog box is displayed (see Figure 9-9).

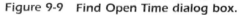

Figure 9-9   Find Open Time dialog box.

3. Key *30* in the Length box. Press the Tab key.

4. Key *11* in the Start Time box.

5. Key *2* in the End Time box.

6. To search for an appointment on Monday or Wednesday, click the Monday and Wednesday boxes in the Day of Week area of the dialog box.

7. Click the Search button to begin looking for an appointment slot. PractiSoft closes the dialog box and locates the first available time slot that meets these specifications. The time slot is outlined on the schedule.

8. Double-click the selected time slot. Click Melanie Sanchez on the drop-down list in the Name box.

9. Press the Tab key until the cursor is in the Length box.

10. Key *30* and press the Tab key.

11. Click the Save button.

12. Verify that the appointment has been entered by looking at the schedule.

EXERCISE 9-6

Schedule Russell Klinger for a 30-minute appointment with Dr. Harold Miller on November 12, 2007. Mr. Klinger is available only between 3:00 p.m. and 5:00 p.m. on that Monday.

1. Click the desired provider in the Provider box.

2. Verify that the date in the calendar is November 12, 2007.

3. Click Find Open Time on the Edit menu to display the Find Open Time dialog box.

4. In the Length box, highlight the number already entered and key *30*. Press the Tab key to move the cursor to the Start Time box.

5. Key *3p* (for 3 p.m.)in the Start Time box to change the start time to 3:00 p.m. Press Tab to move the cursor to the End Time box.

6. Key *5* in the End Time box.

7. In the Day of Week boxes, Monday should already be selected. Click the Wednesday box to deselect Wednesday.

8. Click the Search button. The first available slot that meets the requirements is outlined on the schedule.

9. Double-click in the time slot to open the New Appointment Entry dialog box.

10. Click Russell Klinger from the drop-down list in the Chart box. Press tab several times to move the cursor to the Length box.

11. Key *30* in the Length box, and press the Tab key.

12. Click the Save button. The dialog box closes and Russell Klinger's appointment appears on the schedule.

ENTERING APPOINTMENTS FOR NEW PATIENTS

When a new patient phones the office for an appointment, the appointment can be scheduled in Office Hours before the patient information is entered in PractiSoft. However, while the prospective patient is still on the phone, most offices obtain basic data and enter it in the appropriate PractiSoft dialog boxes (Patient/Guarantor and Case).

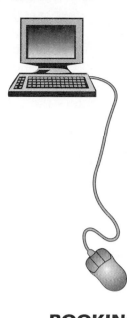

Schedule Louise Grass, a new patient, for a 30-minute appointment with Dr. Harold Miller on November 12, 2007, at 1:45 p.m.

1. Verify that November 12, 2007, is displayed on the schedule and that Dr. Harold Miller is selected as the provider.

2. Double-click the 1:45 p.m. time slot.

3. Click in the Name box and key *Louise Grass*. Press the Tab key to move the cursor to the Phone box.

4. Key *9415553604* in the Phone box and press Tab four times. The cursor should be in the Length box.

5. Key *30* in the Length box.

6. Click the Save button. The appointment is displayed on the November 12, 2007, schedule.

BOOKING REPEATED APPOINTMENTS

Some patients may require or request appointments on a repeated basis, such as every Thursday for four weeks. Repeated appointments are also set up in the New Appointment Entry dialog box. The Repeat feature is located at the bottom of the dialog box. When the Change button is clicked, the Repeat Change dialog box is displayed. The Repeat Change dialog box provides a number of choices for setting up repeating appointments (see Figure 9-10).

The left side of the dialog box contains information about the frequency of the appointments. The default is set to None. Other options include Daily, Weekly, Monthly, and Yearly. When an option other than None is selected, the center section of the dialog box changes and displays additional options for setting up the appointments (see Figure 9-11).

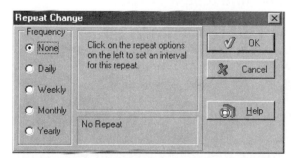

Figure 9-10   Repeat Change dialog box when None is selected.

Figure 9-11   Repeat Change dialog box when an option other than None is selected.

In the center section, an option is provided to indicate how often the appointments should be scheduled, such as every 1 week. Below that there is an option to indicate the day of the week on which the appointment should be scheduled. Finally, there is a box to indicate when the repeating appointments should stop. When all the information has been entered, clicking the OK button closes the Repeat Change dialog box and the New Appointment Entry dialog box is once again visible. Clicking the Save button enters the repeating appointments on the schedule.

EXERCISE 9-8

Schedule Luz Vasquez for a 15-minute appointment with Dr. Harold Miller, once a week for six weeks. Mr. Vasquez has requested that the appointments be at the same time every week, preferably in the early morning, beginning with Wednesday, November 14, 2007.

1. Click the desired provider on the Provider drop-down list.

2. Change the schedule to November 14, 2007.

3. Double-click in the 8:00 a.m. time slot. The New Appointment Entry dialog box is displayed.

4. Select Luz Vasquez from the Chart drop-down list. Press the Tab key until the cursor is in the Length box.

5. Confirm that the entry in the Length box is 15 minutes.

6. Click the Change button to schedule the repeating appointments.

7. In the Frequency column, select Weekly.

8. Accept the default entry of 1 in the Every __ Week(s) box.

9. Accept the default entry of W to accept Wednesday as the day of the week.

10. Click the triangle button to the right of the End On box. A calendar pops up. Change the calendar to display November 14, 2007. Then click the triangle button to open the pop-up calendar again. Counting November 14 as the first week, count six weeks forward. (Note: You will have to change the month to December to count the fourth, fifth, and sixth weeks.) When you find the sixth Wednesday, click in the calendar box for that day. 12/19/2007 appears in the End On box.

11. Click the OK button. Notice that "Every week on Wed" is displayed in the Repeat area of the New Appointment Entry dialog box.

12. Click the Save button to enter the appointments. Notice that "Occurs every week on Wed" appears in the lower left corner of the Office Hours window.

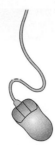

13. Go to December 19, 2007, to verify that Mr. Vasquez is scheduled for an appointment at 8:00 a.m.

14. Go to December 26, 2007, and confirm that Mr. Vasquez is not scheduled. This is the seventh week, and his repeating appointments were only scheduled for six weeks, so no appointment should appear on December 26, 2007.

CHANGING OR DELETING APPOINTMENTS

Very often it is necessary to change a patient's appointment or cancel an appointment. Changing an appointment is accomplished with the Cut and Paste commands on the Office Hours Edit menu.

The following steps are used to reschedule an appointment:

1. Locate the appointment that needs to be changed. Make sure the appointment slot is visible on the schedule.

2. Click on the existing time slot. A dark border surrounds the slot to indicate that it is selected.

3. Click Cut on the Edit menu. The appointment disappears from the schedule.

4. Click the date on the calendar when the appointment is to be rescheduled.

5. Click the desired time slot on the schedule. The slot becomes active.

6. Click Paste on the Edit menu. The patient's name appears in the new time slot.

The following steps are used to cancel an appointment without rescheduling:

1. Locate the appointment on the schedule.

2. Click the time-slot box to select the appointment.

3. Click Cut on the Edit menu. The appointment disappears from the schedule.

TIP . . . Instead of using the Cut and Paste commands to change or delete an appointment, select the appointment and press the right mouse button. A shortcut menu appears with several options, including Cut, Copy, and Delete.

EXERCISE 9-9

Change June Barlow's and Herb Fonagy's appointments.

1. Click Asha Singh on the Provider box drop-down list.

2. Go to Friday, November 16, 2007, on the calendar.

3. Locate June Barlow's 2:00 p.m. appointment on the schedule. Click the 2:00 p.m. time slot. A dark border surrounds the slot.

4. Click Cut on the Edit menu. June Barlow's appointment is removed from the 2:00 p.m. time slot. (You may also use the right mouse click shortcut.)

5. Click the 3:00 p.m. time slot.

6. Click Paste on the Edit menu. June Barlow's name is displayed in the 3:00 p.m. time slot.

7. Click Josephine Wu on the Provider drop-down list.

8. Go to Thursday, November 8, 2007, on the calendar.

9. Locate Herb Fonagy's 9:00 a.m. appointment. Remove his appointment from the 9:00 a.m. time slot.

10. Go to Friday, November 16, 2007, on the calendar.

11. Enter Herb Fonagy's appointment in the 9:15 a.m. time slot.

12. Exit Office Hours.

CREATING A RECALL LIST

Dental offices frequently must keep track of patients who need to return for future appointments. Some offices schedule future appointments when the patient is leaving the office. For example, if a patient has just seen a dentist and needs to return for a follow-up appointment in six weeks, the appointment is usually made before the patient leaves the office. However, when the appointment is needed farther in the future, such as in six months or one year later, it is not always practical to set it up. The patient and the dentist may not know their schedules a year in advance. For this reason, many offices keep a list of patients who need to be contacted for future appointments.

In PractiSoft, the recall feature is located in the main PractiSoft program rather than in the Office Hours scheduling program. A recall list can be created and maintained using the Patient Recall option on the Lists menu in the main PractiSoft window. Patients can also be added to the recall list by clicking the Patient Recall Entry shortcut button on the PractiSoft toolbar. When Patient Recall is selected from the Lists menu, the Patient Recall List dialog box is displayed (see Figure 9-12). This dialog box organizes the recall information in a column format. The scroll bar is used to display the last four columns on the right.

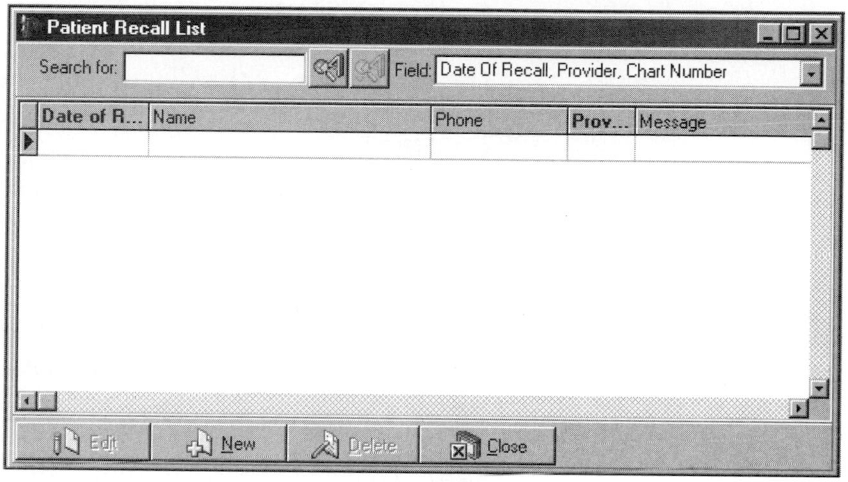

Figure 9-12 *Patient Recall List dialog box.*

◆ **Date of Recall** Lists the date on which the recall is scheduled.

◆ **Name** Displays the patient's name.

◆ **Phone** Lists the patient's phone number, making it easy to call patients for appointments without having to look up phone numbers in another dialog box.

◆ **Provider** Displays the provider code for the patient's provider.

◆ **Message** Displays the entry made in the Message box of the Patient Recall dialog box.

◆ **Extension** Lists the patient's phone extension.

◆ **Chart Number** Displays the patient's chart number.

◆ **Procedure Code** Lists the procedure code for the procedure for which the patient is being recalled.

◆ **Recall Status** Indicates the code for the recall status as follows: 0 - Call; 1 - Call Again; 2 - Appointment Set; 3 - No Appointment. The recall status code can be used to conduct a search based on a patient's recall status.

The Patient Recall List dialog box contains the following boxes to help in locating a patient recall record:

Search For The Search For box is used to locate a specific patient on the recall list. Entering the first few letters or numbers in the Search For box displays the selection that is the closest match to the search criteria.

Field The choices in the Field box determine the order in which patients are listed in the dialog box. There are three sorting options:

- Date of Recall, Provider, Chart Number
- Chart Number, Date of Recall
- Provider, Date of Recall

The first option is the default sort option. Before using the Search For box, the desired sort option should be selected in the Field box.

The Patient Recall List dialog box also contains these buttons: Edit, New, Delete, and Close.

Edit Clicking the Edit button displays the Patient Recall dialog box for the patient whose entry is highlighted. The information on the patient can then be edited by making different selections in the boxes.

New Clicking the New button displays an empty Patient Recall dialog box, in which data on a new recall patient can be entered.

Delete Clicking the Delete button deletes recall data on the patient whose entry is highlighted.

Close The Close button is used to exit the Patient Recall List dialog box.

ADDING A PATIENT TO THE RECALL LIST Patients are added to the recall list by clicking the New button in the Patient Recall List dialog box or by clicking the Patient Recall Entry shortcut button. When either of these actions is performed, the Patient Recall dialog box is displayed (see Figure 9-13). The Patient Recall dialog box contains the following boxes:

Recall Date The date a patient needs to return to see a dentist is entered in the Recall Date box.

Provider A patient's provider is selected from the drop-down list.

Chart A patient's chart number is selected from the drop-down list, or the first few letters of a patient's chart number are entered in the Chart box.

Name, Phone, Extension After a chart number is entered, the system automatically completes the Name, Phone, and Extension boxes.

Procedure If the procedure for which a patient is returning is known, it is entered in the Procedure box in one of two ways. The procedure code can be selected from the drop-down list, or the first few numbers can be entered and the drop-down list will display the entry that most closely matches the entered numbers. This is especially valuable in practices in which there are hundreds of procedure codes, because it eliminates the need to scroll through several hundred codes to locate the desired one.

Message The Message box is used to record any special notes, reminders, or instructions about a patient and his or her appointment.

Recall Status The choices in the Recall Status box are used to indicate the action that needs to be taken. They include:

Call The Call button is used when a patient needs to be telephoned about a future appointment.

Call Again The Call Again button is used when a patient has been called once, but contact was not made and an additional call is necessary.

Appointment Set The Appointment Set button is used when a patient has an appointment already scheduled.

No Appointment The No Appointment button is used when a patient has been contacted for an appointment but has declined for some reason.

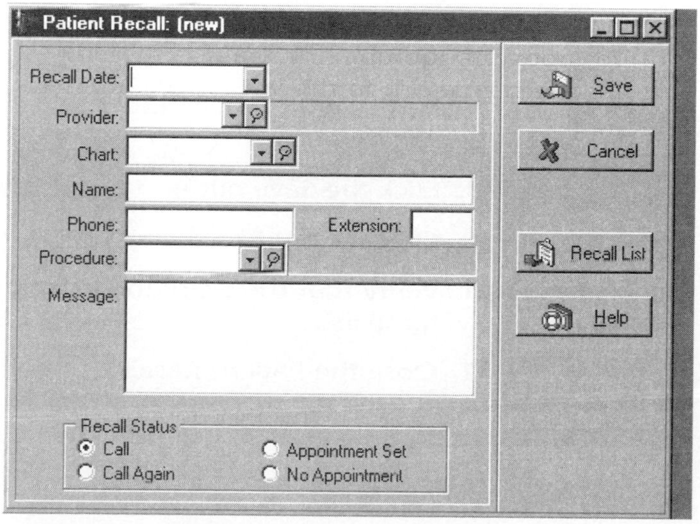

Figure 9-13 Patient Recall (new) dialog box.

After the information has been entered in the dialog box, clicking the Save button saves the data and adds the patient to the recall list. In addition to the Save button, the Patient Recall dialog box contains these buttons: Cancel, Recall List, and Help. The Cancel button exits the dialog box without saving the data entered. The Recall List button in the Patient Recall dialog box is used to display the Patient Recall List dialog box. The Help button displays PractiSoft's online help for the Patient Recall dialog box.

EXERCISE 9-10

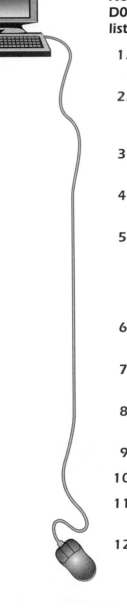

John Ellison needs to receive a phone call one year from November 12, 2007, to set up an appointment for Procedure D0120, periodic oral evaluation. Add John Ellison to the recall list.

1. In PractiSoft, click the Patient Recall Entry shortcut button. The Patient Recall dialog box is displayed.

2. Before filling in the Patient Recall dialog box, determine which dentist is John Ellison's assigned provider. (Look in the Patient/Guarantor dialog box for this information.)

3. In the Recall Date box of the Patient Recall dialog box, enter November 12, 2008.

4. Click John Ellison's provider on the drop-down list in the Provider box.

5. Locate John Ellison's chart number in the Chart box by keying the first few letters of his chart number and pressing Enter. Notice that the system automatically completes the Phone box. (The Extension box would also be completed if there were an extension.)

6. Select procedure code D0120 (periodic oral evaluation) from the drop-down list in the Procedure box.

7. In the Message box, key *Was changing jobs; ask about new insurance coverage.*

8. Verify that the Call radio button in the Recall Status box is selected.

9. Click the Save button to save the entry.

10. Click Patient Recall on the Lists menu.

11. Verify that the entry for John Ellison has been added to the recall list.

12. Close the Patient Recall List dialog box.

CREATING BREAKS

Office Hours break *a block of time when a provider is unavailable for appointments with patients*

Office Hours provides features for inserting standard breaks in dentists' schedules. The **Office Hours break** is a block of time when a provider is unavailable for appointments with patients. Some examples of breaks include Lunch, Meeting, Personal, Emergency, Break, Vacation, Seminar, Holiday, and Trip. In Office Hours, breaks can be created one at a time or on a recurring basis for all providers. One-time breaks, such as those for a vacation, are obviously set up for an individual provider. Other breaks, such as staff meetings, can be entered once for multiple providers.

In the Collier Family Dental Care database, a break has been entered for all providers on Monday morning, from 8:00 a.m. to 9:00 a.m., for a weekly staff meeting. Daily lunch breaks have also been entered for Asha Singh (from noon to 1:00 p.m.) and for Dr. Josephine Wu (from 1:00 p.m. to 2:00 p.m.). Often breaks need to be inserted into a provider's schedule when he or she is not available for appointments with patients. For example, if a dentist will be at an all-day conference the second Thursday of a given month, that whole day must be marked as unavailable on his or her schedule.

To set up a break for a current provider (that is, the provider listed in the Office Hours Provider box), click the Break Entry shortcut button on the Office Hours toolbar. This action causes the New Break Entry dialog box to appear (see Figure 9-14).

Figure 9-14   New Break Entry dialog box.

The New Break Entry dialog box contains the following options:

Name   The name field is used to store a name or description of the break.

Date   The date field displays the current date on the Office Hours calendar. If this is not the correct date for the break entry, a different date can be entered.

Time   The starting time of the break is entered in this box.

Length   This box indicates the length of the break in minutes (from 0 to 720).

Resource   If the practice has assigned codes to various resources, such as an exam room or a piece of equipment, a resource code can be selected from the drop-down list to indicate a resource that is required for the break.

Change   The Change button next to the Repeat box is used to enter breaks that recur at a regular interval.

Color   By selecting a different color from the drop-down list, the color of the break time slot in the schedule can be changed.

Provider(s)   The Provider(s) buttons are used to indicate whether the break is to be set for the current provider (the provider that is selected in the Provider box in Office Hours), some providers, or all providers. If some is selected, a Provider Selection dialog box will be displayed when the Save button is clicked. The appropriate providers can then be selected.

When all the information has been entered, clicking the Save button closes the dialog box and enters the break(s) in PractiSoft.

EXERCISE 9-11

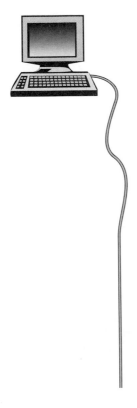

The oral hygienist, Asha Singh, will be away at a seminar from Monday, December 10, 2007, to Wednesday, December 12, 2007. Enter this as a break on her schedule.

1. Start Office Hours.

2. Select Asha Singh from the Provider drop-down list.

3. Change the date on the calendar to December 10, 2007.

4. Click the Break Entry shortcut button on the toolbar. The Edit Break dialog box appears.

5. Key *Seminar* over the existing entry in the Name box and press Tab twice to go to the Time box.

6. If it is not already displayed, change the entry in the Time box to 8:00 am. Press Tab to go to the Length box.

7. Key *540* in the Length box to indicate that the break is all day (9 hours). Press Tab once.

8. Leave the Resource box blank.

9. Click the Change button (to repeat the break for two additional days). The Repeat Change dialog box is displayed.

10. Click the Daily button in the Frequency column. The center of the dialog box changes to display more options (see Figure 9-15).

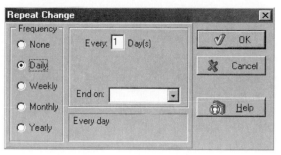

Figure 9-15   Repeat Change dialog box with Daily button selected.

11. Accept the default entry of 1 in the Every __ Day(s) box, since the break occurs every day for a period of three days.

12. Change the date in the End On box to December 12, 2007.

13. Click the OK button. You are returned to the Edit Break dialog box.

14. Click the Save button to enter the break in Office Hours. Notice that December 10, 2007, has been filled in on the calendar and the break name "Seminar" appears next to the 8:00 a.m. time slot.

15. Change the calendar to December 11 and 12, 2007, to verify that the break has been entered correctly.

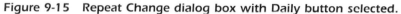

PREVIEWING AND PRINTING SCHEDULES

In most dental offices, providers' schedules are printed on a daily basis. To view a list of all appointments for a provider for a given day, click Appointment List from the Office Hours Reports menu. The report can be previewed on-screen or sent directly to the printer. If the preview option is selected, the appointment list is displayed in a preview window (see Figure 9-16 on page 180). Various buttons are used to view the schedule at different sizes, to move from page to page, to print the schedule, and to save the schedule as a file. Clicking the Close button closes the preview window.

The schedule can also be printed by clicking the Print Appointment List shortcut button, without using the Preview option. (Office Hours prints the schedule for the provider who is listed in the Provider box. To print the schedule of a different provider, change the entry in the Provider box before printing the schedule.)

| | | | ◄ | ◄ | 1 of 1 | ► | ►| | | | Close | Goto Page: 1 |

Collier Family Dental Care   **Friday, November 16, 2007**

Wu, Josephine

Time	Name	Phone	Length	Notes
9:15a	Fonagy, Herb FONAGHE0	(941)444-5555	30	
1:00p	Lunch		60	
				Every day

Figure 9-16   Preview Report window with appointment schedule displayed.

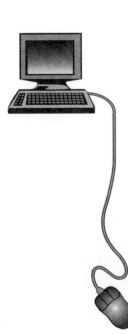

EXERCISE 9-12

Print Dr. Harold Miller's schedule for November 12, 2007.

1. Select Dr. Harold Miller as the provider.

2. Go to Monday, November 12, 2007, on the calendar.

3. Click Appointment List on the Office Hours Reports menu. The Report Setup dialog box appears.

4. Under Print Selection, click the button that prints the report directly to the printer.

5. Under Report Type, click Detail.

6. Click the Start button. The Print dialog box appears.

7. Click OK to print the report.

8. Close Office Hours.

9. Exit PractiSoft.

CHAPTER REVIEW

USING TERMINOLOGY

Define the terms below as they apply to Office Hours.

1. Office Hours schedule

_____

_____

2. Office Hours break

_____

_____

CHECKING YOUR UNDERSTANDING

Answer the questions below in the space provided.

3. What are the different ways of starting Office Hours?

_____

_____

4. In Office Hours, how do you display the schedule for a specific date?

_____

_____

5. If the Office Hours calendar shows October 6, how do you move to November 6?

_____

_____

6. How do you display the schedule for a specific provider for a specific day?

_____

_____

7. How do you schedule a new appointment in Office Hours?

_____

_____

CHAPTER REVIEW

8. How is an appointment deleted?

_____

_____

9. What are the two commands that can be used to move an appointment from one time slot to another? On what menu are they found?

_____

_____

10. Suppose your office has set up Office Hours so that the default appointment length is 30 minutes. If you need to make a one-hour appointment for a patient, in what box do you change 30 to 60?

_____

_____

APPLYING KNOWLEDGE

Answer the questions below in the space provided.

11. After you entered a personal break for Dr. Josephine Wu on February 24, she tells you that she gave you the wrong date. The break should be February 25. How do you correct the schedule?

_____

_____

_____

12. A patient calls to request an appointment on a specific day next week. You determine that the appointment is for a routine checkup with Dr. Harold Miller. What steps should you follow to schedule the appointment?

_____

_____

_____

AT THE COMPUTER

Answer the following questions at the computer.

13. Today is Monday, November 5, 2007. Dr. Miller asks you to find out when Ruby Ellison is coming in for her next appointment and whether the appointment is with him. Change the Office Hours calendar to November 5, 2007. Then use the Appointment List option on the Office Hours Lists menu to locate the required information.

14. Today is November 12, 2007. Samuel Barlow needs to be scheduled as soon as possible for a 30-minute appointment with Dr. Harold Miller, between 10:00 a.m. and 12:00 p.m. When is the next available time slot that meets these requirements? How did you locate the open slot?

CHAPTER 10

Using Claim Management

WHAT YOU NEED TO KNOW

To use this chapter, you need to know how to:

◆ Start PractiSoft, use menus, and enter and edit text.
◆ Work with chart numbers and codes.

OBJECTIVES

When you finish this chapter, you will be able to:

1. Create electronic and paper claims.
2. Review claims for errors and omissions.
3. Review an audit/edit report.

KEY TERMS

filter
navigator buttons

CREATING CLAIMS

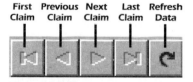

Figure 10-1
Claim Management
shortcut button.

Within the Claim Management area of PractiSoft, insurance claims are created, edited, and submitted for payment. Claims are created from transactions previously entered in PractiSoft. After claims are created, they can either be printed and mailed or transmitted electronically. The Claim Management dialog box is displayed by clicking Claim Management on the Activities menu or by clicking the Claim Management shortcut button on the toolbar (see Figure 10-1). This dialog box (see Figure 10-2) lists all claims that have already been created. In this dialog box, several actions can be performed: existing claims can be reviewed and edited, new claims can be created, the status of existing claims can be changed, and claims can be printed or submitted electronically.

Figure 10-2   Claim Management dialog box.

The Claim Management dialog box contains five **navigator buttons** that simplify the task of moving from one entry to another (see Figure 10-3). The First Claim button selects the first claim in the list and makes it active. The Previous Claim button reactivates the claim that was most recently active. The Next Claim button makes the next claim in the list active. The Last Claim button makes the last claim in the list active. The Refresh Data button is used to restore data when necessary.

First   Previous   Next   Last   Refresh
Claim   Claim   Claim   Claim   Data

Figure 10-3
Navigator buttons.

navigator buttons *buttons that simplify the task of moving from one entry in a list to another*

CREATE CLAIMS DIALOG BOX

filter *in sorting data, a condition that data must meet to be included in the selection*

Claims are created in the Create Claims dialog box. The Create Claims dialog box (see Figure 10-4 on page 186) is accessed by clicking the Create Claims button in the Claim Management dialog box. This dialog box provides several filters to customize the creation of claims. A **filter** is a condition that data must meet to be included in the selection of data. For example, claims can be created for services performed between the first and the fifteenth of the month. If this were the case, the filter would be the condition that services must have been performed between the first and fifteenth of the month. Transactions that meet this criterion would be included in the selection; transactions that do not fall within that date range would not be included. Filters can be used to create claims for a specific patient, for example, or for a specific insurance carrier, or for transactions that exceed a certain dollar amount. The following filters can be applied within the Create Claims dialog box.

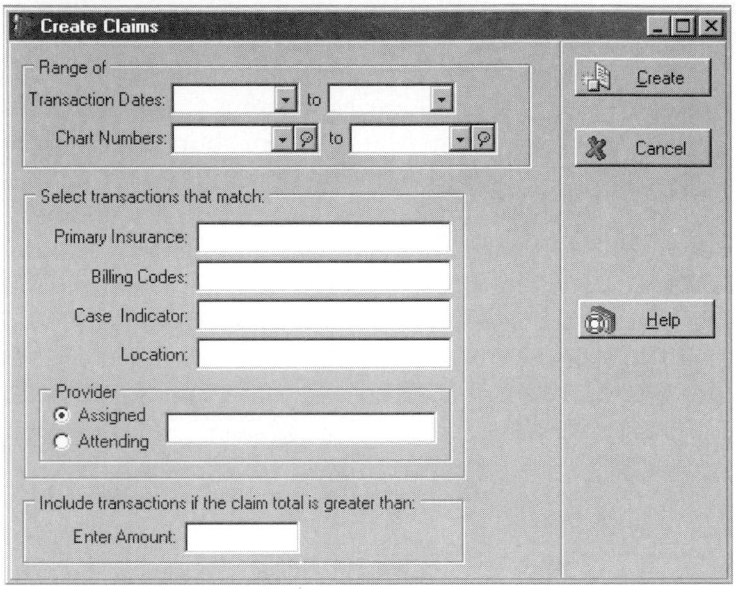

Figure 10-4   Create Claims dialog box.

Range of   The options in this section of the dialog box provide filters for establishing the starting and ending dates as well as the starting and ending chart numbers for the claims that will be created.

Transaction Dates   The Transaction Dates boxes are used to specify the starting and ending dates for which claims will be created. If the boxes are left blank, transactions for all dates will be included.

Chart Numbers   In the Chart Numbers boxes, the starting and ending chart numbers for which claims will be created are entered. If the boxes are left blank, all chart numbers will be included.

Select Transactions That Match   The options in this section of the dialog box provide filters for matching the exact primary insurance carrier(s), billing code(s), case indicator(s), and location(s).

Primary Insurance   The carrier code for the insurance company is entered in the Primary Insurance box. If claims are being sent to a clearinghouse, more than one insurance carrier code can be entered. When more than one code is entered, a comma must be placed between the codes. If claims are being sent directly to the carrier, only that carrier's code is entered.

Billing Codes   The billing code (used to classify and sort patients for billing purposes, for example, by billing cycle) is entered in the Billing Codes box. If more than one code is entered, a comma must be placed between the codes.

Case Indicator   If case indicators are used to classify patients (such as by type of procedure), the case indicator can be listed in the Case Indicator box. If more than one indicator is entered, a comma must be placed between each one.

Location   Sometimes a sort is needed by location, such as all procedures done at a provider's office or in a hospital emergency room. The location code is entered in the Location box. If more than one code is entered, a comma must be placed between the codes.

Provider   The radio buttons in the Provider box indicate whether the provider is the assigned or attending provider. In the box to the right of the radio buttons, the provider code is entered. If more than one code is entered, a comma must be placed between the codes.

Include Transactions if the Claim Total Is Greater Than   The dollar amount entered in this box is the minimum total amount required for a case before a claim can be created.

Any box that is not filled in will default to include all data, and claims with any entry in that box will be included. When all necessary information has been entered, clicking the Create button creates the claims. PractiSoft will create a file of matching claims but will include only those that have not yet been billed.

EXERCISE 10-1

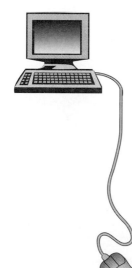

Create insurance claims for all patients who have transactions not already placed on a claim.

Date: November 2, 2007

1. **Start PractiSoft. Change the date if necessary.**

2. **On the Activities menu, click Claim Management. The Claim Management dialog box is displayed. Scroll through the list to view the various batches of already-created claims.**

3. **Click the Create Claims button.**

4. **Leave all boxes in the Create Claims dialog box blank to select all transactions.**

5. **Click the Create button.**

6. **Scroll up to the top of the list to view the claims just created (Batch Ø). Notice their "Ready to Send" status in column 4.**

7. **Click the Close button.**

CLAIM SELECTION

At times it is necessary to select and view specific claims that have already been created. For example, any claims prepared for submission to an insurance carrier must be selected and then reviewed for completeness and accuracy. In addition, all claims that have been rejected by insurance carriers are selected and reviewed before resubmission.

PractiSoft's List Only feature is used when it is necessary to list claims that match certain criteria. Filters are applied in the List Only Claims That Match dialog box. They can be used to view claims selectively, such as claims for a specific insurance carrier or claims created on a certain date. Unlike the filters in the Create Claims dialog box, those in the List Only Claims That Match dialog box do not create claims; they simply list existing claims that meet the specified criteria.

The List Only feature is activated by clicking the List Only... button in the Claim Management dialog box. This causes the List Only Claims That Match dialog box to be displayed (see Figure 10-5). Claims can be sorted by chart number, date the claim was created, insurance carrier, electronic media claim (EMC) receiver, billing method, billing date, batch number, and claim status. Not all the boxes need to be filled in, only the ones that will be used to select the desired claims. Once the filters have been applied, only those claims that match the criteria are listed in the main Claim Management dialog box.

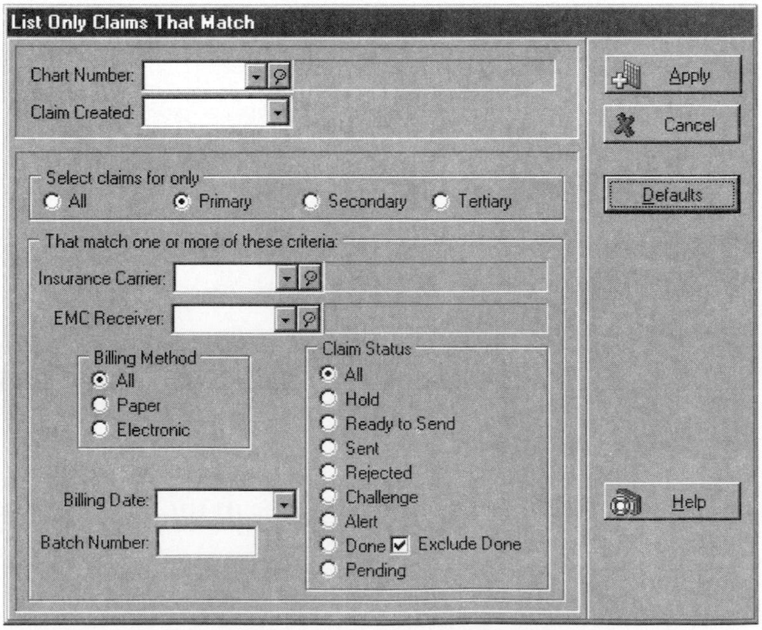

Figure 10-5 List Only Claims That Match dialog box.

The following filters are available in the List Only Claims That Match dialog box.

Chart Number   A patient's chart number is selected from the drop-down list of patients' chart numbers.

Claim Created   The date that a claim was created is entered in MMDDCCYY format.

Select Claims for Only   A radio button is clicked for either all insurance carriers, primary insurance carrier only, secondary insurance carrier only, or tertiary (third) insurance carrier only. When a patient has insurance coverage with more than one carrier, the primary carrier is billed first, and then, if appropriate, the second and third carriers are billed.

Insurance Carrier   An insurance carrier is selected from the drop-down list of choices.

EMC Receiver   An EMC receiver is selected from the choices on the drop-down list.

Billing Method   In the Billing Method box, the radio button for All, Paper, or Electronic is clicked.

Billing Date   The date of billing is entered in the Billing Date box.

Batch Number   A batch number is entered in the Batch Number box.

Claim Status   A claim status is selected from the list of radio buttons provided. If claims that have been billed and accepted (not rejected) are to be excluded from the search, the Exclude Done box is clicked. This causes a check mark to be displayed beside the option.

When the desired boxes have been filled in, clicking the Apply button applies the selected filters to the claims data. The Claim Management dialog box is displayed listing only those claims that match the criteria selected in the List Only Claims That Match dialog box. From the Claim Management dialog box, the claims can now be edited, printed, and mailed or transmitted electronically. To restore the List Only Claims That Match dialog box to its original settings (that is, to remove the filters selected), this dialog box is reopened, the Defaults button is clicked, and then the Apply button is clicked. All of the boxes in the dialog box will become blank, and the full list of claims is displayed again in the Claim Management dialog box.

PractiSoft's Claim Edit feature allows claims to be reviewed and verified on screen before they are submitted to insurance carriers for payment. With careful checking, problems can be solved before claims are sent to insurance carriers. When a claim is active in the Claim Management dialog box, it can be edited by clicking the Edit button or by double-clicking the claim itself. The Claim dialog box is displayed (see Figure 10-6). The top section of the Claim dialog box lists the claim number, the date the claim was created, the chart number, the patient's name, and the case number. This information cannot be edited, although the information in the five tabs can be edited.

CARRIER 1 TAB   The Carrier 1 tab displays information about claims being submitted to a patient's primary insurance carrier.

The following boxes are listed in the Carrier 1 tab:

Claim Status   The Claim Status box indicates the status of a particular claim: Hold, Ready to send, Sent, Rejected, Challenge, Alert, Done, and Pending. The radio button that reflects a claim's status should be clicked.

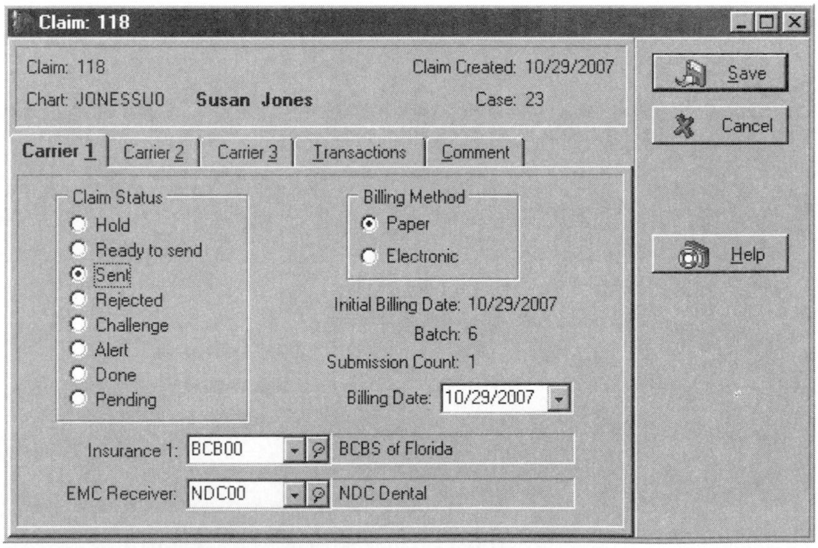

Figure 10-6   Claim dialog box.

Billing Method   The Billing Method box displays two choices: Paper or Electronic. The radio button that describes the billing method should be clicked.

Initial Billing Date   If the bill was sent more than once, this box automatically displays the initial billing date.

Batch   If the claim has been assigned to a batch, the batch number is displayed.

Submission Count   The Submission Count area lists the number of claims submitted.

Billing Date   The Billing Date box lists the date the bill was sent. If the bill was sent more than once, this box lists the most recent billing date.

Insurance 1   The Insurance 1 box lists a patient's primary insurance carrier.

EMC Receiver   The EMC receiver is selected from the drop-down list.

CARRIER 2 AND CARRIER 3 TABS   The Carrier 2 and Carrier 3 tabs display information about claims being submitted to a patient's secondary (Carrier 2) and tertiary (Carrier 3) insurance carriers. The boxes in these tabs are the same as the boxes in the Carrier 1 tab, with the exception of the Claim Status box. In the Carrier 2 and Carrier 3 tabs, there is no Pending radio button in the Claim Status box. Otherwise, the three tabs are the same.

TRANSACTIONS TAB   The Transactions tab lists information about the transactions included in a claim. The scroll bars can be used to view all the information in the Transactions tab (see Figure 10-7).

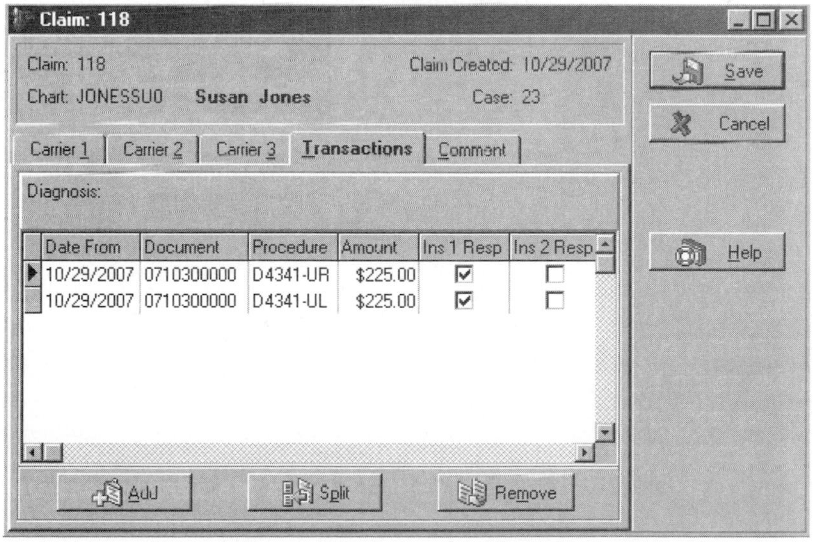

Figure 10-7   Transactions tab.

Date From   The Date From column lists the date on which service was provided.

Document The Document column lists the document number of a transaction.

Procedure The Procedure column displays the procedure code for a procedure performed.

Amount In the Amount column, the dollar cost of a service is displayed.

Ins 1 Resp If the box in this column is checked, the primary insurance carrier is responsible for the claim.

Ins 2 Resp If the box in this column is checked, the secondary insurance carrier is responsible for the claim.

Ins 3 Resp If the box in this column is checked, the tertiary insurance carrier is responsible for the claim.

The Transactions tab also contains three buttons at the bottom of the dialog box: Add, Split, and Remove. The Add button is used to add a transaction to an existing claim. The Split button removes a single transaction from an existing claim and places it on a new claim. The Remove button deletes a transaction from the database.

COMMENT TAB The Comment tab provides a place to include any specific notes or comments about the claim (see Figure 10-8). The comments are for internal use only and are not transmitted or printed elsewhere in the program.

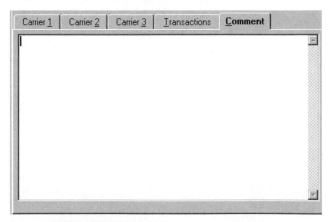

Figure 10-8   Comment tab.

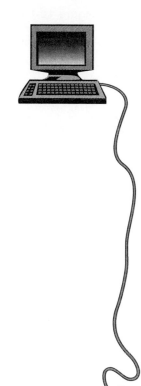

EXERCISE 10-2

Review insurance claims for patients with Aetna as their insurance carrier.

Date: November 2, 2007

1. Open the Claim Management dialog box.

2. Click the List Only... button.

3. Click Aetna in the drop-down list in the Insurance Carrier box.

4. Click the Apply button. You are returned to the Claim Management dialog box. Notice that only claims for patients who have Aetna as their insurance carrier are listed.

5. Double-click Chart Number CHANJOSØ or select this chart number and click the Edit button to review the claim for Josephine Chan. The Claim dialog box is displayed.

6. Review the information in the Carrier 1 tab.

7. Review the information in the Transactions tab.

8. Click the Cancel button to exit the Claim dialog box without saving any changes. (The Cancel button does not cancel the claim; it just cancels any changes that may have been made.)

9. Close the Claim Management dialog box.

PRETREATMENT CLAIM MANAGEMENT

Similar to the Claim Management feature, the Pretreatment/Claim Management option on the Activities menu is used to create and print pretreatment claims. A pretreatment claim is the same as a regular claim except that it is labeled "pretreatment" to indicate that the transactions represented in the claim are projections rather than actual transactions.

The Claim Management—Pretreatment Plan/Estimate dialog box (see Figure 10-9 on page 194) is displayed by clicking Pretreatment Claim Management on the Activities menu or by clicking the Pretreatment Claim Management button on the toolbar (see Figure 10-10 on page 194). The process of creating and printing pretreatment claims is the same as the process for creating and printing claims in the Claim Management dialog box discussed above. Both dialog boxes look and function the same. However, the Claim Management dialog box uses the information in the Transaction Entry dialog box to create claims, while the Claim Management—Pretreatment Plan/Estimate dialog box pulls information from the Pretreatment Plan/Estimate dialog box, which is accessed through the Enter Pretreatment Estimates option on the Activities menu.

Figure 10-9   Claim Management – Pretreatment Plan/Estimate dialog box.

Figure 10-10
Pretreatment Claim
Management button.

The purpose of creating pretreatment claims is to protect the patient by presenting the patient's insurance carrier with an estimate of the costs of dental treatment before beginning the treatment. If the insurance carrier does not agree with the costs outlined by the dentist or if the proposed procedures are not covered by the patient's insurance plan, the patient knows in advance and can work with the dentist to make alternative plans before beginning treatment.

TIP . . . After a pretreatment plan is submitted and approved by the insurance carrier and treatment begins, the pretreatment estimate transactions can be copied to the main Transaction Entry window one transaction at a time. Copying transactions to the Transaction Entry dialog box from the Claim Management – Pretreatment Plan/Estimate dialog box rather than entering them a second time can save time and prevent typing errors.

ELECTRONIC MEDIA CLAIMS

Many of the setup and entry requirements for electronic media claims (EMC) are typically handled by the dental office's systems manager. Insurance carriers and clearinghouses that receive claims electronically have different requirements regarding what information needs to be included on an electronic claim. Each insurance carrier has specific data requirements, indicating which boxes are mandatory and what the data format should be.

The office systems manager maintains detailed information on the EMC requirements of each carrier and updates this information as necessary. However, some basic steps that need to be followed to submit electronic claims are common to most insurance carriers.

STEPS IN SUBMITTING ELECTRONIC CLAIMS

There are a number of steps in the process of submitting electronic claims.

1. Enter information about a patient in the usual manner.

2. Check to make sure all the information required by an insurance carrier is complete; otherwise, the claim will be rejected.

3. Enter transactions and payments as usual.

4. Create claims either through the Transaction Entry dialog box or through the Claim Management feature.

5. Review claims through the Claims Edit and the List Only . . . features to locate any obvious errors.

6. Transmit claims to the clearinghouse.

7. Review the audit/edit report that arrives from the clearinghouse. The audit/edit report lists any problems with the claims. Correct and resubmit any claims that have errors.

8. Allow some time for the claim to be processed. After the clearinghouse transmits the claims to an insurance carrier, the information is received by the insurance carrier and stored in its database, awaiting processing.

TRANSMITTING ELECTRONIC CLAIMS

At present, PractiSoft is set up to send only CMS-1500 (formerly HCFA-1500) claims electronically. All other claims must be marked as paper claims in PractiSoft. To send claims electronically, PractiSoft uses a program called HCFA11 that puts claim data into an MS-DOS text file in the cor-rect format. The file can then be transmitted electronically to a clearinghouse. CMS-1500 claims are used for reporting physician services such as those performed by an oral surgeon.

The following procedure is used to send electronic claims in PractiSoft: After making sure all the information is complete and cor-rect for claims being sent, the Print/Send button in the Claim Management dialog box is clicked. This causes the Print/Send Claims dialog box to be displayed. Within this dialog box, the billing method (paper or electronic) must be indicated (see Figure 10-11). If the claims being sent are paper, the Paper radio button is clicked. If the claims are being submitted electronically, the Electronic radio button is clicked.

When the Electronic radio button is clicked, the Electronic Claim Receiver box becomes active. The EMC receiver is selected from the list of choices in the drop-down list.

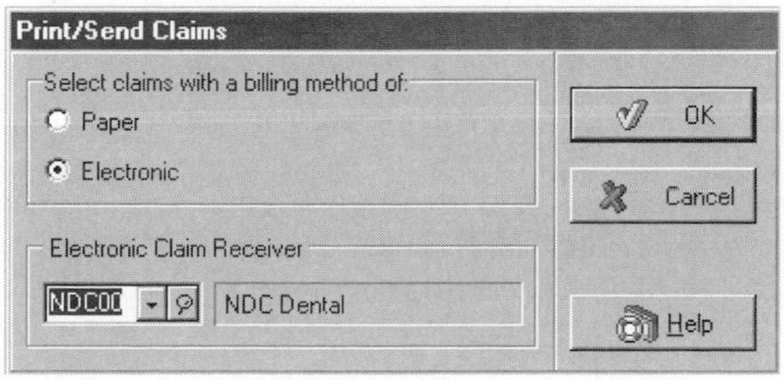

Figure 10-11   Print/Send Claims dialog box.

After the EMC receiver has been selected and the OK button is clicked, the Send Electronic Claims dialog box is displayed (see Figure 10-12). To send electronic claims, the Create File button is clicked. A Save As dialog box appears for naming the new text file, followed by a Data Selection Questions dialog box for applying any filters to the list of claims to be sent. The file is then saved for transmission to a clearinghouse. After claims are sent, the system marks them "Sent" in the Claim Management dialog box.

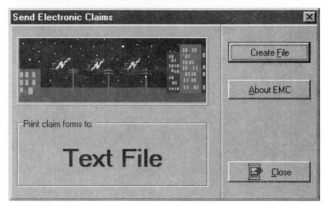

Figure 10-12 Send Electronic Claims dialog box.

TIP . . . An EMC receiver is set up in PractiSoft by selecting the EMC Receivers option on the Lists menu. In the EMC Receiver List dialog box that displays, a code is created for the receiver and the name of the receiver is entered, such as NDC00 for NDC (National Data Corporation) Dental. In the ID and Extra tab, the Program File box must be completed. Because only the standard CMS-1500 claim form can be used in PractiSoft, the Program File box in this tab must contain the program name HCFA11. For the purposes of this text, no CMS-1500 claims are created. For the sake of simulating how to prepare an electronic claim, however, the EMC Receiver NDC Dental has been added to the Collier Family Dental Care database.

EXERCISE 10-3

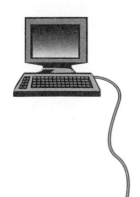

Prepare to send electronic claims to a clearinghouse.

Date: November 2, 2007

1. Open the Claim Management dialog box, and click the Print/Send button.

2. In the Print/Send Claims dialog box, select claims with an electronic billing method by clicking the Electronic radio button.

3. Click NDC Dental on the drop-down list in the Electronic Claim Receiver box.

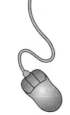

4. Click the OK button. The Send Electronic Claims dialog box is displayed.

5. If you were in a dental office and ready to send a CMS claim form electronically, you would click the Create File button. However, because you are in a school setting and are not actually set up to submit electronic claims, click the Close button.

6. Close the Claim Management dialog box.

7. Exit PractiSoft.

REVIEWING THE AUDIT/EDIT REPORT

When claims are transmitted to a clearinghouse, an audit/edit report is received immediately after claims are sent (see Figure 3-3 on page 35). Options for viewing and printing the report are listed on the screen when the report is received. It is important to print a copy of the report, since some systems do not permit reports to be viewed online at a later time.

The audit/edit report marks each claim as accepted or rejected. Each claim is displayed on a separate line of the report. The Message column queries whether a claim will be sent to an insurance carrier. If a claim cannot be sent, the error is listed in the Message column. In the Flag column of the report, a "P" indicates that the claim will be sent on paper; an "R" indicates that the claim was rejected. A blank Flag column means that the claim will be sent electronically.

The report should be reviewed carefully. Any errors found by a clearinghouse must be corrected before a claim can be sent to an insurance carrier. For example, if an audit/edit report rejects a claim, saying "Missing Insured's ID no.," the following steps should be taken:

1. Go to the Policy 1 tab in the Case dialog box and key the missing number in the Policy Number box.

2. Save the edit, and then close the Patient List dialog box.

3. Open the Claim Management dialog box.

4. Double-click the rejected claim in the Claim Management dialog box to edit the claim.

5. Change the claim status from Rejected to Ready to Send. Click the Save button.

6. Click the Print/Send button in the Claim Management dialog box to begin the process of creating a new file for electronic transmission to the clearinghouse.

CHAPTER REVIEW

USING TERMINOLOGY

Define the terms below.

1. filter

_____

_____

2. navigator buttons

_____

_____

CHECKING YOUR UNDERSTANDING

Answer the questions below in the space provided.

3. A claim needs to be submitted for John Ellison. How would you select only those claims pertaining to John Ellison?

_____

_____

4. On an audit/edit report, what does an "R" in the Flag column indicate?

_____

_____

5. If an error is found on a claim, how is it corrected?

_____

_____

APPLYING KNOWLEDGE

Answer the question below in the space provided.

6. You were asked to create claims for Samuel Barlow. After entering his chart number in the Create Claims dialog box, you receive the message "No new claims were created." Why were no claims created for Samuel Barlow?

_____

_____

AT THE COMPUTER

Answer the following questions at the computer.

7. How many claims were created on September 7, 2007? Whose claims were these?

_____

_____

8. What transactions were included on Gloria Barlow's claim that was created on September 3, 2007?

_____

_____

_____

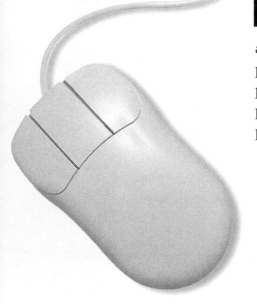

WHAT YOU NEED TO KNOW

To use this chapter, you need to know how to:

◆ Start PractiSoft, use menus, and enter and edit text.
◆ Work with chart numbers and codes.

OBJECTIVES

When you finish this chapter, you will be able to:

1. Select the options available for different reports.
2. Preview and print a variety of PractiSoft reports.
3. Access PractiSoft's Report Designer.

KEY TERMS

aging report
patient day sheet
patient ledger
patient statement
procedure day sheet

REPORTS IN THE DENTAL OFFICE

Reports are an important tool in managing a dental office. They provide useful information about a practice and its patients. Providers and office managers ask for different reports at different times. Some providers want to see a daily report of each day's transactions. Others want to see reports on particular patients' accounts on a weekly or bimonthly basis.

PractiSoft provides a variety of standard reports, and has the ability to create custom reports using the Report Designer. Standard and custom reports are accessed through the Reports menu (see Figure 11-1). The Reports menu lists standard reports and also provides choices for designing custom reports using the Report Designer.

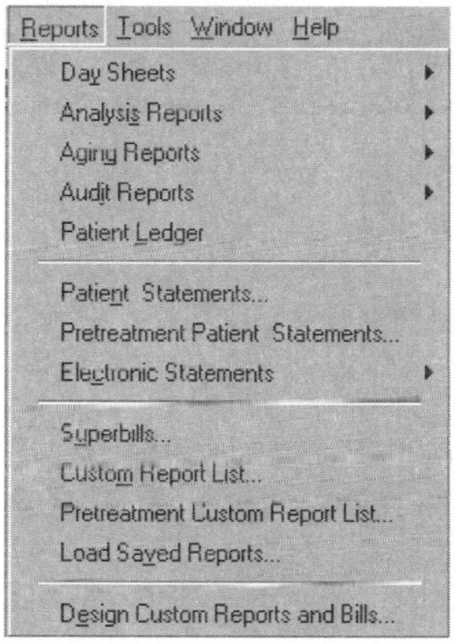

Figure 11-1
Reports menu.

The standard reports are day sheets, analysis reports, aging reports, audit reports, patient ledgers, and patient statements, including pretreatment and electronic patient statements.

PATIENT DAY SHEET

patient day sheet *a summary of the activity of patient accounts on any given day*

At the end of the day, many dental practices print a **patient day sheet**, which is a summary of the activity of patient activity on any given day (see Figures 11-2a and 11-2b on pages 202 and 203). PractiSoft's version of this report lists the procedures for a particular day, grouped by patient, in alphabetical order by chart number. It includes:

◆ Procedures performed for a particular patient or group of patients.

◆ Charges, receipts, adjustments, and balances for a particular patient or group of patients.

◆ A summary of a practice's charges, payments, and adjustments.

Patient Day Sheet
9/3/2007 - 9/3/2007

Entry	Date	Document	POS	Description	Provider	Code	Amount
AXFORSU0		**Susan R Axford**					
1	9/3/2007	0709030000	11		HSM	D2150	120.00
22	9/3/2007	0709030000	11		HSM	CHCOPAY20	-20.00
21	9/3/2007	0709030000	11		HSM	CIGCOPAY	20.00
		Patient's Charges		Patient's Receipts	Adjustments		Patient Balance
		$140.00		-$20.00	$0.00		$0.00
BARLODA0		**Daniel H Barlow**					
4	9/3/2007	0709030000	11		HSM	D1110	60.00
23	9/3/2007	0709030000	11		HSM	CIGCOPAY	20.00
24	9/3/2007	0709030000	11		HSM	CHCOPAY20	-20.00
		Patient's Charges		Patient's Receipts	Adjustments		Patient Balance
		$80.00		-$20.00	$0.00		$0.00
BARLOGL0		**Gloria Barlow**					
13	9/3/2007	0709030000	11		HSM	D1120	45.00
31	9/3/2007	0709030000	11		HSM	CIGCOPAY	20.00
32	9/3/2007	0709030000	11		HSM	CHCOPAY20	-20.00
		Patient's Charges		Patient's Receipts	Adjustments		Patient Balance
		$65.00		-$20.00	$0.00		$0.00
BARLOJI0		**Jimmy Barlow**					
9	9/3/2007	0709030000	11		HSM	D1120	45.00
27	9/3/2007	0709030000	11		HSM	CIGCOPAY	20.00
28	9/3/2007	0709030000	11		HSM	CHCOPAY20	-20.00
		Patient's Charges		Patient's Receipts	Adjustments		Patient Balance
		$65.00		-$20.00	$0.00		$0.00
BARLOJU0		**June Barlow**					
6	9/3/2007	0709030000	11		HSM	D0120	25.00
7	9/3/2007	0709030000	11		HSM	D1110	60.00
25	9/3/2007	0709030000	11		HSM	CIGCOPAY	20.00
26	9/3/2007	0709030000	11		HSM	CHCOPAY20	-20.00
		Patient's Charges		Patient's Receipts	Adjustments		Patient Balance
		$105.00		-$20.00	$0.00		$0.00
BARLOSA0		**Samuel S Barlow**					
17	9/3/2007	0709030000	11		HSM	D1120	45.00
29	9/3/2007	0709030000	11		HSM	CIGCOPAY	20.00
30	9/3/2007	0709030000	11		HSM	CHCOPAY20	-20.00
		Patient's Charges		Patient's Receipts	Adjustments		Patient Balance
		$65.00		-$20.00	$0.00		$0.00

Figure 11-2a   Page 1 of Patient Day Sheet report.

Collier Family Dental Care

Patient Day Sheet

9/3/2007 - 9/3/2007

Total # Patients	6
Total # Procedures	13
Total Procedure Charges	$520.00
Total Product Charges	$0.00
Total Inside Lab Charges	$0.00
Total Outside Lab Charges	$0.00
Total Billing Charges	$0.00
Total Tax Charges	$0.00
Total Charges	$520.00
Total Insurance Payments	$0.00
Total Cash Copayments	$0.00
Total Check Copayments	-$120.00
Total Credit Card Copayments	$0.00
Total Patient Cash Payments	$0.00
Total Patient Check Payments	$0.00
Total Credit Card Payments	$0.00
Total Receipts	-$120.00
Total Credit Adjustments	$0.00
Total Debit Adjustments	$0.00
Total Insurance Debit Adjustments	$0.00
Total Insurance Credit Adjustments	$0.00
Total Insurance Withholds	$0.00
Total Adjustments	$0.00
Net Effect on Accounts Receivable	$400.00

Figure 11-2b   Page 2 of Patient Day Sheet report.

To print a patient day sheet, Day Sheets is clicked on the Reports menu and Patient Day Sheet on the submenu (see Figure 11-3). Then, the Print Report Where? dialog box is displayed, asking whether the report should be previewed on the screen, sent directly to the printer, or exported to a file (see Figure 11-4). Reports that are previewed on the screen can also be printed from the Preview Report window.

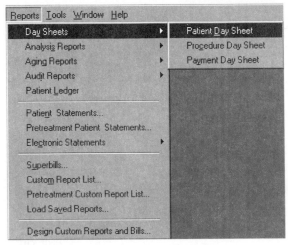

Figure 11-3 Reports menu with Day Sheets submenu displayed.

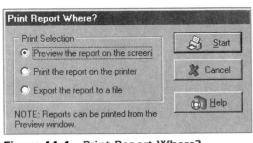

Figure 11-4 Print Report Where? dialog box.

When the Preview the Report on the Screen radio button is selected and the Start button is clicked, the Data Selection Questions dialog box is displayed (see Figure 11-5). This dialog box is used to select the patients, dates, and providers about which a report is being generated. If any box is left blank, all values are included in the report. For example, if no chart numbers are entered, all patients will be included in the report. The selection options in the dialog box are as follows.

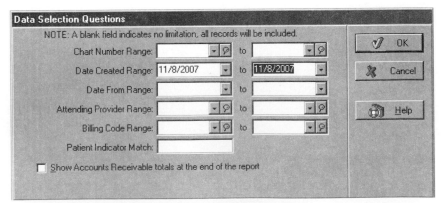

Figure 11-5 Data Selection Questions dialog box.

Chart Number Range   In the Chart Number Range boxes, a range of chart numbers for patients is entered. If a report is needed for just one patient, that patient's chart number is entered in both boxes.

Date Created Range A range of dates when transactions were entered in PractiSoft is entered in the two boxes. The current date is the default entry. If this is not the date desired, it can be changed by selecting new dates and entering them.

Date From Range A range of dates is entered in the Date From Range boxes. For example, if it were necessary to print patient day sheets for the period of May 1 to May 15, 2007, 05012007 would be entered in the first box and 05152007 in the second box. If transactions were needed for the current date, that date would be entered in both boxes.

Attending Provider Range A range of codes for the attending providers is entered in the Attending Provider Range boxes.

Billing Code Range If the practice uses PractiSoft's Billing Code feature, codes can be entered in this box to select only those patients with the designated billing code(s).

Patient Indicator Match If the practice has assigned a Patient Indicator code to each patient, an entry can be made to select only those patients who match a specific code.

Show Accounts Receivable Totals at the End of the Report If this box is checked, accounts receivable totals will appear at the end of the Patient Day Sheet report.

When these selection boxes have been completed, the OK button is clicked. PractiSoft begins creating the report. PractiSoft generates the report and displays it on-screen or sends it to a file or the printer, depending on the selection made in the Print Report Where? dialog box.

The Preview Report window, common to all reports, provides options for viewing or printing a report (see Figure 11-6 on page 206). The buttons on the Preview Report toolbar control how a report is displayed on-screen and how to move from page to page within a report (see Figure 11-7 on page 206).

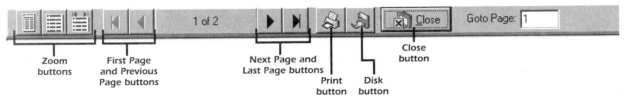

Figure 11-6   Preview Report window.

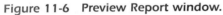

Zoom
buttons

First Page
and Previous
Page buttons

Next Page and
Last Page buttons

Print
button

Disk
button

Close
button

Goto Page: 1

Figure 11-7   Buttons on Preview Report toolbar.

The three zoom buttons at the left of the toolbar are used to adjust the size of the report displayed on-screen. The zoom button farthest to the left reduces a report so that a full page fits on the screen. The middle zoom button displays a report at 100 percent of its size. This option acts like a magnifying glass, allowing a portion of a report to be viewed up close. The zoom button on the right displays the full width of a page on the screen.

A series of four triangle buttons, two on the left and two on the right, are used to move through pages of a multipage report. The First Page button, farthest on the left, moves to the beginning of a report. The Previous Page button moves to the page that precedes the one currently displayed. The bar between the two sets of triangle buttons indicates how many pages are in a report and the number of the current page. To the right of the bar are the other two triangle buttons. The Next Page button moves to the page following the current one. The Last Page button moves to the end of a report.

The remaining buttons include the Print button, which is used to send a report to the printer, and the Disk button, which saves a report to disk. The Close button closes the Preview Report window, redisplaying the main PractiSoft window.

The Preview Report window also contains the Go to Page box, in which the number of a specific page to be displayed in the Preview Report window is entered.

EXERCISE 11-1

Print a patient day sheet report for July 12, 2007.

Date: July 12, 2007

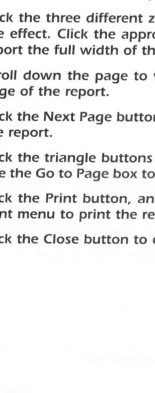

1. Start PractiSoft.

2. On the Reports menu, click Day Sheets and then Patient Day Sheet. The Print Report Where? dialog box is displayed.

3. Click the radio button for previewing the report on-screen if it is not already selected. Click the Start button. The Data Selection Questions dialog box is displayed.

4. Leave the Chart Number Range boxes blank. Key 07122007 in both of the Date Created Range boxes. Do not key any slashes between the numbers; PractiSoft does this automatically. (Today's date—that is, the date on which you are working on this exercise, will most likely appear in both Date Created Range boxes. This is because PractiSoft uses the Windows system date rather than the PractiSoft program date as the default entry when printing reports. Select each entry and enter the July 12, 2007, date instead.) Leave all other boxes blank. This will select data for all patients and attending providers for July 12, 2007.

5. Click the OK button. The patient day sheet report is displayed.

6. Click the three different zoom buttons on the toolbar to see the effect. Click the appropriate zoom button to display the report the full width of the screen so that it is easier to read.

7. Scroll down the page to view additional entries on the first page of the report.

8. Click the Next Page button to advance to the second page of the report.

9. Click the triangle buttons on the toolbar to see their effects. Use the Go to Page box to move back to page 1 of the report.

10. Click the Print button, and then click the OK button on the Print menu to print the report.

11. Click the Close button to exit the Preview Report window.

PROCEDURE DAY SHEET

procedure day sheet   a list of all the procedures performed on a particular day

A **procedure day sheet** lists all the procedures performed on a particular day, and gives the dates, patients, document numbers, places of service, debits, and credits relating to these procedures (see Figure 11-8). Procedures are listed in numerical order. Procedure day sheets are printed by clicking Procedure Day Sheet on the Reports menu. The same Print Report Where? dialog box used for a patient day sheet is displayed. Again, the report can be previewed on-screen, printed directly, or exported to a file.

Collier Family Dental Care
Procedure Code Day Sheet
9/3/2007 - 9/3/2007

Entry	Date	Chart	Name	Document	POS	Debits	Credits
CHCOPAY20		**Check copayment $20**					
22	9/3/2007	AXFORSU0	Axford, Susan R	0709030000	11		-20.00
24	9/3/2007	BARLODA0	Barlow, Daniel H	0709030000	11		-20.00
26	9/3/2007	BARLOJU0	Barlow, June	0709030000	11		-20.00
28	9/3/2007	BARLOJI0	Barlow, Jimmy	0709030000	11		-20.00
30	9/3/2007	BARLOSA0	Barlow, Samuel S	0709030000	11		-20.00
32	9/3/2007	BARLOGL0	Barlow, Gloria	0709030000	11		-20.00
		Total of CHCOPAY20		Quantity:	6	$0.00	-$120.00
CIGCOPAY		**CIGNA Copayment**					
23	9/3/2007	BARLODA0	Barlow, Daniel H	0709030000	11	20.00	
25	9/3/2007	BARLOJU0	Barlow, June	0709030000	11	20.00	
27	9/3/2007	BARLOJI0	Barlow, Jimmy	0709030000	11	20.00	
29	9/3/2007	BARLOSA0	Barlow, Samuel S	0709030000	11	20.00	
31	9/3/2007	BARLOGL0	Barlow, Gloria	0709030000	11	20.00	
21	9/3/2007	AXFORSU0	Axford, Susan R	0709030000	11	20.00	
		Total of CIGCOPAY		Quantity:	6	$120.00	$0.00
D0120		**periodic oral evaluation**					
6	9/3/2007	BARLOJU0	Barlow, June	0709030000	11	25.00	
		Total of D0120		Quantity:	1	$25.00	$0.00
D1110		**prophylaxis--adult**					
4	9/3/2007	BARLODA0	Barlow, Daniel H	0709030000	11	60.00	
7	9/3/2007	BARLOJU0	Barlow, June	0709030000	11	60.00	
		Total of D1110		Quantity:	2	$120.00	$0.00
D1120		**prophylaxis--child**					
9	9/3/2007	BARLOJI0	Barlow, Jimmy	0709030000	11	45.00	
17	9/3/2007	BARLOSA0	Barlow, Samuel S	0709030000	11	45.00	
13	9/3/2007	BARLOGL0	Barlow, Gloria	0709030000	11	45.00	
		Total of D1120		Quantity:	3	$135.00	$0.00
D2150		**amalgam restor., 2 surf., prim. or perm.**					
1	9/3/2007	AXFORSU0	Axford, Susan R	0709030000	11	120.00	
		Total of D2150		Quantity:	1	$120.00	$0.00

Figure 11-8   Procedure Day Sheet report.

Once the decision to preview, print, or export is made, the data selection criteria must be determined. The Data Selection Questions dialog box provides options to select by procedure codes, dates, and providers (see Figure 11-9). A procedure day sheet will be generated only for the data that meet the selection criteria. If any box is left blank, all values are included in the report.

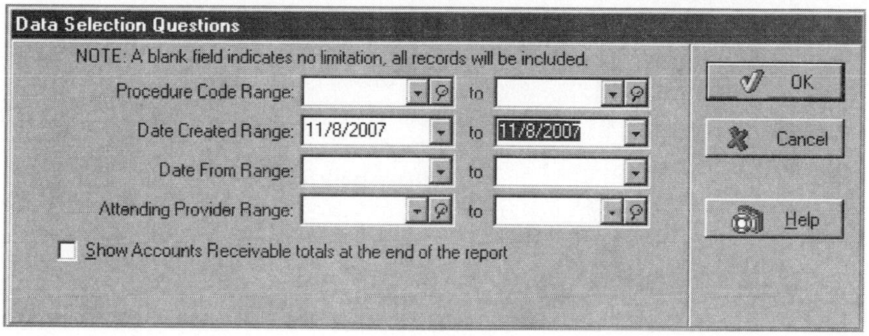

Figure 11-9   Data Selection Questions dialog box.

The following boxes are listed in the Data Selection Questions dialog box.

Procedure Code Range   In the Procedure Code Range box, a range of procedure codes is entered. If a report is needed for a single code, it is entered in both boxes.

Date Created Range   A range of dates when transactions were entered in PractiSoft is entered in the two boxes. The Windows system date is the default entry. If this is not the date desired, it can be changed by selecting new dates and entering them.

Date From Range   A range of dates when each transaction occurred is entered in the Date From Range boxes.

Attending Provider Range   Codes for attending providers are entered in the Attending Provider Range boxes.

Show Accounts Receivable Totals at the End of the Report   If this box is checked, accounts receivable totals will appear at the end of the report.

Print a procedure day sheet report for July 12, 2007, with the entire range of procedure codes, dates from, and attending providers.

Date: July 12, 2007

1. On the Reports menu, click Day Sheets and then Procedure Day Sheet. The Print Report Where? dialog box is displayed.

2. Click the radio button option for previewing the report on-screen. Click the Start button. The Data Selection Questions dialog box is displayed.

3. Leave the Procedure Code Range boxes blank.

4. Key *07122007* in both Date Created Range boxes. Leave the other boxes blank. Click the OK button. The procedure day sheet report is displayed.

5. Send the report to the printer.

6. Exit the Preview Report window.

PRACTICE ANALYSIS REPORT

PractiSoft's practice analysis report analyzes the revenue of a practice for a specified period of time, usually a month or a year (see Figures 11-10a and 11-10b). The report can be used to generate dental practice financial statements. It can also be used for profit analysis. The summary at the end of the report breaks down the report into total charges, including procedure, product, inside lab, outside lab, and billing charges; total insurance and patient payments and copayments; and total debit and credit adjustments by both patients and insurance carriers. The following boxes are listed in the Data Selection Questions dialog box (see Figure 11-11 on page 212).

Practice Analysis

From September 1, 2007 to September 30, 2007

Code	Description	Amount	Units	Average	Cost	Net
CACOPAY15	Cash copayment $15	-30.00	2	-15.00	0.00	-30.00
CHCOPAY15	Check copayment $15	-30.00	2	-15.00	0.00	-30.00
CHCOPAY20	Check copayment $20	-160.00	8	-20.00	0.00	-160.00
CIGCOPAY	CIGNA Copayment	160.00	8	20.00	0.00	160.00
D0120	periodic oral evaluation	25.00	1	25.00	0.00	25.00
D0274	bitewings--four X rays	25.00	1	25.00	0.00	25.00
D1110	prophylaxis--adult	310.00	5	62.00	0.00	310.00
D1120	prophylaxis--child	180.00	4	45.00	0.00	180.00
D2150	amalgam restor., 2 surf., prim. or	120.00	1	120.00	0.00	120.00
D2750	crown restoration, porcelain-metal	2990.00	3	996.67	0.00	2990.00
D3330	root canal 3	760.00	1	760.00	0.00	760.00
D5213	upper partial denture--cast	1120.00	1	1120.00	0.00	1120.00
D5214	lower partial denture--cast	1120.00	1	1120.00	0.00	1120.00
D7111	extraction--coronal remnants	280.00	2	140.00	0.00	280.00
DELCOPAY	Delta Dental Copayment	30.00	2	15.00	0.00	30.00
PACHECPAY	Patient check payment	-15.00	1	-15.00	0.00	-15.00
SUNCOPAY	Sunshine Copayment	45.00	3	15.00	0.00	45.00

Figure 11-10a   Page 1 of Practice Analysis report.

Collier Family Dental Care

Practice Analysis

From September 1, 2007 to September 30, 2007

Code	Description	Amount	Units	Average	Cost	Net
			Total Procedure Charges			$7,165.00
			Total Product Charges			$0.00
			Total Inside Lab Charges			$0.00
			Total Outside Lab Charges			$0.00
			Total Billing Charges			$0.00
			Total Tax Charges			$0.00
			Total Insurance Payments			$0.00
			Total Cash Copayments			-$30.00
			Total Check Copayments			-$190.00
			Total Credit Card Copayments			$0.00
			Total Patient Cash Payments			$0.00
			Total Patient Check Payments			-$15.00
			Total Credit Card Payments			$0.00
			Total Debit Adjustments			$0.00
			Total Credit Adjustments			$0.00
			Total Insurance Debit Adjustments			$0.00
			Total Insurance Credit Adjustments			$0.00
			Total Insurance Withholds			$0.00
			Net Effect on Accounts Receivable			$6,930.00

Figure 11-10b   Page 2 of Practice Analysis report.

Procedure Code Range A range of procedure codes is entered in the Procedure Code Range boxes.

Date Created Range A range of dates when transactions were entered in PractiSoft is entered in the two boxes.

Date From Range A range of dates is entered in the Date From Range boxes. The system enters a default entry in the second of the two boxes. To change this date, highlight the default entry and enter the new date in MMDDCCYY format.

Attending Provider Range Codes for attending providers are entered in the Attending Provider Range boxes.

Place of Service Range Codes for place of service are entered in the Place of Service Range boxes. If a report is needed for a single code, it is entered in both boxes.

Show Accounts Receivable Totals at the End of the Report If this box is checked, accounts receivable totals will appear at the end of the report.

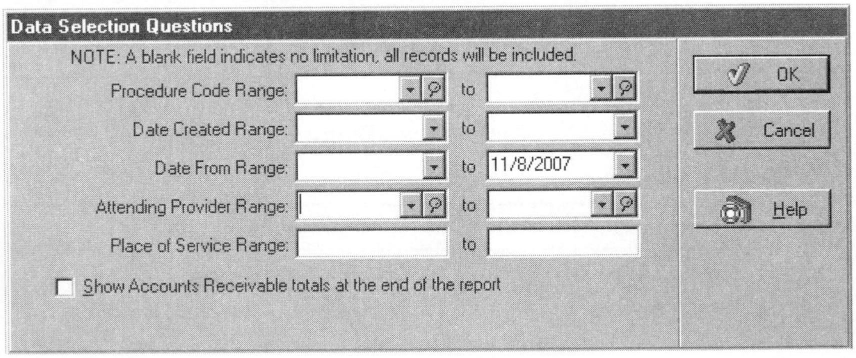

Figure 11-11 Data Selection Questions dialog box.

EXERCISE 11-3

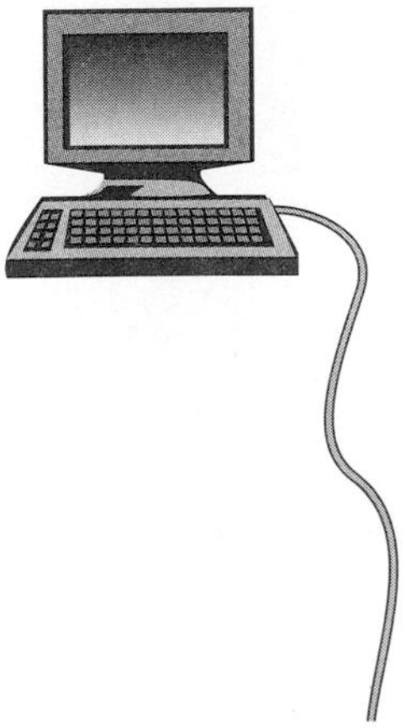

Print a practice analysis report for July 2007.

Date: July 31, 2007

1. On the Reports menu, click Analysis Reports and then Practice Analysis.

2. Click the radio button for previewing the report on-screen. Click the Start button.

3. Leave the Procedure Code Range boxes and the Date Created Range boxes blank.

4. In the first Date From Range box, key *07012007*. In the second box, key *07312007*.

5. Leave the other boxes blank. Click the OK button.

6. View the report on-screen.

7. Go to the second page of the report.

8. Send the report to the printer.

9. Exit the Preview Report window.

PATIENT AGING REPORT

aging report a report that lists the amounts owed to the practice, categorized by the number of days late

An **aging report** lists the amount of money owed to the practice, organized by the amount of time the money has been owed. A patient aging report lists a patient's balance by age, the date and amount of the last payment, and the telephone number. The columns display the amounts that are current and those that are 31–60, 61–90, and more than 90 days past due (see Figure 11-12). The aging begins on the date of the transaction. Patient aging reports are printed by clicking Aging Reports and then Patient Aging on the Reports menu. After making a selection in the Print Report Where? dialog box, the data must be selected. The boxes in the Data Selection Questions dialog box are as follows (see Figure 11-13).

Collier Family Dental Care
Patient Aging
As of October 31, 2007

Chart	Name	Current 0 - 30	Past 31 - 60	Past 61 - 90	Past 91 ----->	Total Balance
KLINGRU0	Russell R Klinger		2,380.00			2,380.00
Last Pmt: -15.00	On: 9/4/2007	(941)777-1111				
	Report Aging Totals	$0.00	$2,380.00	$0.00	$0.00	2,380.00
	Percent of Aging Total	0.0 %	100.0 %	0.0 %	0.0 %	100.00 %

Figure 11-12 Patient Aging report.

Figure 11-13 Data Selection Questions dialog box.

Chart Number Range In the Chart Number Range boxes, a range of chart numbers for patients is entered. If the report is needed for just one patient, that patient's chart number is entered in both boxes.

Date From Range   A range of dates is entered in the Date From Range boxes.

Attending Provider Range   A range of codes for the attending providers is entered in the Attending Provider Range boxes.

Billing Code Range   If the practice uses PractiSoft's Billing Code feature, codes can be entered in this box to select only those patients with the designated billing code(s).

Patient Indicator Match   If the practice has assigned a Patient Indicator code to each patient, an entry can be made to select only those patients who match a specific code.

EXERCISE 11-4

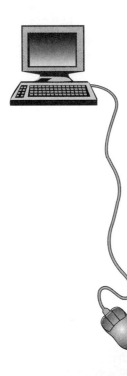

Print a patient aging report for Rosina Vasquez.

Date: October 1, 2007

1. On the Reports menu, click Aging Reports and then Patient Aging.
2. Click the radio button for previewing the report on-screen. Click the Start button.
3. Select Rosina Vasquez's chart number in both boxes of the Chart Number Range boxes.
4. Leave the starting date in the first of the Date From Range boxes blank, and key *09302007* in the second of the boxes.
5. Leave the other boxes blank. Click the OK button.
6. View the report on-screen.
7. Print the report.
8. Exit the Preview Report window.

INSURANCE AGING REPORT   An insurance aging report permits tracking of claims filed with insurance carriers. The report lists claims that have been on file 0–30 days, 31–60 days, 61–90 days, and 91–999 days (see Figure 11-14). This information is used to follow up on overdue payments from insurance carriers. Printing the aging report and following up on overdue claims speeds the collection process. The aging begins on the initial date of billing. PractiSoft provides three insurance aging reports: primary, secondary, and tertiary. Boxes in the Data Selection Questions dialog box for the Primary Insurance Aging report are as follows (see Figure 11-15).

Collier Family Dental Care
Primary Insurance Aging
As of 3/31/2008

Date of Service	Procedure	-- Past -- 0 - 30	-- Past -- 31 - 60	-- Past -- 61 - 90	-- Past -- 91 - 120	-- Past -- 121 ---->	Total Balance
Aetna (AET00)							**(800)554-1700**
CHANJOS0	**Josephine Chan**		**SS: 189-45-3782**		**Policy: 189453782C**	**Group: 3014**	
Claim: 119	Initial Billing Date: 10/30/2007		Last Billing Date: 10/30/2007				
10/30/2007	D3310					$500.00	500.00
10/30/2007	D0220					$20.00	20.00
		0.00	0.00	0.00	0.00	520.00	520.00
VASQURO0	**Rosina Vasquez**		**SS: 780-65-1231**		**Policy: 780651231M**	**Group: 3334**	
Claim: 110	Initial Billing Date: 9/7/2007		Last Billing Date: 9/7/2007				
9/7/2007	D2750					$1,150.00	1150.00
		0.00	0.00	0.00	0.00	1150.00	1150.00
	Insurance Totals	$0.00	$0.00	$0.00	$0.00	$1,670.00	$1,670.00

Figure 11-14 *Primary Insurance Aging report.*

Insurance Carrier 1 Range   A range of codes for insurance carriers is entered in the Insurance Carrier 1 Range boxes.

Initial Billing Date 1 Range   A range of billing dates for the primary insurance carrier is entered in the Initial Billing Date 1 Range boxes. The program displays the Windows system date as the default entry in the second of these boxes.

Attending Provider Range   Codes for attending providers are entered in the Attending Provider Range boxes.

Boxes in the Data Selection Questions dialog box for the Secondary and Tertiary Insurance Aging report are the same except for the difference in the carrier number and billing date number.

Figure 11-15 *Data Selection Questions dialog box.*

PATIENT LEDGER

patient ledger *a listing of financial activity in a patient's account*

A **patient ledger** lists the financial activity in each patient's account, including charges, payments, and adjustments (see Figure 11-16). This information is especially useful if there is a question about a patient's account. A full set of patient ledgers details the status of every patient's account.

Collier Family Dental Care
Patient Account Ledger
As of October 31, 2007

Entry	Date	POS	Description	Procedure	Document	Provider	Amount
ELLISJO0	John Ellison			(941)444-4444			
	Last Payment:	-140.00	On: 10/1/2007				
99	9/4/2007			D7111	0709040000	HSM	140.00
108	9/4/2007			DELCOPAY	0709040000	HSM	15.00
109	9/4/2007			CHCOPAY15	0709040000	HSM	-15.00
120	10/1/2007			D5211	0710010000	HSM	720.00
121	10/1/2007			DELCOPAY	0710010000	HSM	15.00
122	10/1/2007			D5212	0710010000	HSM	720.00
124	10/1/2007			CHCOPAY15	0710010000	HSM	-15.00
139	10/1/2007		#412877429 DeltaDental PPO	DELPAY	0709040000	HSM	-140.00
	Patient Totals						1,440.00
	Ledger Totals						1,440.00

Figure 11-16 Patient Account Ledger report.

Patient ledgers are printed by clicking Patient Ledger on the Reports menu. The Print Report Where? dialog box is displayed. After the preview, print, or export selection is made, the Data Selection Questions dialog box is displayed, as it is with the other reports (see Figure 11-17). It provides options to select by chart numbers, patient reference balances, dates, and providers. A patient ledger is generated only for data that meet the selection criteria. If any selection box is left blank, all values are included in the report.

Chart Number Range   In the Chart Number Range box, a range of chart numbers for patients is entered. If a report is needed for just one patient, that patient's chart number is entered in both boxes.

Patient Reference Balance Range   Minimum and maximum dollar amounts are entered in the Patient Reference Balance Range boxes to delineate the dollar amount of an outstanding balance. The amounts are entered with decimal points.

Date From Range   A range of dates is entered in the Date From Range boxes. For example, if it were necessary to print patient day sheets for the period of May 1 to May 15, 2007, 05012007 would be entered in the first box and 05152007 in the second box. If transactions were needed for the current date, that date would be entered in both boxes.

Attending Provider Range   A range of codes for the attending providers is entered in the Attending Provider Range boxes.

Billing Code Range   If the practice uses PractiSoft's Billing Code feature, codes can be entered in this box to select only those patients with the designated billing code(s).

Patient Indicator Match   If the practice has assigned a Patient Indicator code to each patient, an entry can be made to select only those patients who match a specific code.

Print One Patient Per Page   If this box is checked, each patient's ledger will be printed on a separate page.

Show Accounts Receivable Totals at the End of the Report   If this box is checked, accounts receivable totals will appear at the end of the report.

Data Selection Questions

NOTE: A blank field indicates no limitation, all records will be included.

Chart Number Range:		to
Patient Reference Balance Range:	0.01	to 99999
Date From Range:		to 11/8/2007
Attending Provider Range:		to
Billing Code Range:		to
Patient Indicator Match:		

☐ Print one patient per page

☐ Show Accounts Receivable totals at the end of the report

✓ OK   ✗ Cancel   Help

Figure 11-17   Data Selection Questions dialog box.

EXERCISE 11-5

Print patient ledgers for July 2007 for patients whose last names begin with the letters *R* through *W*.

Date: July 31, 2007

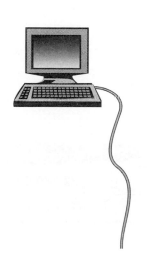

1. On the Reports menu, click Patient Ledger.

2. If necessary, click the radio button for previewing the report on-screen. Click the Start button.

3. Key *R* in the first box of the Chart Number Range box and press Tab. Key *W* in the second box. Notice that the program stopped at the first patient with a last name beginning with *W*. To include all patients with last names beginning with *W*, key *WI* to select Hannah Wilson, the last patient, and press Tab.

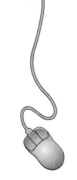

4. Press Tab twice to keep the default settings in the Patient Reference Balance Range boxes.

5. In the first Date From Range box, key *07012007* for July 1, 2007. In the second box, key *07312007* for July 31, 2007.

6. Leave the other boxes blank.

7. Click the OK button.

8. Send the report to the printer.

9. Exit the Preview Report window.

PATIENT STATEMENTS

patient statement *a listing of the amount of money a patient owes*

A **patient statement** lists the amount of money a patient owes, the procedures performed, and the dates the procedures were performed. The bottom of the report lists total charges, total payments, total adjustments, and the balance due (see Figure 11-18). Patient statements are printed and sent out on a regular basis to patients who have an outstanding balance. Statements are not printed for patients with a zero balance on their account.

Collier Family Dental Care
Medical/Dental Arts Building
Naples, FL 34104-8756
(941)555-8900

Statement Date		Page
10/1/2007		1

Chart Number
KLINGRU0

Russell R. Klinger
503 Raphael Drive
Naples, FL 34109

Date	Document	Description	Case Number	Amount
Date of Last Payment: 9/4/2007	Amount:	-15.00	Previous Balance:	0.00
Patient: Russell R. Klinger		Chart #: KLINGRU0	Case Description: Dentures	
9/4/2007	0709040000	upper partial denture--cast	24	1,120.00
9/4/2007	0709040000	lower partial denture--cast	24	1,120.00
9/4/2007	0709040000	extraction--coronal remnants	24	140.00
9/4/2007	0709040000	Sunshine Copayment	24	15.00
9/4/2007	0709040000	Patient check payment	24	-15.00

Total Charges	Total Payments	Total Adjustments	Balance Due
$2395.00	-$15.00	$0.00	**2,380.00**

Figure 11-18 Patient statement.

When Patient Statements is clicked on the Reports menu, the Open Report dialog box appears (see Figure 11-19). There are several options in the Open Report dialog box.

- Patient Statement (30, 60, 90)
- Patient Statement (Color)
- Patient Statement (Color) (30, 60, 90)
- Patient Statement (w/ Charges Only)
- Patient Statement
- Pre Printed Statement
- Remainder Statement (All Payments)
- Remainder Statement (All Pmts/Deduct)
- Remainder Statement (Combined Payments)
- Sample Statement w/ Image
- Sample Statement w/ Logo

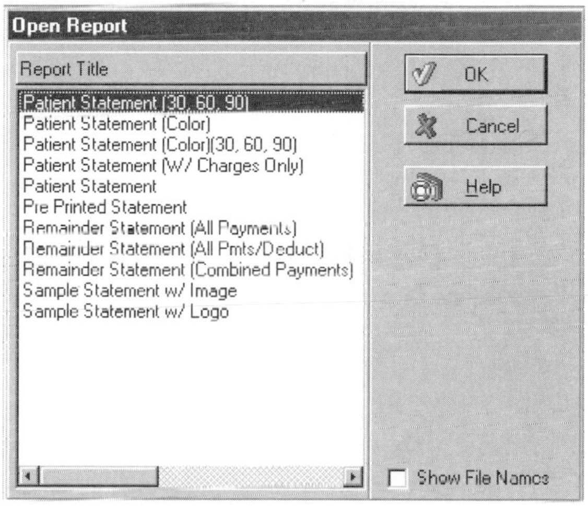

Figure 11-19   Open Report dialog box.

The Patient Statement (30, 60, 90) option prints the standard PractiSoft patient statement with aging boxes for displaying the amount that is 30, 60, or 90 days past due. The Patient Statement (Color) option prints a color version of the standard PractiSoft patient statement, assuming a color printer is used. The Pre Printed Statement option is chosen when a dental practice uses its own preprinted forms for patient statements. The Remainder Statements are used to print patient statements after all insurance carrier payments have been received. The Sample Statements illustrate the Patient Statement option with a colored image or logo in the upper right corner of each statement. Using PractiSoft's Report Designer, an image or logo can be added to a patient statement to customize its appearance. Like any of the standard reports in PractiSoft, patient statements can be customized in a number of ways using PractiSoft's Report Designer, discussed later in this chapter.

After the statement type is selected, the OK button is clicked. The Print Report Where? dialog box is displayed. After the choice to preview, print, or export is made, the Data Selection Questions dialog box is displayed (see Figure 11-20). The following selections can be made.

Data Selection Questions

NOTE: A blank field indicates no limitation, all records will be included.

Chart Number Range:	to	
Billing Code Range:	to	
Date From Range:	to	
Patient Indicator Match:		
Statement Total Range: 0.01	to 999999.99	

OK

Cancel

Help

Figure 11-20 Data Selection Questions dialog box.

Chart Number Range   In the Chart Number Range boxes, a range of chart numbers for patients is entered. If a report is needed for just one patient, that patient's chart number is entered in both boxes.

Billing Code Range   A range of billing codes to be included is entered in the Billing Code Range boxes.

Date From Range   A range of dates is entered in the Date From Range boxes.

Patient Indicator Match   If indicator codes are used by a practice, a range of codes can be entered to select only those patients who match the indicator criteria. For example, if an indicator code has been set up to track patients receiving treatment for a certain condition, it could be entered here to print statements only for those patients.

Statement Total Range   The Statement Total Range boxes are used to filter claims that are below a certain dollar amount. For example, the practice might have a policy of not billing patients whose account balances are less than $1.00.

EXERCISE 11-6

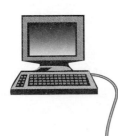

Print patient statements for July 2007 for patients whose last names begin with the letters _R_ through _W_.

Date: July 31, 2007

1. **On the Reports menu, click Patient Statements.**

2. **In the Open Report dialog box, click Patient Statement (30, 60, 90) if it is not already selected. Then click the OK button.**

3. Click the radio button for previewing the report on-screen. Click the Start button.

4. Key *R* in the first Chart Number Range box and *WI* in the second box.

5. Leave the Billing Code Range boxes blank.

6. Enter July 1, 2007, to July 31, 2007, in the Date From Range boxes.

7. Leave the other boxes as they are. Click the OK button.

8. View the report at the full width of the screen. Notice that only one statement appears. This is because the other patients who appeared on the Patient Ledger report in Exercise 11-5 have zero balances—the amount of payments equals the amount of the charges.

9. Send the report to the printer.

10. Exit the Preview Report window.

PRETREATMENT PATIENT STATEMENTS

The difference between pretreatment patient statements and patient statements is that pretreatment patient statements contain suggested procedures and costs, rather than actual procedures and costs. The Pretreatment Patient Statements option on the Reports menu is used to print patient statements using data entered in the Pretreatment Plan/Estimate dialog box. In creating a pretreatment patient statement, the same options exist in the Open Report dialog box and the Data Selection Questions dialog box as in the boxes for creating a patient statement. Although the two types of reports draw on different databases, the procedures used in creating both reports are the same.

EXERCISE 11-7

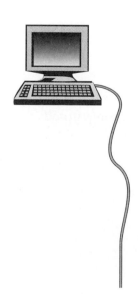

Print a pretreatment patient statement for Sheila Rossi for her visit in September 2007.

Date: October 1, 2007

1. On the Reports menu, click Pretreatment Patient Statements.

2. In the Open Report dialog box, click Patient Statement. Then click the OK button.

3. Click the radio button for previewing the report on-screen. Click the Start button.

4. In both Chart Number Range boxes, key *R* and press Tab to select Sheila Rossi.

5. Leave the Billing Code Range boxes blank.

6. Enter September 1, 2007, to September 30, 2007, in the Date From Range boxes.

7. Leave the other boxes as they are. Click the OK button.

8. View the report on-screen.

9. Print the report.

10. Exit the Preview Report window.

ELECTRONIC STATEMENTS

The Electronic Statements option on the Reports menu is used to transfer patient statements electronically with the help of a modem. This option requires enrollment in MedPrint, a service offered through MediSoft. Unlike other standard PractiSoft reports, MedPrint statement formats cannot be customized using the Report Designer.

The Electronic Statements submenu contains three MedPrint statement formats (see Figure 11-21).

◆ Patient Statement

◆ Patient Statement (30 60 90)

◆ Remainder Statement (All Payments)

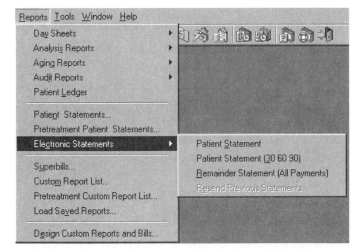

Figure 11-21 *Reports menu with Electronic Statements submenu displayed.*

The fourth option on the submenu, Resend Previous Statements, is used when the initial data transfer fails or is interrupted.

A user name, password, client ID, and billing ID, the information needed to use the Electronic Statements option, is provided by MedPrint after enrollment. A series of dialog boxes guides the user through the required steps for sending patient statements electronically.

CUSTOM REPORTS   PractiSoft has already created a number of custom reports using the built-in Report Designer. These reports include:

♦ The ADA dental claim form, the ADA 2000 dental claim form, the CMS-1500 (formerly HCFA 1500), and the Medicare claim form in a variety of printer formats.

♦ Lists of addresses, billing codes, EMC receivers, patients, patient recalls, procedure codes, providers, and referring providers.

♦ A dental superbill.

♦ Patient statements and walkout receipts.

When Custom Report List is clicked on the Reports menu, the Open Report dialog box is displayed, listing a variety of custom reports already created in PractiSoft using the Report Designer (see Figure 11-22). Additional custom reports can be created using the Report Designer. When a new custom report is created, it is added to the list of custom reports displayed on-screen.

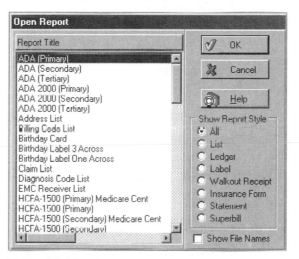

Figure 11-22   Open Report dialog box.

The Open Report dialog box also contains seven radio buttons that are used to control the list of reports displayed in the dialog box. When the All radio button is clicked, all types of custom reports are listed in the dialog box. However, when one of the other radio buttons is clicked, only reports of that style are listed. For example, if the Insurance Form radio button is clicked, only reports that are insurance forms are listed.

To print a custom report, the title of the report is highlighted by clicking it, and then the OK button is clicked. The same options that are available with standard reports for previewing the report on-screen, sending it directly to the printer, and exporting it to a file are available with custom reports.

SHORT CUT To print a custom report, double-click the report title.

EXERCISE 11-8

Print a list of all patients.

Date: October 31, 2007

TIP . . . For the reports generated in this and the remaining two exercises in this chapter, PractiSoft prints the Windows system date under the report title. However, it is not necessary to change the Windows system date for the sake of the exercises. The dates in the remaining exercises are provided for simulation purposes only. Any date printed on the reports will serve the purpose.

1. **On the Reports menu, click Custom Report List.**

2. **Scroll down the list of report titles and select Patient List. Click the OK button.**

3. **Click the radio button to preview the report on-screen. Click the Start button.**

4. **Leave the Chart Number Range boxes blank to select all patients.**

5. **Click the OK button.**

6. **View the report on-screen.**

7. **Send the report to the printer.**

8. **Exit the Preview Report window.**

EXERCISE 11-9

Print a list of all the procedure codes in the database.

Date: October 31, 2007

1. **On the Reports menu, click Custom Report List.**

2. **In the Show Report Style section of the dialog box, click the List radio button.**

3. **Select Procedure Code List. Click the OK button.**

4. **Click the radio button to preview the report on-screen. Click the Start button.**

5. **Leave the Code 1 Range boxes blank to select all procedure codes. Click the OK button.**

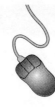

6. **View the report on-screen.**

7. **Send the report to the printer.**

8. **Exit the Preview Report window.**

USING REPORT DESIGNER

PractiSoft's Report Designer allows the user maximum flexibility and control over data in the report and how they are displayed. Report styles include list, ledger, label, walkout receipt, insurance form, statement, and superbill. Reports can be created from scratch, or an existing report can be used as a starting point. The details of how to create new custom reports with the Report Designer are beyond the coverage of this book, but Exercise 11-10 offers practice working with the Report Designer to modify an existing report. The Report Designer is accessed by clicking Design Custom Reports and Bills on the Reports menu. This action causes the Report Designer window to be displayed (see Figure 11-23).

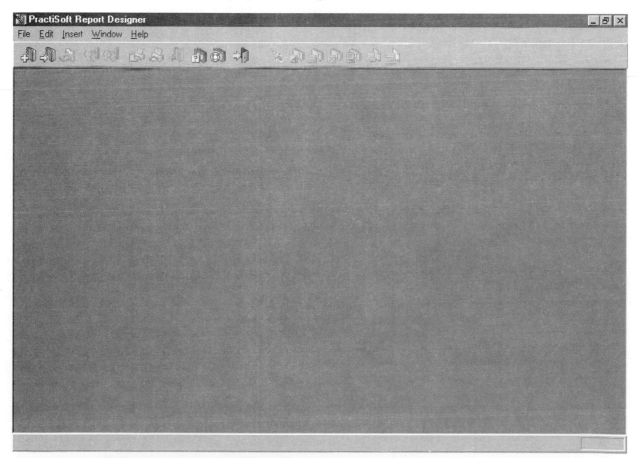

Figure 11-23   *PractiSoft's Report Designer window.*

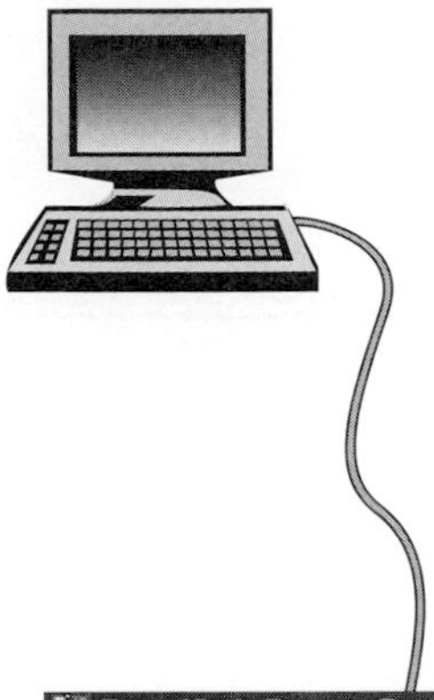

Modify the Patient List report so that a work telephone number replaces a home telephone number in the report.

Date: October 31, 2007

1. On the Reports menu, click Design Custom Reports and Bills. The Report Designer window is displayed.

2. Click Open Report on the File menu. The Open Report dialog box is displayed.

3. Double-click Patient List in the list. The Patient List report is displayed (see Figure 11-24).

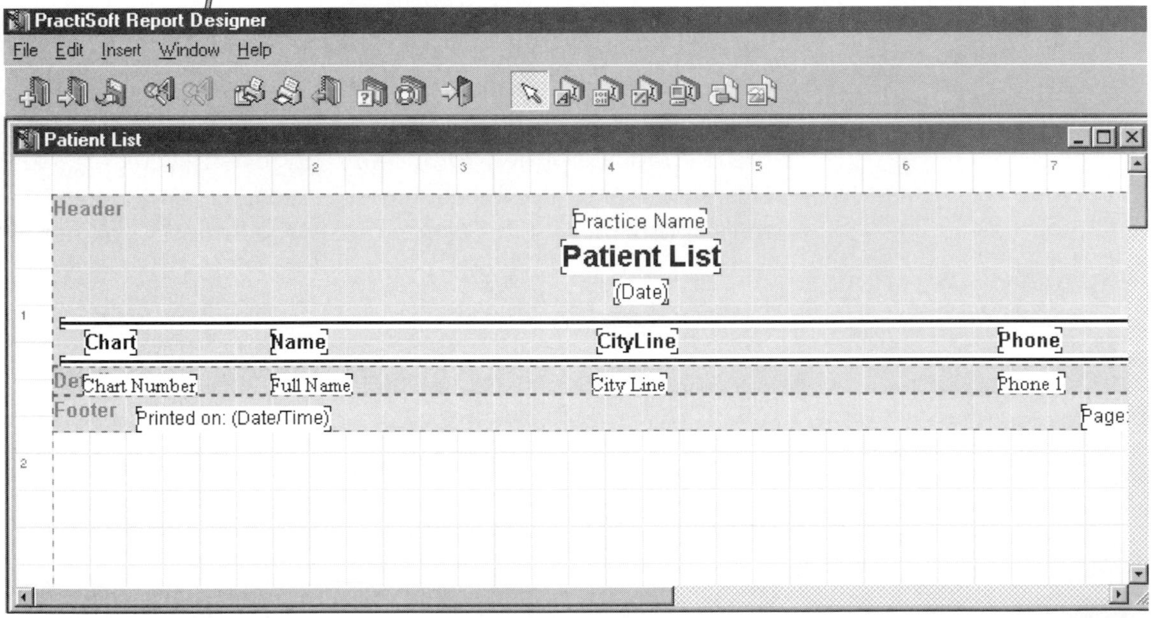

Figure 11-24   Patient List report in the PractiSoft Report Designer.

4. Notice the black horizontal lines that run across the width of the window. That band contains column labels. Use the scroll bar to scroll right (or change the width of the window) until the Phone column label is in view. Double-click Phone inside the black band to select it. Then double-click Phone again to edit it. The Text Properties dialog box is displayed (see Figure 11-25).

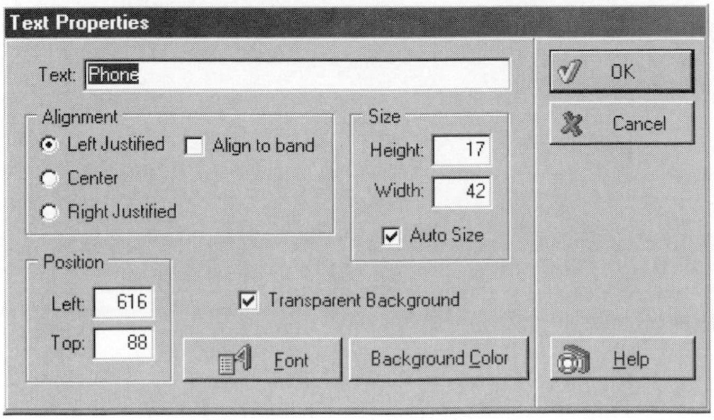

Figure 11-25   Text Properties dialog box.

5. Key *Work Phone* in the text box that currently reads Phone.

6. Since Work Phone contains more letters than Phone, it is necessary to lengthen the space allotted for the label on the report so that all the letters can be displayed. This is done in the section of the dialog box labeled Size. Click in the Auto Size box to deselect that option. In the Width box, key *80* to replace the current entry.

7. Click the OK button. Work Phone is displayed inside the black band where Phone used to be.

8. In the green band below the black band, click the Phone 1 box to select it. Then double-click the Phone 1 box again to edit its contents. The Data Field Properties dialog box is displayed (see Figure 11-26).

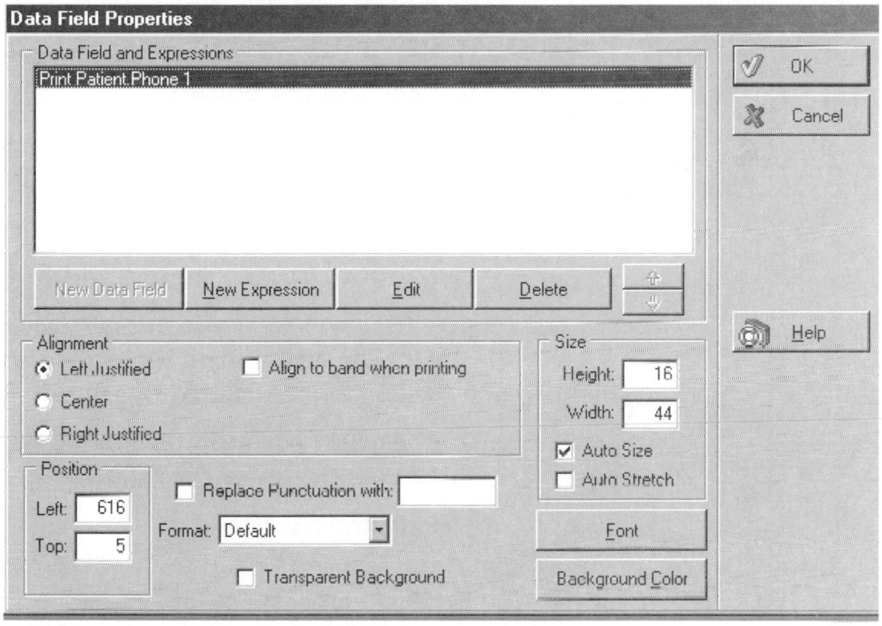

Figure 11-26   Data Field Properties dialog box.

9. The current data box, Print Patient Phone 1, is active in the Data Field and Expressions box. Click the Edit button to change this box. The Select Data Field dialog box is displayed (see Figure 11-27).

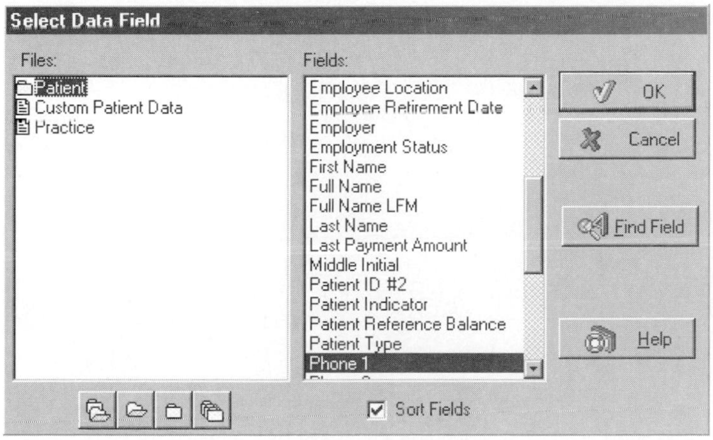

Figure 11-27   Select Data Field dialog box.

10. In the Fields column, highlight Work Phone, and click OK. The Data Field and Expressions box now lists Print Patient Work Phone.

11. To increase the space allotted in the report for this new value (perhaps to allow for phone extensions in the future), click the Auto size box to deselect it. Then go to the Width box and key *100*. Click the OK button. Work Phone is displayed where Phone 1 used to be.

12. On the Report Designer File menu, click Preview Report to see how the report will look when printed. The Save Report As... dialog box is displayed.

13. Key *Patient List - Work* in the Report Title box. Click the OK button. The Data Selection Questions dialog box is displayed.

14. Leave the Chart Number Range boxes blank to select all patients for the report.

15. Click the OK button.

16. The Preview Report dialog box is displayed, showing the report.

17. Click the Print button to print the report.

18. Exit the Preview Report window.

19. Click Close on the Report Designer File menu, or click the Close button in the top right corner of the Patient List – Work dialog box, to close the report file.

20. Click Exit on the File menu, or click the Exit button on the toolbar, to leave PractiSoft's Report Designer.

21. Exit PractiSoft.

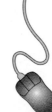

CHAPTER REVIEW

USING TERMINOLOGY

Match the terms on the left with the definitions on the right.

_____ **1.** aging report

_____ **2.** patient day sheet

_____ **3.** patient ledger

_____ **4.** patient statement

_____ **5.** procedure day sheet

a. A summary of the activity of a patient on any given day.

b. A report that lists procedures performed on a particular day and the dates, patients, document numbers, places of service, debits, and credits relating to these procedures.

c. A report that lists the amount of money owed, organized by the length of time the money has been owed.

d. A report that lists the financial activity in each patient's account, including charges, payments, and adjustments.

e. A printed document that informs the patient of the amount of money owed.

CHECKING YOUR UNDERSTANDING

Answer the questions below in the space provided.

6. Which report shows the status of each patient's account on a separate page by default? Which report contains the option Print One Patient Per Page?

_____

_____

7. What is the name of the dialog box, used while generating reports, that contains one or more options for including data on only those patients who fall within certain ranges?

_____

8. Which report indicates how far past due a patient's account is?

_____

9. Which entries print in a report if the boxes in the Data Selection Questions dialog box are left blank?

_____

_____

APPLYING KNOWLEDGE

Answer the questions below in the space provided.

10. One of the providers in a practice asks for a report of yesterday's transactions for his patients only. How would this report be created?

_____

_____

_____

_____

11. A patient is unsure whether she mailed a check last month to pay an outstanding balance on her account. How could you use PractiSoft's Reports feature to help answer the question?

_____

_____

_____

_____

12 Using Utilities

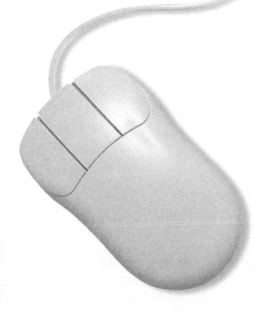

WHAT YOU NEED TO KNOW

To use this chapter, you need to know how to:

◆ Start PractiSoft and use menus.

◆ Enter and edit text.

OBJECTIVES

When you finish this chapter, you will be able to:

1. **Make backup copies of data.**
2. **View and restore backed up data.**
3. **Use PractiSoft's file maintenance features.**

KEY TERMS

packing data
purging data
rebuilding indexes
removable media device
restoring data

PRACTISOFT'S UTILITY FEATURES

PractiSoft provides a number of built-in utilities to manage and maintain the data stored in the system. The utilities in PractiSoft are used for saving and storing data, retrieving data, maintaining data files, and deleting data that are no longer needed. All PractiSoft's utilities are accessed through the File menu.

Whenever information is stored on a computer, it is possible to lose data. The cause can be a machine failure, sometimes called a hard disk crash, or the cause can be human error, such as when data are erased accidentally by pressing the wrong key. PractiSoft's backup utility can minimize the amount of data that has to be reentered should a loss occur. If copies of computer data files, called backups (see Chapter 4), are created on a regular basis, the amount of actual data gone from a system when a data loss occurs is minimal. It is limited to the amount entered between the time of the loss and the time the last backup was performed.

SHORT CUT Warning! Do not attempt to perform the utility functions listed in this chapter on your computer. They are for reference only. If the utility functions are performed, the data on the Student Data Disk or in the C:\PractiData\Collier folder on the hard drive could be accidentally erased.

BACKING UP DATA

removable media device a device that stores data but is not a permanent part of a computer

Dental offices generally have a regular schedule for backing up data. Depending on the volume of information, backups may be done as often as once a day or as infrequently as once a week. When data are backed up, they are stored on a removable media device. A **removable media device** is one that stores data but is not a permanent part of a computer. Examples of removable media devices include disks, cartridges, tapes, and CD-ROMs. Removable media devices may be stored at a location other than the office to protect them from fire or theft.

To perform a data backup in an office situation, you would complete the following steps.

1. Insert the removable media device in the drive.

2. Click Backup Data on the File menu. The PractiSoft Backup dialog box is displayed (see Figure 12-1).

3. In the Destination File Path and Name box at the top of the PractiSoft Backup dialog box, key the drive, directory, and filename of the location where the backup copy of the data is to

be stored. This should correspond to the drive that contains the removable media device, and should include a name for the backup file, such as A:\Collier.mbk.

SHORT CUT The Find button to the right of the Destination File Path and Name box can be used to browse through and locate a destination drive and directory on your system. When you click Find, the Browse for Folder dialog box appears (see Figure 12-2). Locate the appropriate destination drive and directory name in the dialog box and then click the OK button. The Browse for Folder dialog box closes, and the selected drive and directory name are copied to the Destination File Path and Name box for you. The name of the backup file is added to the drive and directory name to complete the entry in the Destination File Path and Name box.

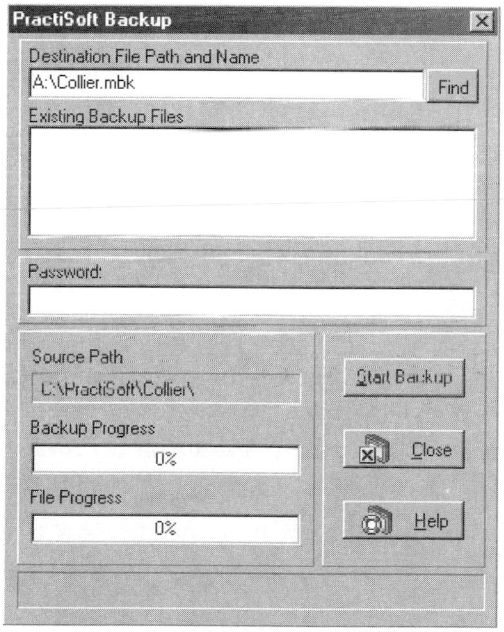

Figure 12-1 PractiSoft Backup dialog box.

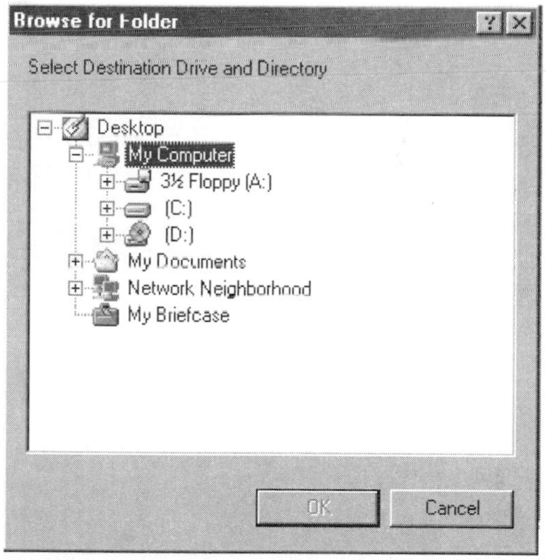

Figure 12-2 Browse for Folder dialog box.

4. After the Destination File Path and Name box is complete, click the Start Backup button. The program copies the data from the source (indicated in the Source Path box in the lower half of the PractiSoft Backup dialog box) to the location indicated in the Destination File Path and Name box. In the backup process, the source path is the drive and directory of the file that is being backed up.

5. When the backup is complete, an Information dialog box appears with the message "Backup complete." Click the OK button to continue.

6. The PractiSoft Backup dialog box disappears. Eject the removable media device, and label it with the date and time of the backup and with any other information required by the dental office.

As a security feature for protecting data, the PractiSoft Backup dialog box also contains a Password box. If a password is assigned to a backup file, the password must be used to restore the data to the system. Each backup file can be assigned a different password.

Viewing Backup Data

PractiSoft provides a feature that allows a list of files on a backup device to be viewed on-screen or in a printed format. Information about the backup files is listed in the Backup View dialog box. In the top section of the dialog box, the following information is displayed: the name of the backup file and its location, the time and date it was created, the original data path, and the total number of files. The middle of the dialog box contains information about each file in the backup. File names, dates, times, original and compressed sizes, and the percentage of disk space saved by compression are listed.

To view backup data in an office situation, you would complete the following steps.

1. Click View Backup Disks on the File menu. The View Backup dialog box is displayed.

2. In the Source Path box, key the drive, directory, and filename of the disk or the device with the backup files.

TIP . . . The Find button to the right of the Source Path box can be used to browse and locate the source drive and directory.

3. Click the View Backup button. The Backup View dialog box is displayed (see Figure 12-3).

4. Review the information on-screen, or print it by clicking the Print button.

5. Click the Close button to exit the Backup View dialog box.

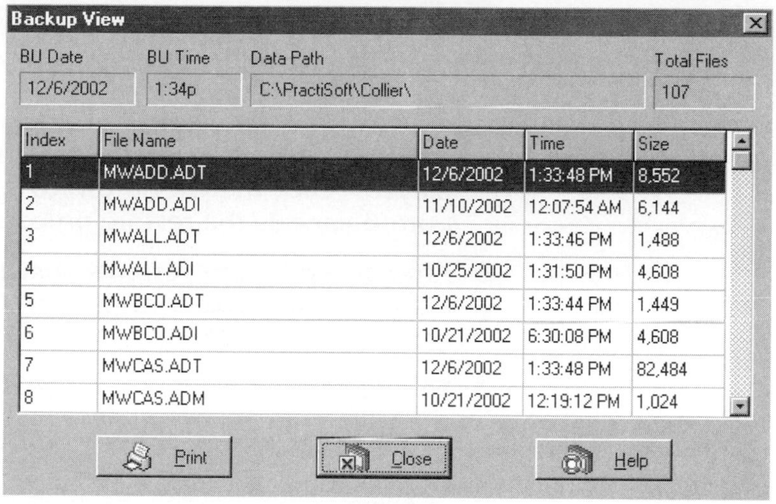

Figure 12-3 Backup View dialog box.

RESTORING DATA

restoring data the process of retrieving data from backup storage devices

The process of retrieving data from backup storage devices is called **restoring data**. Restoring data replaces all other data in the database. Since backup data are typically at least one day old, all the transactions, patient data, and appointments that were entered since the backup was made need to be reentered. This is one reason why it is important to print daily reports of activity in the practice. These reports can be used to reenter data when data need to be restored.

Under normal working conditions, data are not restored very often. In an office, only if there were serious problems with the current data would it be necessary to use PractiSoft's restore feature. However, in an instructional environment where computers are shared by many people, a program's restore feature is often used in combination with a backup feature to save students' work. In this text, data are restored from the Student Data Disk to the hard drive at the beginning of each session and then backed up again to the Student Data Disk at the end of each session. By restoring their files before each session, students are certain to be working on their own data.

To restore data, you would complete the following steps.

1. **Insert the removable media device that contains the backup data in the drive.**

2. **Click Restore Data on the File menu. A Warning dialog box is displayed, stating that the current files are about to be overwritten. Click the OK button. (Clicking the Cancel button cancels the Restore process.)**

3. **The Restore dialog box is displayed (see Figure 12-4 on page 236).**

4. **In the Backup File Path and Name box at the top of the dialog box, key the drive, directory, and filename of the disk or the device containing the backup file that is to be restored, for example, *A:\Collier.mbk*.**

TIP . . . The Find button to the right of the Backup File Path and Name box can be used to browse and locate the source drive and directory.

5. **Click the Start Restore button. A Confirm dialog box is displayed. Click the OK button to continue. (Clicking the Cancel button cancels the restore process.)**

6. **After the program restores the data to the system, an information dialog box is displayed, indicating that the restore is complete. Click OK.**

7. **The Restore dialog box disappears.**

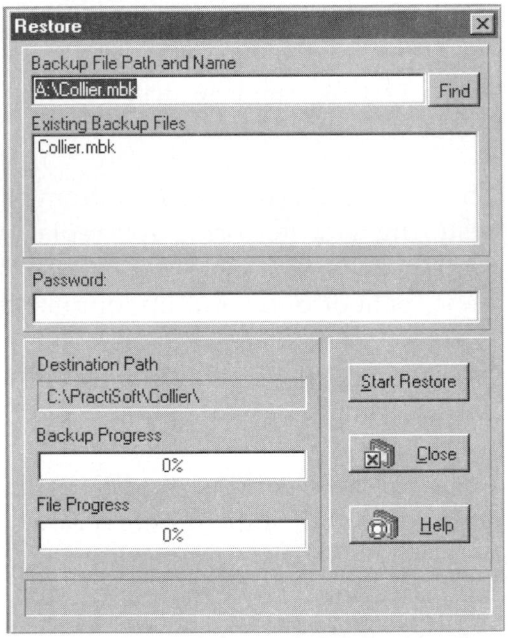

Figure 12-4   Restore dialog box.

FILE MAINTENANCE UTILITIES

PractiSoft provides four features to assist in maintaining data files stored in a system. These four features are found on tabs in the File Maintenance dialog box (see Figure 12-5).

◆ Rebuild Indexes

◆ Pack Data

◆ Purge Data

◆ Recalculate Balances

The dialog box is accessed by clicking File Maintenance on the File menu.

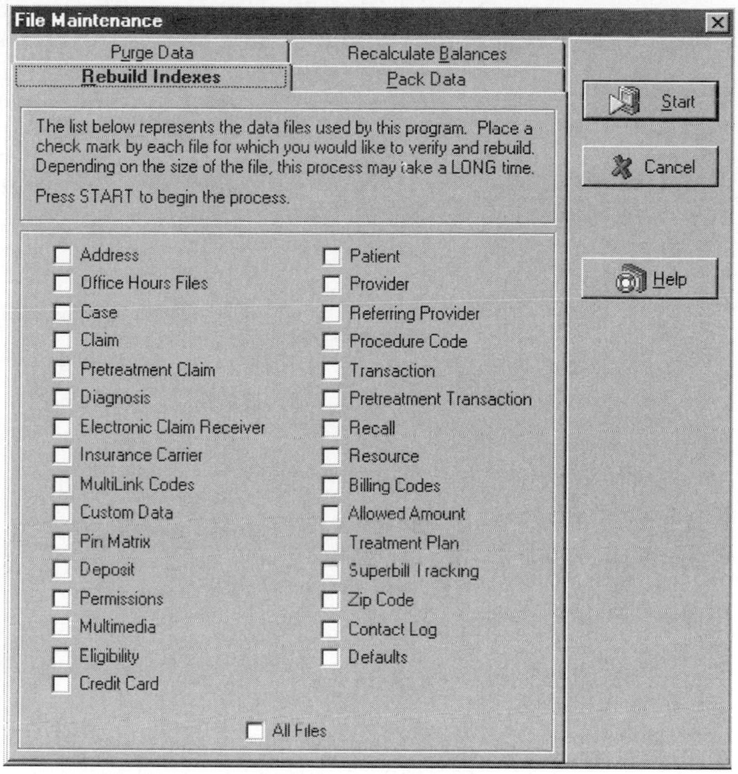

Figure 12-5   File Maintenance dialog box.

If the dental office's database is large, PractiSoft's utilities may take a long time to finish. For this reason, it is usually a good idea to use the utility functions at the end of the day or when the system will not be needed for a while.

Rebuilding Indexes

rebuilding indexes   a process that checks and verifies data and corrects any internal problems with the data

Rebuilding indexes is a process that checks and verifies data and corrects any internal problems. The rebuild does not check or verify the content of the data. For example, the system will not check whether John Ellison paid $50 on his last visit. Rebuilding does not change the content of any data files. To keep files working efficiently, files should be rebuilt about once a month. Files to be rebuilt are selected from the list of files in the Rebuild Indexes tab (see Figure 12-6 on page 238). If the database is large, rebuilding indexes could take a long time.

To rebuild files in PractiSoft in an office, you would complete the following steps.

1. **Click File Maintenance on the File menu. The File Maintenance dialog box is displayed with the Rebuild Indexes tab active.**

2. **Click in each check box next to the files that are to be verified and rebuilt. If all files are to be rebuilt, click the All Files box at the bottom of the list of files. This saves the time it would take to click a box for every PractiSoft file.**

3. Click the Start button. The Confirm dialog box is displayed with the message "All of the checked file processes will be performed. Do you want to continue?" Click the OK button to continue. (Clicking the Cancel button aborts the process.)

4. The rebuild process is performed automatically. When the process is complete, an Information dialog box displays the message "All checked file processes are complete." Click the OK button.

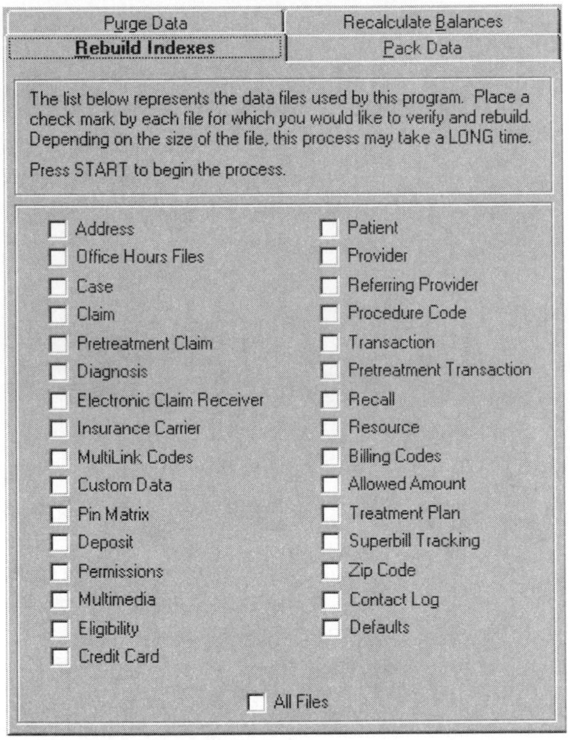

Figure 12-6 Rebuild Indexes tab.

Packing Data

When data are deleted in PractiSoft, the system empties the data from the record but keeps the empty slot in the database so it is available when new data need to be entered in the system. For example, if a patient were deleted in the Patient List dialog box, the system would delete all the records pertaining to that patient but would maintain an empty slot in the patient database. Then, the next time a new patient is entered, the data for the new patient would occupy the vacant slot in the database. In cases in which there is not much space available on the hard disk, it is sometimes desirable to delete the vacant slots to make more disk space available. The deletion of vacant slots from the database is known as **packing data.** Data for packing can be selected from the list of files in the Pack Data tab (see Figure 12-7). (Only transaction files with a zero balance can be deleted.) If the database is large, packing data can take a long time.

packing data the deletion of vacant slots from a database

To pack files in an office situation, you would complete the following steps.

1. **Click File Maintenance on the File menu. The File Maintenance dialog box is displayed with the Rebuild Indexes tab active. Make the Pack Data tab active.**

2. **Click in each check box next to the files that are to have deleted data removed. If all files are to be checked for deleted data, click the All Files box at the bottom of the list of files.**

3. **Click the Start button. The Confirm dialog box is displayed with the message "All of the checked file processes will be performed. Do you want to continue?" Click the OK button to continue. (Clicking the Cancel button aborts the process.)**

4. **The pack process is performed automatically. When the process is complete, an Information dialog box displays the message "All checked file processes are complete." Click the OK button.**

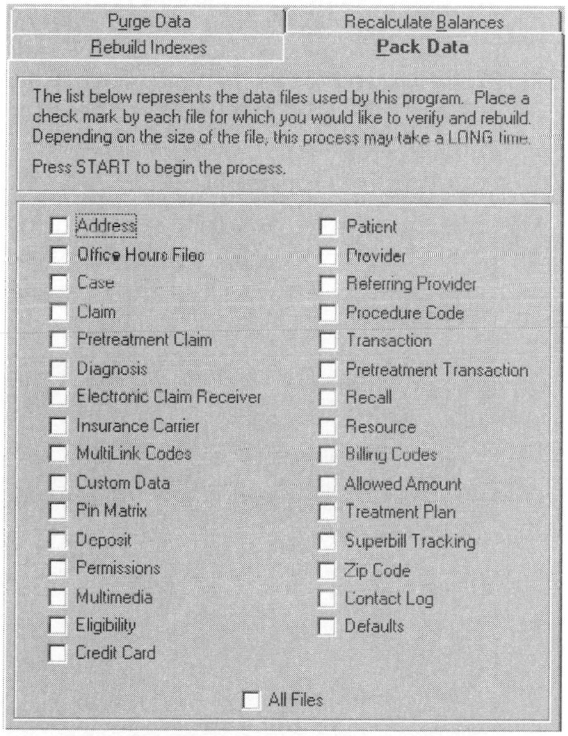

Figure 12-7 Pack Data tab.

Purging Data

purging data the process of deleting files of patients who are no longer seen by a provider in a practice

The process of deleting files of patients who are no longer seen by a provider in a practice is called **purging data.** Purging data frees space on the computer and permits the system to run more efficiently. *However, purging should be done with great caution.* Once data are purged from the system, the information cannot be retrieved, except from a backup file. As a safety precaution, always perform a backup before purging.

The Purge Data tab offers several options (see Figure 12-8). Data can be purged for appointments, claims, pretreatment claims, appointment recalls, audits, and closed cases. All options except Purge Closed Cases are purged by date. A cutoff date is entered, and PractiSoft deletes all data up to that date. For example, if all the data entered prior to December 31, 1997, are to be purged, that date would be entered as the cutoff date. Data entered in cases that have been closed are purged by clicking the check box labeled "Purge Closed Cases."

To purge data in an office situation, you would complete the following steps.

1. Click File Maintenance on the File menu. The File Maintenance dialog box is displayed with the Rebuild Indexes tab active. Make the Purge Data tab active.

2. Click in each check box next to the files that are to be purged. Enter a cutoff date in the Cutoff Dates box.

3. Click the Start button. The Confirm dialog box is displayed with the message "All of the checked file processes will be performed. Do you want to continue?" Click the OK button to continue. (Clicking the Cancel button aborts the process.)

4. The purge process is performed automatically. When the process is complete, an Information dialog box displays the message "All checked file processes are complete." Click the OK button.

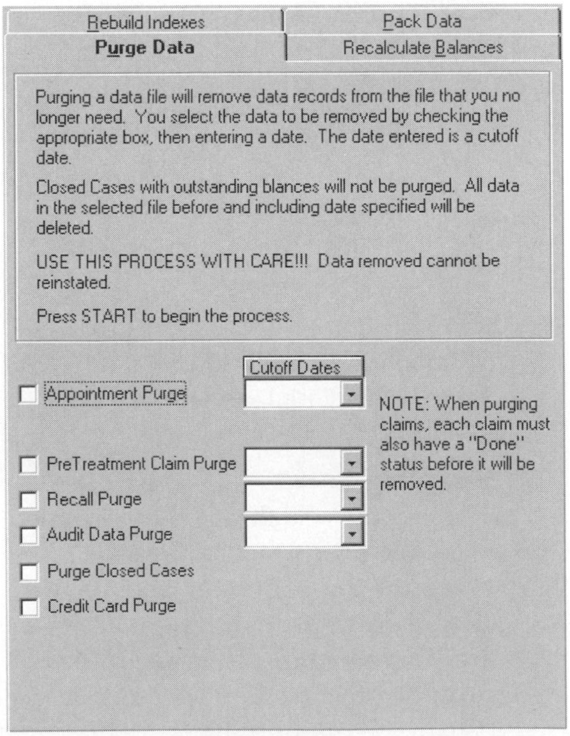

Figure 12-8 Purge Data tab.

Recalculating Patient Balances

As transaction entries are changed or deleted, there are times when the balance listed on-screen is not accurate. To update balances to reflect the most recent changes made to the data, the Recalculate Balances feature is used. This feature is accessed through the Recalculate Balances tab on the File Maintenance dialog box (see Figure 12-9).

When balances are recalculated, the system reviews every patient's data and recalculates the balances. The process of recalculating balances can be time-consuming. Individual patient balances can be recalculated in the Transaction Entry dialog box by clicking the New button in the Charges section or the Payments section.

To recalculate balances in an office situation, you would complete the following steps.

1. Click File Maintenance on the File menu. The File Maintenance dialog box is displayed with the Rebuild Indexes tab active. Make the Recalculate Balances tab active.

2. Click to place a check mark in the Recalculate Balances box.

3. Click the Start button. The Confirm dialog box is displayed with the message "All of the checked file processes will be performed. Do you want to continue?" Click the OK button to continue. (Clicking the Cancel button aborts the process.)

4. The recalculate process is performed automatically. When the process is complete, an Information dialog box displays the message "All checked file processes are complete." Click the OK button.

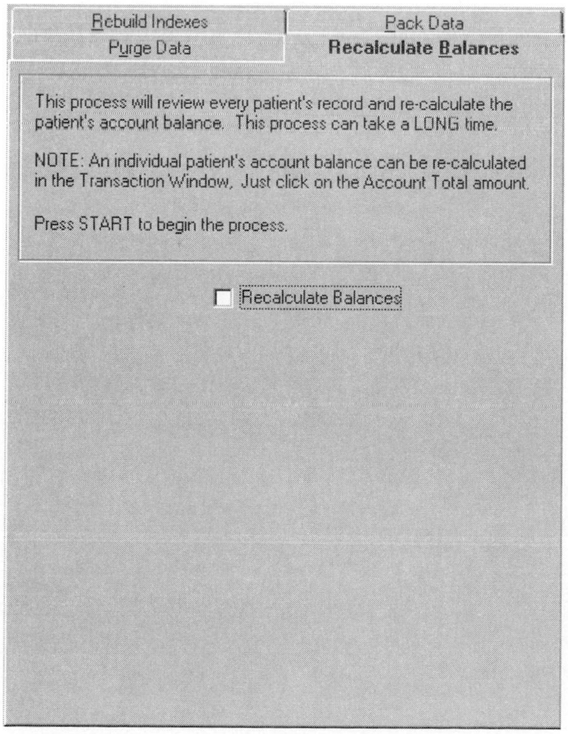

| Rebuild Indexes | Pack Data |
| Purge Data | Recalculate Balances |

This process will review every patient's record and re-calculate the patient's account balance. This process can take a LONG time.

NOTE: An individual patient's account balance can be re-calculated in the Transaction Window. Just click on the Account Total amount.

Press START to begin the process.

☐ Recalculate Balances

Figure 12-9 Recalculate Balances tab.

CHAPTER REVIEW

USING TERMINOLOGY

Match the terms on the left with the definitions on the right.

_____ 1. packing data

_____ 2. purging data

_____ 3. rebuilding indexes

_____ 4. removable media device

_____ 5. restoring data

a. A device that stores data but is not a permanent part of a computer.

b. A process that checks and verifies data and corrects any internal problems with the data.

c. The process of retrieving data from backup storage devices.

d. The deletion of vacant data slots from a database.

e. The process of deleting files of patients who are no longer seen by a provider of a practice.

CHECKING YOUR UNDERSTANDING

Answer the questions below in the space provided.

6. Why is it important to back up data regularly?

_____

_____

7. Why is extra caution required when purging data?

_____

_____

8. When is a data restore performed in an office setting?

_____

_____

9. In PractiSoft, where are the two places a patient's balance can be recalculated?

_____

_____

APPLYING KNOWLEDGE

Answer the question below in the space provided.

10. You come to work on a Monday morning and find that the office computer is not working. The systems manager informs everyone that the computer's hard disk crashed, and that all data that were not backed up are lost. What do you do?

_____

_____

_____

_____

Applying Your Knowledge

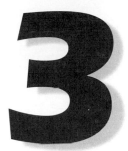

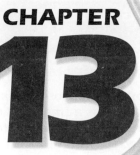

CHAPTER
13
Handling Patient Records and Transactions

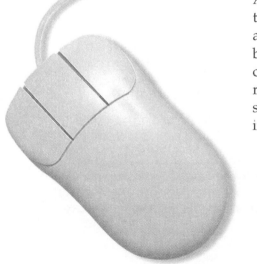

WHAT YOU NEED TO KNOW

To complete the exercises in this chapter, you need to know how to:

◆ Locate patient information.

◆ Change the PractiSoft Program Date.

◆ Assign a new chart number and enter information on a new patient.

◆ Create a new case for a patient.

◆ Change information on an established patient.

◆ Add an insurance company to the database.

◆ Enter procedures and charges.

◆ Record payments from patients and insurance carriers.

◆ Print walkout receipts.

All office personnel at Collier Family Dental Care know how to input patient information in the Patient/Guarantor dialog box and in the Case dialog box. Whenever possible, all information for both dialog boxes is entered into the computer as soon as patients complete the handwritten information sheet and return it to the receptionist. On busy days, however, or when the office is understaffed because one of the dental assistants is sick or on vacation, input operations may be delayed.

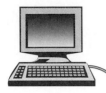

EXERCISE 13-1: INPUTTING PATIENT INFORMATION

For this exercise, you need Source Documents 11–14.

It is Monday, November 12, 2007. You are a records billing clerk at Collier Family Dental Care. On your desk is a small pile of information sheets and encounter forms from Friday afternoon, November 9. You decide to input all patient information first, and then go back and record the transactions. First, you arrange the papers alphabetically:

Arrez

Chan

Fondo

Walsh

Then you begin. (Remember to change the PractiSoft Program Date to November 12, 2007.)

Patient 1: Anthony Arrez

Record the address and phone number changes that are written on Mr. Arrez's encounter form (Source Document 11).

1. Click Patients/Guarantors and Cases on the Lists menu. The Patient List dialog box is displayed.

2. Select Anthony Arrez from the list of patients.

3. Click the Edit Patient button. The Patient/Guarantor dialog box is displayed, with the Name, Address tab active.

4. Enter the new address and phone number.

5. Click the Save button.

Patient 2: Josephine Chan

You can see from the encounter form (Source Document 12) that Ms. Chan is an established patient. There are no changes to be made for her in the Patient/Guarantor dialog box. The work you need to do must take place in the Case dialog box. Ms. Chan's crown has fallen out, so a new case must be created.

1. After you have saved the changes for Mr. Arrez in the Patient/Guarantor dialog box, the Patient List dialog box is redisplayed.

2. In the list of patients, click the listing for Chan to select her as the patient. In the list of cases, click the Endodontics case. (You will not enter new information in the Endodontics case; instead, you will copy information from the Endodontics case to create a new case.)

3. Click the Copy Case button to copy the information from the existing case into a new case. A duplicate case is displayed.

4. Using Source Document 12, edit the information that appears in the PractiSoft boxes listed below. If a box is not listed, either the information in that box does not need to be changed, or the box is to remain blank.

Personal Tab
Description

Account Tab
Assigned Provider
Referring Provider (delete existing entry)
Authorized Number of Visits (delete existing entry)
ID (delete existing entry)
Last Visit Date (delete existing entry)
Last Visit Number (delete existing entry)

5. Save your work.

TIP . . . When entering information on different tabs within a dialog box, it is not necessary to click the Save button after completing each tab. However, once all the tabs are complete, the Save button must be clicked before exiting the dialog box.

Patient 3: Jeffrey Fondo

1. The information you need to make the necessary changes to the Patient/Guarantor dialog box for Jeffrey Fondo is on Source Documents 13 and 14. The new insurance company, SouthWest Florida HMO, is not on the patient information form, nor is it in Collier Family Dental Care's database. Jeffrey Fondo does not have his insurance card. You look up SouthWest Florida HMO in the phone book, find the correct zip code on the map in the front of the phone book, and call the insurance company to find out what percentage of charges are covered by the plan. SouthWest pays 80 percent after a $20 copayment.

2. After you have saved the new case for Chan, you are in the Patient List dialog box. Select Jeffrey Fondo, and click the Edit Patient button.

3. Move to the Street box, and enter the new address.

4. Move to the Phones 1 box and enter the new phone number.

5. Save the information you just entered.

6. Now the new insurance carrier must be added to the database. From the Lists menu, click Insurance Carriers.

TIP . . . If the entire dialog box is not visible on your screen, resize the dialog box or use the scroll bars to see the additional entries.

7. The Insurance Carrier List dialog box is displayed.

8. Click the New Button to add information for SouthWest Florida HMO.

9. Using the information on Source Document 14, enter the information in the following boxes.

   Address Tab
   Code
   Name
   Street
   City
   State
   Zip Code
   Phone

   Options Tab
   Plan Name
   Type
   Procedure Code Set
   Diagnosis Code Set
   Patient/Insured/Physician Signature on File
   Print PINs on Forms
   Default Billing Method

   EMC, Codes Tab
   EMC Receiver
   EMC Payor Number
   EMC Sub ID
   NDC Record Code

   Notice that there are no Default Payment Application Codes for SouthWest Florida, so these must be created. With the Payment drop-down list visible, press the F8 key to display the Procedure/Payment/Adjustment: (new) dialog box.

   In the Code 1 box, key *SOUPAY*. Key *SouthWest Florida Payment* in the Description box. Press the Tab key. Accept the default entries in the other boxes. No entries need to be made in the Amounts and Allowed Amounts tabs.

   Click the Save button. The Procedure/Payment/Adjustment dialog box closes, and SOUPAY is displayed in the Payment box on the EMC, Codes tab for SouthWest Florida HMO.

   Follow the same procedure to create Adjustment, Withhold, and Deductible codes for SouthWest Florida HMO.

10. Click the Save button. SouthWest Florida HMO is now displayed on the list of insurance carriers.

11. With SouthWest Florida HMO highlighted, click the Edit button. Using Source Document 14, complete the following boxes in the PINs tab.

Provider	PIN	Group ID
Singh		
Miller		
Wu		

12. Click the Save button.

13. Close the Insurance Carrier List dialog box. The Patient List dialog box is still displayed. Jeffrey Fondo is still the selected patient.

14. A procedure code must be created for the Southwest Florida HMO copayment. To do so, click Procedure/Payment/Adjustment codes on the Lists menu. The Procedure/Payment/Adjustment dialog box opens.

    Click the New button. Enter *SOUCOPAY* in the Code 1 box. Enter Southwest Florida Copayment in the Description box.

    Click the Amounts tab. Enter *20* in the Charge Amount box B and press Tab.

    Click the Save button. Verify that the Southwest Florida HMO copayment charge appears in the Procedure/Payment/Adjustment List dialog box.

    Close the Procedure/Payment/Adjustment List dialog box.

15. Create a new case for Jeffrey Fondo by copying his existing case.

16. Using Source Documents 13 and 14, edit the information in the copied case to reflect the information relevant to the new case. Change information in the following boxes:

    Personal Tab
    Description

    Account Tab
    Price Code: B

    Policy 1 Tab
    Insurance 1
    Policy Number
    Group Number
    Policy Dates, Start
    Capitated Plan
    Copayment Amount
    Insurance Coverage Percents by Service Classification: Enter
        100 in box A (leave boxes B through H as they are)

17. Click the Save button to save the new case.

TIP . . . Do not change the insurance carrier in the restorative case for Jeffrey Fondo, because at the time he was treated for that condition, Fondo was covered by DeltaDental PPO, not SouthWest Florida HMO.

Patient 4: Michelle Walsh

Use Source Documents 15 and 16 to enter information on a new patient, Michelle Walsh. Michelle is the daughter of Brad and Myrna Walsh, who are patients of Dr. Harold Miller. Michelle has been seeing her own dentist, Dr. Lopez, who does a lot of pediatric work, but is now switching to Collier Family Dental Care. Michelle's father is the guarantor on her account.

1. Go to the Patient List dialog box, and click the New Patient button.

2. Key *WALSHMIØ* in the Chart Number box.

3. Complete the boxes for name, address, phone, birth date, sex, and Social Security number.

4. Complete the following boxes in the Other Information tab.

   Type
   Assigned Provider
   Signature on File
   Signature Date

5. Save your work.

6. Click the Case radio button to make the Case portion of the Patient List dialog box active.

7. Click the New Case button to open a new Case dialog box.

8. Complete the following tabs in the Case dialog box.

   Personal Tab
   Description
   Guarantor
   Marital Status
   Student Status (full time)

   Account Tab
   Referring Provider
   Price Code (make sure Price Code A is indicated)

   Policy 1 Tab
   When you attempt to complete the Policy 1 tab, you notice that Michelle has not filled in her insurance company, but since she would be covered by her father's insurance, you know that information will be easy to find if necessary.

   First save your work on Michelle's case. Then open the Case dialog box for Brad Walsh's crown repair. Go to the Policy 1 tab. Notice that Brad Walsh has no insurance coverage. Therefore, Michelle's Policy 1 tab does not need to be filled in. However, if you open the Personal tab in Brad Walsh's Case dialog box you will notice that the Cash Case box is checked. You will need to go back to Michelle's Case dialog box and check the Cash Case box in the Personal tab.

9. Close Brad Walsh's Case dialog box.

10. Open Michelle's Case dialog box, make the required edit, and save your work.

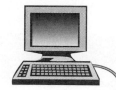

EXERCISE 13-2: A VISIT FROM PAUL LAMPARSKI

You will need Source Document 17 for this exercise.

It is still Monday morning, November 12, 2007. Paul Lamparski has just seen Dr. Wu for a root canal. You need to enter the procedure charges, accept his payment, and print a walkout receipt. Make sure all transaction information is properly recorded in the database.

1. Verify that the PractiSoft Program Date is November 12, 2007.

2. From the Patient List dialog box, create a new case for Paul Lamparski by copying the information in the case that already exists.

3. Using Source Document 17, complete the following box.

   Personal Tab
   Description

4. Save your work.

5. Click Enter Transactions on the Activities menu.

6. Select Mr. Lamparski in the Chart box.

7. Select the case you just created in the Case box.

8. If necessary, change the number in the Document box to 0711120000 to reflect the correct date.

9. Click the New button in the Charges section to create a new transaction.

10. Make sure 11/12/2007 appears in the Date box.

11. Enter the first procedure number checked on the encounter form and press Tab.

12. Click the New button again to enter the other procedure number from the encounter form. An Information dialog box opens with the reminder that the case requires a $15.00 copay. Click the OK button to close the dialog box.

13. Click the New button again, and then enter the procedure code for the $15 copay charge (SUNCOPAY) and press Tab.

14. Click the New button again, and enter the procedure code and tooth number for the second procedure listed on the encounter form.

15. Now enter Lamparski's copayment in the Payment, Adjustments, and Comments section of the dialog box.

    Hint: In the Pay/Adj Code box, select the option that reads "CHCOPAY15—Check Copayment $15" and press Tab. Remember to tab over to the Check Number box and enter the check number listed in Source Document 17.

16. Click the Apply button, and apply the payment to the charges.

17. Click the Print Receipt button to print a walkout receipt.

18. Select the All Transactions option for the walkout receipt.

19. Close the Transaction Entry dialog box.

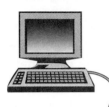

EXERCISE 13-3: INPUTTING TRANSACTION DATA

For this exercise, you need Source Documents 11, 12, 13, and 16.

You are now ready to record the transactions from Friday's four encounter forms. Before you begin, set the PractiSoft Program Date to November 9, 2007.

Anthony Arrez

1. Click Enter Transactions on the Activities menu.

2. Select Anthony Arrez in the Chart box.

3. Verify that Restoration is displayed to the right of the Case box.

4. Record the procedures one at a time.

5. Check your work.

Josephine Chan

Follow essentially the same steps to enter the transaction data. Remember to check your work.

Jeffrey Fondo

Follow essentially the same steps to enter the transaction data. You need to record the date and the code for the procedure as well as for the copayment charge, and then enter Fondo's payment. Apply the payment to the charges, and check your work.

Michelle Walsh

Follow essentially the same steps to enter the transaction data. You need to record the date and the procedures, and then Walsh's payment. Apply the payment to the charges, and check your work.

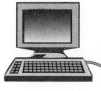

EXERCISE 13-4: ENTERING A NEW PATIENT AND TRANSACTIONS

For this exercise, you need Source Documents 18 and 19.

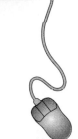

The date is November 9, 2007. Enter patient information and all transactions for Ian McCubbin, a new patient of Dr. Miller. When adding Mr. McCubbin's employer (First Florida Bank) to the Address list, use code EFR00, as code EFI00 already exists.

Hint: To determine DeltaDental PPO's price code and insurance coverage percents by service classification, look in the Account and Policy 1 tabs of another patient covered by DeltaDental PPO, for example, John Ellison. Delta Dental PPO requires a $15 copay. Remember to enter a copayment charge and payment for the visit.

EXERCISE 13-5: ENTERING AND APPLYING AN INSURANCE CARRIER PAYMENT

For this exercise, you need Source Document 20.

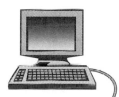

The date is November 9, 2007. A remittance advice has just been received from BCBS of Florida with a check attached. Enter the deposit in PractiSoft, and apply the payment to the appropriate patient accounts.

1. Open the Deposit List dialog box.

2. Change the date in the Deposit Date box to November 9, 2007.

3. Enter the deposit.

4. Apply the payment to the patient charges. Be sure to click the Save Payments/Adjustments button after each patient. Notice that as you enter and save payments, the amount listed in the Unapplied box decreases.

5. When you are finished, verify that the amount in the Un-applied column in the Deposit List dialog box for the deposit on 11/9/2007 is 0.00.

6. Payments entered in the Deposit List dialog box are automatically linked to data in the Transaction Entry dialog box. Open the Transaction Entry dialog box and confirm that the insurance company payments and adjustments appear in the transaction list at the bottom of the window for each patient in this exercise.

WHAT YOU NEED TO KNOW

To complete the exercises in this chapter, you need to know how to:

◆ Start Office Hours.

◆ Move around in the schedule.

◆ Enter appointments.

◆ Change appointment information.

◆ Move or copy an appointment.

◆ Schedule a recall appointment.

◆ Create a new case record for a patient.

◆ Change a transaction record.

Collier Family Dental Care uses Office Hours as the primary tool for recording appointments. For the simulations in this chapter, assume that you are the front-desk receptionist and are responsible for most of Collier Family Dental Care's scheduling tasks. Remember, you can access Office Hours at any time, no matter what you are working on. For example, suppose a patient who wants to make an appointment calls while you are preparing a letter for one of the dentists. All you have to do is click the Start button on the task bar; select Programs—PractiSoft, and then Office Hours; enter the appointment; exit Office Hours; and return to your word-processing program. Office Hours can also be accessed from within PractiSoft, either by clicking the shortcut button or by clicking Appointment Book on the Activities menu.

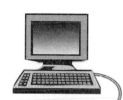

EXERCISE 14-1: SCHEDULING APPOINTMENTS

It is Monday, November 12, 2007. In Office Hours, schedule the following patient appointments for December 7, 2007.

Patient	Provider	Time	Length
Nancy Thompson	H. S. Miller	9:30	30 minutes
Georgette Foncet	H. S. Miller	10:00	45 minutes
Fran Mitchell-Dean	H. S. Miller	2:45	30 minutes

1. Open Office Hours.

2. Go to December 7, 2007.

3. Select each patient's provider from the Provider drop-down list, and enter each appointment.

EXERCISE 14-2: MAKING AN APPOINTMENT CHANGE

Paul Lamparski has just called to say that he has lost his appointment card and cannot remember the time of his December 3 appointment. He thinks it may conflict with a meeting he has that day. If the appointment is in the morning, he wants you to change it to 2:00 p.m. that same day. If the 2:00 p.m. slot is not available, he needs to make the appointment for the next day at the earliest possible time.

1. Open Office Hours if it is not already open.

2. Go to December 3, 2007.

3. Find out who Lamparski's dentist is by calling up the Patient/Guarantor dialog box in PractiSoft. Select the Other Information tab, and check the Assigned Provider box. Then select Lamparski's provider from the Provider drop-down list in Office Hours.

4. Locate Mr. Lamparski's appointment.

5. Check to see whether 2:00 p.m., the time he wanted to change the appointment to, is available.

6. Since 2:00 is not available, move to December 4 on the calendar and see if 8:00 a.m. is available.

7. Go back to December 3. Move Mr. Lamparski's appointment from December 3 to December 4. (If you do not remember how to move an appointment, see Chapter 9.)

EXERCISE 14-3: JUGGLING SCHEDULES

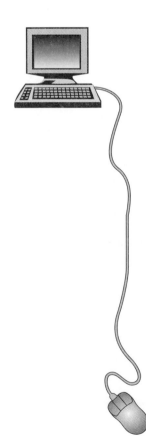

Mrs. Hersen is on the phone. She needs to make an appointment for herself and her seventeen-year-old daughter Georgette on Friday, December 7, 2007, sometime after 3:00 p.m. That is the only day they can come in, so she hopes you can accommodate her. Mrs. Hersen needs an appointment with the hygienist for a cleaning, and her daughter needs a checkup.

1. Find out who Georgette's dentist is by looking up the information in PractiSoft.

2. Go into Office Hours, and check her provider's schedule for December 7. He is booked from 9:30 a.m. until 4:00 p.m. but is available from 4:00 to 5:00 p.m.

3. Check the schedule of the hygienist, Asha Singh, from 4:00 to 5:00 p.m. on the same day. Since the hygienist is also available at this time, first book Mrs. Hersen for a cleaning with Asha Singh from 4:00 to 4:30 p.m., and then book Georgette for an appointment with Dr. Miller at the same time.

EXERCISE 14-4: ADDING PATIENTS TO THE RECALL LIST

Mrs. Hersen and her daughter need to be called back for follow-up appointments with the hygienist in six months. Add both of them to the Recall list for six months from December 7, 2007.

1. Click Patient Recall on the Lists menu in PractiSoft. The Patient Recall List dialog box is displayed.

2. Click the New button.

3. Enter June 7, 2008, in the Recall Date box.

4. Select Asha Singh in the Provider box.

5. Key the first few letters of Mrs. Hersen's chart number in the Chart box, and then select her name from the drop-down list.

6. In the Message box, key *Six-month follow-up appointment needed.*

7. Verify that the Call radio button in the Recall Status box is selected.

8. Click the Save button to save the entry.

9. Repeat the steps to add Georgette Hersen to the Patient Recall List.

10. Close the Patient Recall List dialog box.

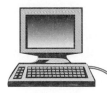

EXERCISE 14-5: DIANA FONDO AND BRAD WALSH

For this simulation, you will need Source Documents 14, 21, and 22.

It is Monday, November 12, 2007. Diana Fondo and Brad Walsh are leaving the office after their appointments. Use the information on Source Documents 21 and 22 to perform the following tasks.

1. Create new cases for both patients by copying existing cases.

   For Fondo, copy the preventive case. Complete the boxes listed below in the Personal, Account, and Policy 1 tabs. When completing the Account and Policy 1 tabs for Fondo, remember that her husband changed insurance carriers to SouthWest Florida HMO. Since Diana Fondo is covered under her husband's policy, the new insurance company information must be used. This information can be found in Jeffrey Fondo's periodontal case (see also Source Document 14).

   Personal Tab
   Description

   Account Tab
   Price Code

   Policy 1 Tab
   Insurance 1
   Policy Number
   Group Number
   Policy Dates, Start
   Capitated Plan
   Copayment Amount
   Insurance Coverage Percents by Service Classification

2. While looking up Diana Fondo's new insurance information, it occurs to you that Diana's patient information also needs to be updated because of the Fondo's recent change in address. After saving the new case for Diana Fondo, you are in the Patient List dialog box. Reselect Diana Fondo's chart number, and then click the Edit Patient button.

3. Move to the Street box, and enter the Fondo's new address (located in Source Document 14).

4. Move to the Phones 1 box, and enter the new phone number.

5. Save the information you just entered.

6. For Walsh's new case, complete the following box in the Personal tab.

   Personal Tab
   Description

7. Record the charges in the Transaction Entry dialog box for Fondo.

8. Record the payments, and apply the payments to the charges.

9. Print a walkout receipt.

10. Record Walsh's transactions in the same way, and print a walkout receipt.

11. Using Office Hours, make the appointment indicated on Mrs. Fondo's encounter form. Do not exit PractiSoft.

EXERCISE 14-6: CHANGING A TRANSACTION RECORD

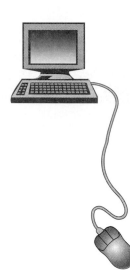

Just as you finish making Mrs. Fondo's appointment, Dr. Harold Miller comes to the desk to say that he thinks he forgot to note on Ian McCubbin's November 9, 2007, encounter form that he performed an X ray (intraoral—first X-ray). He asks you to check and add the charge if necessary.

1. Go to the Transaction Entry dialog box. Check through the entries to find out whether the charge was entered. (It was not.)

2. Enter the new charge. (*Hint:* Remember to change the default date entries in the Document and Date boxes to November 9, 2007.)

3. Check your work.

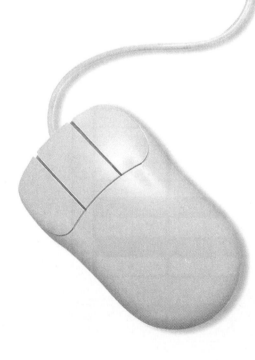

15 Printing Lists and Reports

WHAT YOU NEED TO KNOW

To complete the exercises in this chapter, you need to know how to:

◆ Create a patient ledger.

◆ Create a day sheet report.

◆ Understand what aging means, in an accounting sense.

◆ Create a patient aging report.

◆ Enter transactions.

◆ Print an appointment list.

◆ Print a patient ledger report.

Because PractiSoft is an accounting package, its most powerful features involve computerized manipulation of patients account data. PractiSoft uses information in the system to produce reports on any facet of patients' or insurers' accounts and to generate bills for patients and insurance companies. For example, as long as the office personnel in Collier Family Dental Care have entered transactions correctly and have performed basic accounting procedures, the PractiSoft program can be used to print current reports on the practice's finances. You can print a report showing details of a day's transactions for any one of the practice's dentists or for all dentists. You can print a report of late accounts for a particular patient, for all patients, for one insurance company, or for all insurance companies.

Before starting the exercises in this chapter, you should understand some basic aspects of dental office accounting procedures.

Every dental office must keep a daily record of charges and payments for every patient of every provider. For charges, the record usually includes the name of the patient, the type of service provided, and the amount of the charge. For payments, the record usually includes the name of the patient whose account is being credited and the amount of the payment. Whereas day sheets record information on charges and payments for a single day, ledgers show all current information up to and including the date shown on the ledger.

As the name suggests, aging reports show how long unpaid charges have been due. In PractiSoft, aging reports are divided into four columns, showing, in order, accounts that are currently due, accounts that have been due for 31 to 60 days, accounts that have been due for 61 to 90 days, and accounts that have been due for more than 90 days.

EXERCISE 15-1: FINDING A PATIENT'S BALANCE

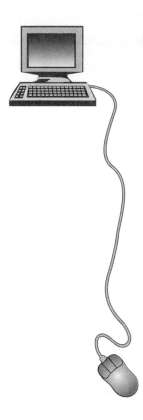

It is still Monday, November 12, 2007. Anthony Arrez calls. He would like to know the amount of the charges from November 9 that he is responsible for, assuming his insurance carrier pays its portion of the total charges. How can you find the amount he is responsible for?

PractiSoft Program Date: November 12, 2007

1. On the Activities menu, click Enter Transactions.

2. In the Chart box, select Anthony Arrez's chart number.

3. Verify that the Restoration case is active in the Case box.

4. Click the ellipses in the Document box, and select the document number associated with the procedures performed on November 9, 2007.

5. Look at the middle panel at the top of the Transaction Entry dialog box, where the information about estimated financial responsibility (Est. Resp.) is listed. Determine the insurance carrier's portion of the charges for the procedures performed on 11/9/2007, and then determine what amount of the charges is the guarantor's responsibility for that day.

EXERCISE 15-2: PRINTING A SCHEDULE

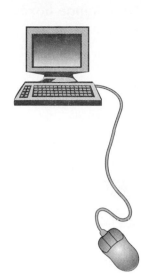

Print Dr. Harold Miller's appointment schedule for Monday, December 10, 2007.

1. Open Office Hours.

2. Select Dr. Harold Miller as the Provider.

3. Go to December 10, 2007, in the calendar.

4. Click Appointment List on the Office Hours Reports menu.

5. Select the option to print the report on the printer, and select Summary as the report type.

6. Click the Start button.

7. Exit Office Hours

EXERCISE 15-3: PRINTING DAY SHEET REPORTS

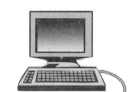

Patient day sheets and procedure day sheets can be viewed and/or printed using options on the Reports menu.

PractiSoft Program Date: November 9, 2007

Creating a Patient Day Sheet Report

1. On the Reports menu, click Day Sheets and then Patient Day Sheet.

2. Select the option to preview the report on-screen. Click the Start button.

3. Leave the Chart Number Range boxes blank, to include all patients.

4. Delete the entries in both Date Created Range boxes.

5. Key *11092007* in both Date From Range boxes.

6. Leave all the other boxes blank.

7. Click the OK button.

8. The patient day sheet report is displayed on-screen.

9. Close the Preview Report window.

Creating a Procedure Day Sheet Report

10. On the Reports menu, click Day Sheets and then Procedure Day Sheet.

11. Select the option to preview the report on-screen. Click the Start button.

12. Leave the Procedure Code Range boxes blank.

13. Delete both entries in the Date Created Range boxes.

14. Key *11092007* in both of the Date From Range boxes.

15. Leave the Attending Provider boxes blank.

16. Click the OK button.

17. The procedure day sheet report appears on-screen.

18. Close the Preview Report window.

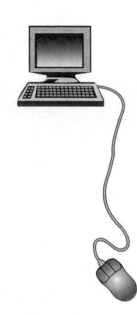

EXERCISE 15-4: CREATING A PATIENT AGING REPORT

Print a patient aging report as a first step in the billing process. The aging report shows which accounts are overdue and how long they have been overdue.

PractiSoft Program Date: December 31, 2007

1. On the Reports menu, click Aging Reports and then Patient Aging.

2. Select the option to preview the report on-screen. Click the Start button.

3. Leave all data selection fields blank except the second Date From Range box. Key *12312007* in this box.

4. Click the OK button.

5. View the report.

6. Close the Preview Report window.

EXERCISE 15-5: STEWART SCHOBER, A NEW PATIENT

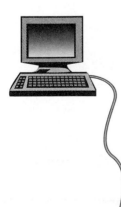

You need Source Documents 23 and 24 for this exercise, which consists of two parts. For the first part, assume that it is December 7, 2007. A new patient of Dr. Miller, Stewart Schober, has stopped by to fill out a patient information form. He wants an appointment for December, specifically for the third Wednesday of the month, as early as possible. Schedule him for a one-hour appointment.

Part One – December 7, 2007

PractiSoft Program Date: December 7, 2007

1. Using Source Document 23, enter the patient information for Mr. Schober. Complete the Patient/Guarantor dialog box and the Case dialog box. You will need to add Schober's employer to the database. You will also need to create a new case.

Schober's insurance company is BCBS of Florida. Therefore, the Price Code box in his Account tab should be A. In his Policy 1 tab, Box A of the Insurance Coverage Percents by Service Classification should be 80.

2. In Office Hours, schedule Schober for his appointment.

Part Two – December 19, 2007

PractiSoft Program Date: December 19, 2007

1. Using Source Document 24, enter the charges for Stewart Schober's visit.

EXERCISE 15-6: BRAD WALSH, AN EMERGENCY VISIT

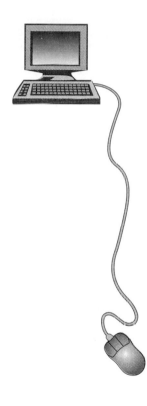

PractiSoft Program Date: December 14, 2007

1. Read the following account of Brad Walsh's visit to Collier Family Dental Care on December 14, 2007.

   On the way out of the door of his house to go to his daughter Michelle's soccer game, Walsh had a minor accident. As a result, his fixed partial denture has come out. He has come in to see Dr. Miller on an emergency basis. Dr. Miller is unavailable, so he is treated by Dr. Wu. She takes an X ray, recements the denture, and asks Walsh to come back in a week so she can check on it.

   At the reception desk, Brad Walsh realizes that he left his checkbook at home. Therefore, he pays for the X ray with cash and explains that he will pay the balance due with a check when he returns next week. He schedules an appointment for Friday, December 21, at 2:00 p.m.

2. In PractiSoft, enter all the information pertaining to this visit using Source Document 25. Remember to print a walkout receipt.

16 Printing Statements and Creating Claims

WHAT YOU NEED TO KNOW

To complete the exercises in this chapter, you need to know how to:

◆ Print patient statements.

◆ Create insurance claims.

◆ Print insurance claim forms.

Different dental practices have different billing procedures. Collier Family Dental Care collects copayments from patients at the time service is rendered. The practice then bills the insurance company. Once a remittance advice is received from the carrier, the patient is billed for the remainder. Bills for remainder balances are mailed out on the fifteenth of the month for patients whose last names begin with A through L, and on the thirtieth of the month for patients whose last names begin with M through Z.

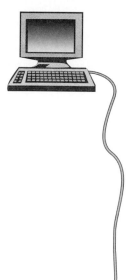

EXERCISE 16-1: PRINTING PATIENT STATEMENTS

Today's date is December 21, 2007. Brad Walsh has arrived in the office for a follow-up appointment. He remembers he did not pay in full last week (Exercise 15-6). He would like a copy of his patient statement before he sees Dr. Wu.

PractiSoft Program Date: December 21, 2007

1. Click Patient Statements on the Reports menu.

2. Select Patient Statement (30, 60, 90) in the Open Report dialog box. Click the OK button.

3. Click the appropriate radio button to preview the statement on-screen. Click the Start button.

4. Enter Walsh's chart number in both Chart Number Range boxes.

5. Enter December 21, 2007, in the second Date From Range box. Leave the first Date From Range box and the other data selection boxes blank.

6. Click the OK button.

7. Preview the statement. Notice that because Brad is guarantor on his daughter Michelle's account, her charges appear on his statement.

8. Print the statement.

9. Close the Preview Report window.

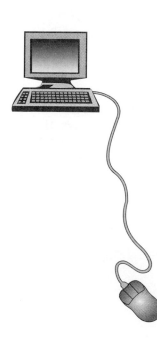

EXERCISE 16-2: CREATING INSURANCE CLAIMS

Create insurance claims for patients who have had transactions from November 9, 2007, to November 30, 2007.

PractiSoft Program Date: November 30, 2007

1. Click Claim Management on the Activities menu.

2. Click the Create Claims button.

3. Key *11092007* in the first Transaction Dates box and *11302007* in the second.

4. Leave the rest of the boxes blank.

5. Click the Create button.

6. The new claims are recorded at the top of the list in the Claim Management dialog box, indicated by the "Ready to Send" message in the Status 1 column.

7. Do not exit the Claim Management dialog box.

EXERCISE 16-3: PRINTING INSURANCE CLAIM FORMS

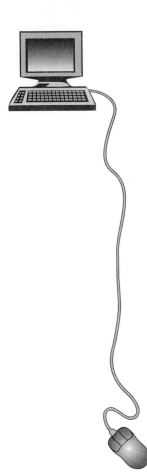

Print an insurance claim form for Paul Lamparski.

PractiSoft Program Date: November 30, 2007

1. In the Claim Management dialog box, select Lamparski's claim.

2. Click the Print/Send button.

3. Click the Paper radio button to select claims with a default billing method of paper, if it is not already selected. Click the OK button.

4. Select ADA (Primary) from the list of reports in the Open Report dialog box. Click the OK button.

5. Select the option to preview the form on-screen. Click the Start button.

6. Enter Lamparski's chart number in both Chart Number Range boxes.

7. Click the OK button.

8. Preview the form on-screen, and then print it.

9. Close the Preview Report window.

10. In the Claim Management dialog box, notice that the Lamparski claim has been moved to the bottom of the list and that the status has changed from "Ready to Send" to "Sent." Close the Claim Management dialog box.

EXERCISE 16-4: PRINTING REMAINDER STATEMENTS FOR PATIENTS WITH OUTSTANDING BALANCES

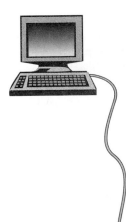

PractiSoft Program Date: November 30, 2007

Print remainder statements for all patients whose last names begin with the letters A through L and who have outstanding balances as of November 30, 2007. Figure 16-1 shows the Open Report dialog box with the appropriate report highlighted. Figure 16-2 shows the Data Selection Questions dialog box for this task.

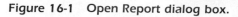

Figure 16-1   Open Report dialog box.

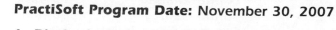

Figure 16-2   Data Selection Questions dialog box.

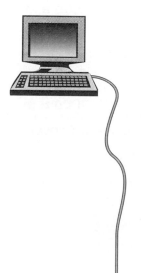

EXERCISE 16-5: VIEWING CLAIMS FOR PATIENTS WITH DELTADENTAL PPO AS THEIR PRIMARY INSURANCE CARRIER

PractiSoft Program Date: November 30, 2007

1. Display insurance claims for all patients who have DeltaDental PPO as their primary insurance carrier. Figure 16-3 on page 270 shows the List Only Claims That Match dialog box for this task.

List Only Claims That Match

Chart Number: [▼ 🔍]

Claim Created: [▼]

Apply

Cancel

Select claims for only
○ All ● Primary ○ Secondary ○ Tertiary

Defaults

That match one or more of these criteria:

Insurance Carrier: [DEL00 ▼ 🔍] DeltaDental PPO

EMC Receiver: [▼ 🔍]

Billing Method
● All
○ Paper
○ Electronic

Claim Status
● All
○ Hold
○ Ready to Send
○ Sent
○ Rejected
○ Challenge
○ Alert
○ Done ☑ Exclude Done
○ Pending

Billing Date: [▼]

Batch Number: [ ]

Help

Figure 16-3   List Only Claims That Match dialog box.

2. Use the Edit feature to review the transaction information contained in Ruby Ellison's claim.

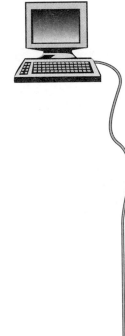

EXERCISE 16-6: PUTTING IT ALL TOGETHER

For this exercise, you need to use almost all the skills you have practiced in the preceding material.

1. Enter January 2, 2008, as the program date in PractiSoft.

2. Schedule appointments for January 2, 2008, for the following patients. Make sure they are scheduled for the right dentists.

Hersen, Joshua	30 minutes	9:00 a.m.
Fondo, Diana	60 minutes	9:00 a.m.
Fondo, Jeffrey	30 minutes	9:30 a.m.
Schubert-Seku, Juliet	60 minutes	10:00 a.m.
Thompson, Nancy	60 minutes	11:00 a.m.
Walsh, Myrna	30 minutes	1:30 p.m.
Foncet, Georgette	60 minutes	3:00 p.m.
Arrez, Paula	45 minutes	4:00 p.m.

3. Switch the appointment times for Walsh and Foncet.

4. Cancel both of the Fondos' appointments.

5. Print the appointment lists for January 2, 2008, for Dr. Miller and Dr. Wu.

6. Create new cases for all patients with appointments on January 2, 2008. All patients involved have existing cases that can be copied. Fill in the following box on the Personal tab using the information found on Source Documents 26 through 31.

   Personal Tab
   Description

7. Using Source Documents 26 through 31, record the charge and payment transactions for all of the patients who had appointments. Print walkout receipts for patients who made payments.

8. Print a patient day sheet that includes all the patients with transactions on January 2, 2008.

9. Create insurance claims for the day's transactions.

Source Documents

Collier Family Dental Care
Medical/Dental Arts Building
2890 Palm Avenue
Naples, FL 34104-8756
941-555-8900

PATIENT INFORMATION FORM

PERSONAL INFORMATION

Name (last, first): Hannah Wilson

Address: 37 Pine Ridge

Naples, FL 34101

Sex: ☐ Male
☒ Female

Date of Birth: 8-17-1981

Social Security No.: 459-33-8945

Home Phone No.: (941) 555-8888
(   )

Marital Status: ☐ Married   ☒ Single
☐ Separated   ☐ Divorced
☐ Widowed

Employer: East Collier County Schools

Address: 2500 Golden Gate Avenue

Naples, FL 34102

Work Phone No.: (941) 555-1001

Reason for visit: Extraction

Name of
Referring Dentist: Sheila R. Lopez

SPOUSE/PARENT INFORMATION

Name (last, first): _____

Social Security No.: _____

Employer: _____

Address: _____

EMERGENCY CONTACT

Name (last, first): Colleen Wilson Quigley

Relationship: sister

Phone No.: (941) 555-8833

INSURANCE INFORMATION

Insurance Company: CIGNA PPO (Price Code B)

Policy No.: 43-98

Copayment: $20

Plan/Group No.: Collier County Schools / 12

Name of Responsible Party: _____

Relationship to Patient:

☒ Self   ☐ Spouse   ☐ Child   ☐ Other

PHYSICIAN INFORMATION

Name (last, first): George Parker, MD

Specialty: Family Practice

Phone No.: (941) 555-9922

Location/City: North Naples, FL

PAYMENT INFORMATION

Check all that apply: ☒ Insurance   ☐ Cash   ☐ Check   ☐ Credit Card   ☐ Other

Assignment and Release: I hereby authorize any insurance benefits to be paid directly to the dentist. I am financially responsible for the services provided, regardless of insurance coverage. I also authorize the dentist to release any information required.

Hannah Wilson

Patient's signature/Parent or guardian's signature

10/1/2007

Date

Name of Referring Provider   Shelly Zurich, DDS

Address   Unit 216D, Collier Building
Naples, FL 34107-2836

Phone   941-555-3904

Fax   941-555-3905

License Number   7711547

Specialty   Dentistry

Social Security Number   199-46-0733

Dentist's Notes for Hannah Wilson
Date: 10/1/2007

Case: Extraction

Referring Provider: Sheila R. Lopez, DDS

Tooth 15 extraction—coronal remnant   D7111

Tooth 18 extraction—erupted tooth or exposed root   D7140

Last X rays 6/12/2007. X rays received from office of Dr. Lopez on September 27, 2007.

Collier Family Dental Care
Medical/Dental Arts Building
2890 Palm Avenue
Naples, FL 34104-8756
941-555-8900

| Patient Name: | Hannah Wilson | Chart Number: | WILSOHAO | Dentist: | Dr. Miller | Date of Service: | 10/1/2007 |

	SERVICE		FEE
	DIAGNOSTIC/PREVENTIVE		
	D1110 Prophylaxis – adult		
	D0120 Periodic oral evaluation		
	D0274 Bitewings – four X rays		
	D1120 Prophylaxis – child		
	D0210 Intraoral – complete series (including bitewings)		
	D0220 Intraoral – first X ray		
	D0230 Intraoral – each additional X ray		
	D0321 TMJ film		
	D0470 Diagnostic casts		

	ENDODONTICS	Tooth #s	
	D3310 Root canal 1		
	D3320 Root canal 2		
	D3330 Root canal 3		
	D3110 Pulp cap		
	D3220 Pulpotomy		
	D0460 Pulp vitality test		
	D2940 Sedative filling		

	RESTORATIVE Amalgam Restorations:	Surface	Tooth #s	
	D2140 One surface, primary or permanent			
	D2150 Two surfaces, primary or permanent			
	D2160 Three surfaces, primary or permanent			
	D2161 Four or more surfaces, primary or permanent			

	Resin-based Composite Restorations Anterior:	Surface	Tooth #s	
	D2330 One surface			
	D2331 Two surfaces			
	D2332 Three surfaces			
	D2335 Four or more surfaces			

	Posterior:	Surface	Tooth #s	
	D2391 One surface			
	D2392 Two surfaces			
	D2393 Three surfaces			
	D2394 Four or more surfaces			

	Crown Restorations:	Tooth #s	
	D2740 Porcelain		
	D2750 Porcelain–metal		

Collier Family Dental Care
Medical/Dental Arts Building
2890 Palm Avenue
Naples, FL 34104-8756
941-555-8900

Patient Name: Hannah Wilson   **Chart Number:** WILSOHAO   **Dentist:** Dr. Miller   **Date of Service:** 10/1/2007

	Crown Restorations:	Tooth #s	
	D2920 Recement Crown		
	D2950 Core buildup		
	D2980 Repair		
	PROSTHETICS Complete Dentures:		
	D5110 Upper denture		
	D5120 Lower denture		
	D5130 Immediate upper denture		
	D5140 Immediate lower denture		
	Partial Dentures:		
	D5211 Upper partial denture—resin		
	D5212 Lower partial denture—resin		
	D5213 Upper partial denture—cast		
	D5214 Lower partial denture—cast		
	D5750 Reline full upper denture		
	D6930 Recement fixed partial denture		
	PERIODONTICS/SURGERY	**Tooth/Quad**	
	D4341 Periodontal scaling and root planing,		
	per quadrant		
	Upper right		
	Upper left		
	Lower right		
	Lower left		
	D4210 Gingivectomy		
	D4240 Gingival flap		
	D4260 Osseous surgery		
	Upper right		
	Upper left		
	Lower right		
	Lower left		
X	D7111 Extraction—Coronal remnant	15 / upper left	
X	D7140 Extraction—erupted tooth or exposed root	18 / lower left	
	D7210 Surgical extraction		
	ADJUNCTIVE GENERAL SERVICES	**Tooth #s**	
	D9951 Occlusal adjustment—limited		
	OTHER		

Payments: $20 copay, check #123   **Total charge:**

Remarks:

Collier Family Dental Care
Medical/Dental Arts Building
2890 Palm Avenue
Naples, FL 34104-8756
941-555-8900

Patient Name: Luz Vasquez   **Chart Number:** VASQULUO   **Dentist:** Dr. Miller   **Date of Service:** 10/1/2007

	SERVICE DIAGNOSTIC/PREVENTIVE			FEE
	D1110 Prophylaxis – adult			
	D0120 Periodic oral evaluation			
	D0274 Bitewings – four X rays			
	D1120 Prophylaxis – child			
	D0210 Intraoral – complete series (including bitewings)			
	D0220 Intraoral – first X ray			
	D0230 Intraoral – each additional X ray			
	D0321 TMJ film			
	D0470 Diagnostic casts			
	ENDODONTICS		**Tooth #s**	
	D3310 Root canal 1			
	D3320 Root canal 2			
	D3330 Root canal 3			
	D3110 Pulp cap			
	D3220 Pulpotomy			
	D0460 Pulp vitality test			
	D2940 Sedative filling			
	RESTORATIVE Amalgam Restorations:	**Surface**	**Tooth #s**	
	D2140 One surface, primary or permanent			
	D2150 Two surfaces, primary or permanent			
	D2160 Three surfaces, primary or permanent			
	D2161 Four or more surfaces, primary or permanent			
	Resin-based Composite Restorations Anterior:	**Surface**	**Tooth #s**	
	D2330 One surface			
	D2331 Two surfaces			
	D2332 Three surfaces			
	D2335 Four or more surfaces			
	Posterior:	**Surface**	**Tooth #s**	
	D2391 One surface			
	D2392 Two surfaces			
	D2393 Three surfaces			
	D2394 Four or more surfaces			
	Crown Restorations:		**Tooth #s**	
	D2740 Porcelain			
	D2750 Porcelain–metal			

Collier Family Dental Care
Medical/Dental Arts Building
2890 Palm Avenue
Naples, FL 34104-8756
941-555-8900

Patient Name: Luz Vasquez   **Chart Number:** VASQULUO   **Dentist:** Dr. Miller   **Date of Service:** 10/1/2007

	Crown Restorations:	Tooth #s	
X	D2920 Recement Crown	32	
	D2950 Core buildup		
	D2980 Repair		
	PROSTHETICS **Complete Dentures:**		
	D5110 Upper denture		
	D5120 Lower denture		
	D5130 Immediate upper denture		
	D5140 Immediate lower denture		
	Partial Dentures:		
	D5211 Upper partial denture–resin		
	D5212 Lower partial denture–resin		
	D5213 Upper partial denture–cast		
	D5214 Lower partial denture–cast		
	D5750 Reline full upper denture		
	D6930 Recement fixed partial denture		
	PERIODONTICS/SURGERY	**Tooth/Quad**	
	D4341 Periodontal scaling and root planing,		
	per quadrant		
	Upper right		
	Upper left		
	Lower right		
	Lower left		
	D4210 Gingivectomy		
	D4240 Gingival flap		
	D4260 Osseous surgery		
	Upper right		
	Upper left		
	Lower right		
	Lower left		
	D7111 Extraction–Coronal remnant		
	D7140 Extraction–erupted tooth or exposed root		
	D7210 Surgical extraction		
	ADJUNCTIVE GENERAL SERVICES	**Tooth #s**	
	D9951 Occlusal adjustment–limited		
	OTHER		

Payments: **Total charge:**

Remarks:

Collier Family Dental Care
Medical/Dental Arts Building
2890 Palm Avenue
Naples, FL 34104-8756
941-555-8900

Patient Name: John Ellison **Chart Number:** ELLISJOO **Dentist:** Dr. Miller **Date of Service:** 10/1/2007

	SERVICE			FEE
	DIAGNOSTIC/PREVENTIVE			
	D1110 Prophylaxis – adult			
	D0120 Periodic oral evaluation			
	D0274 Bitewings – four X rays			
	D1120 Prophylaxis – child			
	D0210 Intraoral – complete series (including bitewings)			
	D0220 Intraoral – first X ray			
	D0230 Intraoral – each additional X ray			
	D0321 TMJ film			
	D0470 Diagnostic casts			
	ENDODONTICS		**Tooth #s**	
	D3310 Root canal 1			
	D3320 Root canal 2			
	D3330 Root canal 3			
	D3110 Pulp cap			
	D3220 Pulpotomy			
	D0460 Pulp vitality test			
	D2940 Sedative filling			
	RESTORATIVE Amalgam Restorations:	**Surface**	**Tooth #s**	
	D2140 One surface, primary or permanent			
	D2150 Two surfaces, primary or permanent			
	D2160 Three surfaces, primary or permanent			
	D2161 Four or more surfaces, primary or permanent			
	Resin-based Composite Restorations Anterior:	**Surface**	**Tooth #s**	
	D2330 One surface			
	D2331 Two surfaces			
	D2332 Three surfaces			
	D2335 Four or more surfaces			
	Posterior:	**Surface**	**Tooth #s**	
	D2391 One surface			
	D2392 Two surfaces			
	D2393 Three surfaces			
	D2394 Four or more surfaces			
	Crown Restorations:		**Tooth #s**	
	D2740 Porcelain			
	D2750 Porcelain–metal			

Collier Family Dental Care
Medical/Dental Arts Building
2890 Palm Avenue
Naples, FL 34104-8756
941-555-8900

Patient Name: John Ellison	**Chart Number:** ELLISJOO	**Dentist:** Dr. Miller	**Date of Service:** 10/1/2007

	Crown Restorations:	**Tooth #s**	
	D2920 Recement Crown		
	D2950 Core buildup		
	D2980 Repair		
	PROSTHETICS Complete Dentures:		
	D5110 Upper denture		
	D5120 Lower denture		
	D5130 Immediate upper denture		
	D5140 Immediate lower denture		
	Partial Dentures:		
X	D5211 Upper partial denture–resin		
X	D5212 Lower partial denture–resin		
	D5213 Upper partial denture–cast		
	D5214 Lower partial denture–cast		
	D5750 Reline full upper denture		
	D6930 Recement fixed partial denture		
	PERIODONTICS/SURGERY	**Tooth/Quad**	
	D4341 Periodontal scaling and root planing,		
	per quadrant		
	Upper right		
	Upper left		
	Lower right		
	Lower left		
	D4210 Gingivectomy		
	D4240 Gingival flap		
	D4260 Osseous surgery		
	Upper right		
	Upper left		
	Lower right		
	Lower left		
	D7111 Extraction–Coronal remnant		
	D7140 Extraction–erupted tooth or exposed root		
	D7210 Surgical extraction		
	ADJUNCTIVE GENERAL SERVICES	**Tooth #s**	
	D9951 Occlusal adjustment–limited		
	OTHER		

Payments: $15 copay, check #456	**Total charge:**

Remarks:

DeltaDental

No. 412877429

Date OCT. 1, 2007

PAYABLE
TO: COLLIER FAMILY DENTAL CARE

$ $140.00

ONE HUNDRED FORTY & NO CENTS

Dollars

Naples Bank
Naples, FL 34104

For CLAIM #67035A

SIGNATURE

⑈120302743⑈ ⑉412877429⑉ ⑈9730 466 20⑈

Sunshine State HMO

No. 98721043

Date OCT. 1, 2007

PAYABLE
TO: COLLIER FAMILY DENTAL CARE

$ $2500.00

TWO THOUSAND FIVE HUNDRED & NO CENTS

Dollars

Naples Bank
Naples, FL 34104

For 9/2007

SIGNATURE

⑈120302743⑈ ⑉98721043⑉ ⑈9730 223 40⑈

Aetna
8000 Coral Drive, Suite 500
Naples, FL 34506-7613

Collier Family Dental Care
Medical/Dental Arts Building
2890 Palm Avenue
Naples, FL 34104-8756

Practice ID: 706FB8A

Date Prepared: 11/15/2007   **RA Number:** 100432

Patient's Name	Dates of Service From – Thru	POS	Proc	Qty	Proc Charge	Amt Paid Provider
Foncet, Georgette	10-30-07 – 10-30-07	11	D2740	1	1050.00	840.00
Foncet, Georgette	10-30-07 – 10-30-07	11	D2920	1	60.00	48.00
Foncet, Georgette	10-30-07 – 10-30-07	11	D2980	1	175.00	140.00
Schubert-Seku, Juliet	10-30-07 – 10-30-07	11	D4341-LR	1	225.00	180.00
Schubert-Seku, Juliet	10-30-07 – 10-30-07	11	D4341-LL	1	225.00	180.00

* * * * * * * *   *Check #1098 is attached in the amount of $1388.00.*   * * * * * * * *

CIGNA PPO
5 First Avenue, Building D
Tampa, FL 33607-6657

Collier Family Dental Care
Medical/Dental Arts Building
2890 Palm Avenue
Naples, FL 34104-8756

Practice ID: 10-432765

Date Prepared: 10/01/2007

RA Number: 010101

Patient's Name	Dates of Service From – Thru	POS	Proc	Qty	Proc Charge	Amt Paid Provider
Axford, Susan	09-03-07 – 09-03-07	11	D2150	1	120.00	120.00
Barlow, Daniel	09-03-07 – 09-03-07	11	D1110	1	60.00	60.00
Barlow, June	09-03-07 – 09-03-07	11	D0120	1	25.00	25.00
Barlow, June	09-03-07 – 09-03-07	11	D1110	1	60.00	60.00
Barlow, Jimmy	09-03-07 – 09-03-07	11	D1120	1	45.00	45.00
Barlow, Samuel	09-03-07 – 09-03-07	11	D1120	1	45.00	45.00
Barlow, Gloria	09-03-07 – 09-03-07	11	D1120	1	45.00	45.00

* * * * * * * *   *Check #6549870 is attached in the amount of $400.00.*   * * * * * * * *

Collier Family Dental Care
Medical/Dental Arts Building
2890 Palm Avenue
Naples, FL 34104-8756
941-555-8900

Patient Name: Anthony Arrez **Chart Number:** ARREZANO **Dentist:** Dr. Miller **Date of Service:** 11/9/2007

	SERVICE	FEE
	DIAGNOSTIC/PREVENTIVE	
	D1110 Prophylaxis – adult	
	D0120 Periodic oral evaluation	
	D0274 Bitewings – four X rays	
	D1120 Prophylaxis – child	
	D0210 Intraoral – complete series (including bitewings)	
X	D0220 Intraoral – first X ray	
X	D0230 Intraoral – each additional X ray	
	D0321 TMJ film	
	D0470 Diagnostic casts	

	ENDODONTICS	Tooth #s
	D3310 Root canal 1	
	D3320 Root canal 2	
	D3330 Root canal 3	
	D3110 Pulp cap	
	D3220 Pulpotomy	
	D0460 Pulp vitality test	
	D2940 Sedative filling	

	RESTORATIVE Amalgam Restorations:	Surface	Tooth #s
	D2140 One surface, primary or permanent		
	D2150 Two surfaces, primary or permanent		
	D2160 Three surfaces, primary or permanent		
	D2161 Four or more surfaces, primary or permanent		

	Resin-based Composite Restorations Anterior:	Surface	Tooth #s
	D2330 One surface		
	D2331 Two surfaces		
	D2332 Three surfaces		
	D2335 Four or more surfaces		

	Posterior:	Surface	Tooth #s
	D2391 One surface		
	D2392 Two surfaces		
	D2393 Three surfaces		
	D2394 Four or more surfaces		

	Crown Restorations:	Tooth #s
	D2740 Porcelain	
	D2750 Porcelain–metal	

Collier Family Dental Care
Medical/Dental Arts Building
2890 Palm Avenue
Naples, FL 34104-8756
941-555-8900

Patient Name: Anthony Arrez **Chart Number:** ARREZANO **Dentist:** Dr. Miller **Date of Service:** 11/9/2007

	Crown Restorations:	Tooth #s	
	D2920 Recement Crown		
X	D2950 Core buildup	13	
	D2980 Repair		
	PROSTHETICS Complete Dentures:		
	D5110 Upper denture		
	D5120 Lower denture		
	D5130 Immediate upper denture		
	D5140 Immediate lower denture		
	Partial Dentures:		
	D5211 Upper partial denture—resin		
	D5212 Lower partial denture—resin		
	D5213 Upper partial denture—cast		
	D5214 Lower partial denture—cast		
	D5750 Reline full upper denture		
	D6930 Recement fixed partial denture		
	PERIODONTICS/SURGERY	**Tooth/Quad**	
	D4341 Periodontal scaling and root planing,		
	per quadrant		
	Upper right		
	Upper left		
	Lower right		
	Lower left		
	D4210 Gingivectomy		
	D4240 Gingival flap		
	D4260 Osseous surgery		
	Upper right		
	Upper left		
	Lower right		
	Lower left		
	D7111 Extraction—Coronal remnant		
	D7140 Extraction—erupted tooth or exposed root		
	D7210 Surgical extraction		
	ADJUNCTIVE GENERAL SERVICES	**Tooth #s**	
	D9951 Occlusal adjustment—limited		
	OTHER		

Payments: **Total charge:**

Remarks: New address: 333 25th Street, Naples, FL, 34104, (941) 444-1010

Collier Family Dental Care
Medical/Dental Arts Building
2890 Palm Avenue
Naples, FL 34104-8756
941-555-8900

Patient Name: Josephine Chan **Chart Number:** CHANJOSO **Dentist:** Dr. Miller **Date of Service:** 11/9/2007

	SERVICE DIAGNOSTIC/PREVENTIVE			FEE
	D1110 Prophylaxis – adult			
	D0120 Periodic oral evaluation			
	D0274 Bitewings – four X rays			
	D1120 Prophylaxis – child			
	D0210 Intraoral – complete series (including bitewings)			
X	D0220 Intraoral – first X ray			
	D0230 Intraoral – each additional X ray			
	D0321 TMJ film			
	D0470 Diagnostic casts			
	ENDODONTICS		**Tooth #s**	
	D3310 Root canal 1			
	D3320 Root canal 2			
	D3330 Root canal 3			
	D3110 Pulp cap			
	D3220 Pulpotomy			
	D0460 Pulp vitality test			
	D2940 Sedative filling			
	RESTORATIVE Amalgam Restorations:	**Surface**	**Tooth #s**	
	D2140 One surface, primary or permanent			
	D2150 Two surfaces, primary or permanent			
	D2160 Three surfaces, primary or permanent			
	D2161 Four or more surfaces, primary or permanent			
	Resin-based Composite Restorations Anterior:	**Surface**	**Tooth #s**	
	D2330 One surface			
	D2331 Two surfaces			
	D2332 Three surfaces			
	D2335 Four or more surfaces			
	Posterior:	**Surface**	**Tooth #s**	
	D2391 One surface			
	D2392 Two surfaces			
	D2393 Three surfaces			
	D2394 Four or more surfaces			
	Crown Restorations:		**Tooth #s**	
	D2740 Porcelain			
	D2750 Porcelain–metal			

Collier Family Dental Care
Medical/Dental Arts Building
2890 Palm Avenue
Naples, FL 34104-8756
941-555-8900

| Patient Name: | Josephine Chan | Chart Number: | CHANJOSO | Dentist: | Dr. Miller | Date of Service: | 11/9/2007 |

	Crown Restorations:		Tooth #s	
X	D2920 Recement Crown		30	
	D2950 Core buildup			
X	D2980 Repair		30	
	PROSTHETICS **Complete Dentures:**			
	D5110 Upper denture			
	D5120 Lower denture			
	D5130 Immediate upper denture			
	D5140 Immediate lower denture			
	Partial Dentures:			
	D5211 Upper partial denture–resin			
	D5212 Lower partial denture–resin			
	D5213 Upper partial denture–cast			
	D5214 Lower partial denture–cast			
	D5750 Reline full upper denture			
	D6930 Recement fixed partial denture			
	PERIODONTICS/SURGERY	Tooth/Quad		
	D4341 Periodontal scaling and root planing,			
	per quadrant			
	Upper right			
	Upper left			
	Lower right			
	Lower left			
	D4210 Gingivectomy			
	D4240 Gingival flap			
	D4260 Osseous surgery			
	Upper right			
	Upper left			
	Lower right			
	Lower left			
	D7111 Extraction–Coronal remnant			
	D7140 Extraction–erupted tooth or exposed root			
	D7210 Surgical extraction			
	ADJUNCTIVE GENERAL SERVICES	Tooth #s		
	D9951 Occlusal adjustment–limited			
	OTHER			

| Payments: | | Total charge: | |

Remarks:

Collier Family Dental Care
Medical/Dental Arts Building
2890 Palm Avenue
Naples, FL 34104-8756
941-555-8900

Patient Name: Jeffrey Fondo **Chart Number:** FONDOJEO **Dentist:** Dr. Miller **Date of Service:** 11/9/2007

SERVICE DIAGNOSTIC/PREVENTIVE		FEE
D1110 Prophylaxis – adult		
D0120 Periodic oral evaluation		
D0274 Bitewings – four X rays		
D1120 Prophylaxis – child		
D0210 Intraoral – complete series (including bitewings)		
D0220 Intraoral – first X ray		
D0230 Intraoral – each additional X ray		
D0321 TMJ film		
D0470 Diagnostic casts		

ENDODONTICS	Tooth #s
D3310 Root canal 1	
D3320 Root canal 2	
D3330 Root canal 3	
D3110 Pulp cap	
D3220 Pulpotomy	
D0460 Pulp vitality test	
D2940 Sedative filling	

RESTORATIVE Amalgam Restorations:	Surface	Tooth #s
D2140 One surface, primary or permanent		
D2150 Two surfaces, primary or permanent		
D2160 Three surfaces, primary or permanent		
D2161 Four or more surfaces, primary or permanent		

Resin-based Composite Restorations Anterior:	Surface	Tooth #s
D2330 One surface		
D2331 Two surfaces		
D2332 Three surfaces		
D2335 Four or more surfaces		

Posterior:	Surface	Tooth #s
D2391 One surface		
D2392 Two surfaces		
D2393 Three surfaces		
D2394 Four or more surfaces		

Crown Restorations:	Tooth #s
D2740 Porcelain	
D2750 Porcelain–metal	

Collier Family Dental Care
Medical/Dental Arts Building
2890 Palm Avenue
Naples, FL 34104-8756
941-555-8900

Patient Name: Jeffrey Fondo   **Chart Number:** FONDOJEO   **Dentist:** Dr. Miller   **Date of Service:** 11/9/2007

	Crown Restorations:	Tooth #s	
	D2920 Recement Crown		
	D2950 Core buildup		
	D2980 Repair		
	PROSTHETICS Complete Dentures:		
	D5110 Upper denture		
	D5120 Lower denture		
	D5130 Immediate upper denture		
	D5140 Immediate lower denture		
	Partial Dentures:		
	D5211 Upper partial denture–resin		
	D5212 Lower partial denture–resin		
	D5213 Upper partial denture–cast		
	D5214 Lower partial denture–cast		
	D5750 Reline full upper denture		
	D6930 Recement fixed partial denture		
	PERIODONTICS/SURGERY °	Tooth/Quad	
	D4341 Periodontal scaling and root planing,		
	per quadrant		
	Upper right		
	Upper left		
	Lower right		
	Lower left		
X	D4210 Gingivectomy		
	D4240 Gingival flap		
	D4260 Osseous surgery		
	Upper right		
	Upper left		
	Lower right		
	Lower left		
	D7111 Extraction–Coronal remnant		
	D7140 Extraction–erupted tooth or exposed root		
	D7210 Surgical extraction		
	ADJUNCTIVE GENERAL SERVICES	Tooth #s	
	D9951 Occlusal adjustment–limited		
	OTHER		

Payments: $20 copay, check #1066   **Total charge:**

Remarks: see case notes

SOURCE DOCUMENT 14

Jeffrey Fondo – Case Notes

Date: 11/9/2007
Description: Periodontal

Change Patient's Address

New Address:

691 Palm Run Road
Naples, FL 34104
941-444-7070

Add New Insurance Carrier to Database

Code:	SOU00
Name:	SouthWest Florida HMO
Address:	2020 Ave. U
	North Naples, FL 34110
Phone:	941-555-6200

Plan Name:	SOU HMO
Type:	Dental
Procedure Code Set:	1
Diagnosis Code Set:	1
Patient / Insured / Physician Signature on File:	—
Print PINS on Forms:	—
Default Billing Method:	Paper

EMC Receiver:	NDC00 (NDC Dental)
EMC Payor Number:	1000
EMC Sub ID:	7000
NDC Record Code:	01
Payment:	SOUPAY – SouthWest Florida Payment
Adjustment:	SOUADJ – SouthWest Florida Adjustment
Withhold:	SOUWIT – SouthWest Florida Withhold
Deductible:	SOUDED – SouthWest Florida Deductible

Miller PIN / Group ID:	5678 / 6000
Wu PIN / Group ID:	9012 / 6000
Singh / Group ID:	3456 / 6000

Create New Case

Price Code:	B

Policy Number:	022981333P
Group Number:	1049
Policy Dates, Start:	11/1/2007
Assignment of Benefits / Accept Assignment:	Yes
Capitated Plan:	Yes
Annual Deductible:	0
Copayment Amount:	20.00
Insurance Coverage Percents by Service Classification:	A: 100% (leave boxes B through H as they are)

Collier Family Dental Care
Medical/Dental Arts Building
2890 Palm Avenue
Naples, FL 34104-8756
941-555-8900

PATIENT INFORMATION FORM

PERSONAL INFORMATION

Name (last, first): _Michelle Walsh_

Address: _450-A Arlington Road_
North Naples, FL 34110

Sex: ☐ Male
☒ Female

Date of Birth: _12-4-1988_

Social Security No.: _789-56-9876_

Home Phone No.: _(941) 555-1111_
( )

Marital Status: ☐ Married ☒ Single
☐ Separated ☐ Divorced
☐ Widowed

Employer: _____

Address: _____

Work Phone No.: ( )

Reason for visit: _Preventive_

Name of
Referring Dentist _Dr. Sheila Lopez_

SPOUSE/PARENT INFORMATION

Name (last, first): _Brad Walsh_

Social Security No.: _450-67-8890_

Employer: _Landscapes of Naples_

Address: _540 Collier Street_
Naples, FL 34509

EMERGENCY CONTACT

Name (last, first): _Myrna Walsh_

Relationship: _mother_

Phone No.: _(941) 555-1111_

INSURANCE INFORMATION

Insurance Company: _____

Policy No.: _____

Copayment: _____

Plan/Group No.: _____

Name of Responsible Party: _____

Relationship to Patient:
☐ Self ☐ Spouse ☐ Child ☐ Other

PHYSICIAN INFORMATION

Name (last, first): _____

Specialty: _____

Phone No.: ( )

Location/City: _____

PAYMENT INFORMATION

Check all that apply: ☐ Insurance ☐ Cash ☐ Check ☐ Credit Card ☐ Other

Assignment and Release: I hereby authorize any insurance benefits to be paid directly to the dentist. I am financially responsible for the services provided, regardless of insurance coverage. I also authorize the dentist to release any information required.

Brad Walsh

Patient's signature/Parent or guardian's signature

_11/9/2007_

Date

Collier Family Dental Care
Medical/Dental Arts Building
2890 Palm Avenue
Naples, FL 34104-8756
941-555-8900

Patient Name: Michelle Walsh   **Chart Number:** WALSHMIO   **Dentist:** Dr. Miller   **Date of Service:** 11/9/2007

	SERVICE DIAGNOSTIC/PREVENTIVE			FEE
	D1110 Prophylaxis – adult			
X	D0120 Periodic oral evaluation			
	D0274 Bitewings – four X rays			
X	D1120 Prophylaxis – child			
	D0210 Intraoral – complete series (including bitewings)			
	D0220 Intraoral – first X ray			
	D0230 Intraoral – each additional X ray			
	D0321 TMJ film			
	D0470 Diagnostic casts			
	ENDODONTICS		Tooth #s	
	D3310 Root canal 1			
	D3320 Root canal 2			
	D3330 Root canal 3			
	D3110 Pulp cap			
	D3220 Pulpotomy			
	D0460 Pulp vitality test			
	D2940 Sedative filling			
	RESTORATIVE Amalgam Restorations:	Surface	Tooth #s	
	D2140 One surface, primary or permanent			
	D2150 Two surfaces, primary or permanent			
	D2160 Three surfaces, primary or permanent			
	D2161 Four or more surfaces, primary or permanent			
	Resin-based Composite Restorations Anterior:	Surface	Tooth #s	
	D2330 One surface			
	D2331 Two surfaces			
	D2332 Three surfaces			
	D2335 Four or more surfaces			
	Posterior:	Surface	Tooth #s	
	D2391 One surface			
	D2392 Two surfaces			
	D2393 Three surfaces			
	D2394 Four or more surfaces			
	Crown Restorations:		Tooth #s	
	D2740 Porcelain			
	D2750 Porcelain–metal			

Collier Family Dental Care
Medical/Dental Arts Building
2890 Palm Avenue
Naples, FL 34104-8756
941-555-8900

Patient Name: Michelle Walsh   **Chart Number:** WALSHMI0   **Dentist:** Dr. Miller   **Date of Service:** 11/9/2007

	Crown Restorations:	Tooth #s	
	D2920 Recement Crown		
	D2950 Core buildup		
	D2980 Repair		
	PROSTHETICS Complete Dentures:		
	D5110 Upper denture		
	D5120 Lower denture		
	D5130 Immediate upper denture		
	D5140 Immediate lower denture		
	Partial Dentures:		
	D5211 Upper partial denture–resin		
	D5212 Lower partial denture–resin		
	D5213 Upper partial denture–cast		
	D5214 Lower partial denture–cast		
	D5750 Reline full upper denture		
	D6930 Recement fixed partial denture		
	PERIODONTICS/SURGERY	Tooth/Quad	
	D4341 Periodontal scaling and root planing, per quadrant		
	Upper right		
	Upper left		
	Lower right		
	Lower left		
	D4210 Gingivectomy		
	D4240 Gingival flap		
	D4260 Osseous surgery		
	Upper right		
	Upper left		
	Lower right		
	Lower left		
	D7111 Extraction–Coronal remnant		
	D7140 Extraction–erupted tooth or exposed root		
	D7210 Surgical extraction		
	ADJUNCTIVE GENERAL SERVICES	Tooth #s	
	D9951 Occlusal adjustment–limited		
	OTHER		

Payments: $95, check #3019   **Total charge:**

Remarks:

Collier Family Dental Care
Medical/Dental Arts Building
2890 Palm Avenue
Naples, FL 34104-8756
941-555-8900

| **Patient Name:** | Paul Lamparski | **Chart Number:** | LAMPAPAO | **Dentist:** Dr. Wu | **Date of Service:** | 11/12/2007 |

	SERVICE			FEE
	DIAGNOSTIC/PREVENTIVE			
	D1110 Prophylaxis – adult			
	D0120 Periodic oral evaluation			
	D0274 Bitewings – four X rays			
	D1120 Prophylaxis – child			
	D0210 Intraoral – complete series (including bitewings)			
X	D0220 Intraoral – first X ray			
	D0230 Intraoral – each additional X ray			
	D0321 TMJ film			
	D0470 Diagnostic casts			

	ENDODONTICS		**Tooth #s**	
	D3310 Root canal 1			
X	D3320 Root canal 2		29	
	D3330 Root canal 3			
	D3110 Pulp cap			
	D3220 Pulpotomy			
	D0460 Pulp vitality test			
	D2940 Sedative filling			

	RESTORATIVE Amalgam Restorations:	**Surface**	**Tooth #s**	
	D2140 One surface, primary or permanent			
	D2150 Two surfaces, primary or permanent			
	D2160 Three surfaces, primary or permanent			
	D2161 Four or more surfaces, primary or permanent			

	Resin-based Composite Restorations Anterior:	**Surface**	**Tooth #s**	
	D2330 One surface			
	D2331 Two surfaces			
	D2332 Three surfaces			
	D2335 Four or more surfaces			

	Posterior:	**Surface**	**Tooth #s**	
	D2391 One surface			
	D2392 Two surfaces			
	D2393 Three surfaces			
	D2394 Four or more surfaces			

	Crown Restorations:		**Tooth #s**	
	D2740 Porcelain			
	D2750 Porcelain–metal			

Collier Family Dental Care
Medical/Dental Arts Building
2890 Palm Avenue
Naples, FL 34104-8756
941-555-8900

Patient Name: Paul Lamparski **Chart Number:** LAMPAPAO **Dentist:** Dr. Wu **Date of Service:** 11/12/2007

	Crown Restorations:	Tooth #s	
	D2920 Recement Crown		
	D2950 Core buildup		
	D2980 Repair		
	PROSTHETICS **Complete Dentures:**		
	D5110 Upper denture		
	D5120 Lower denture		
	D5130 Immediate upper denture		
	D5140 Immediate lower denture		
	Partial Dentures:		
	D5211 Upper partial denture–resin		
	D5212 Lower partial denture–resin		
	D5213 Upper partial denture–cast		
	D5214 Lower partial denture–cast		
	D5750 Reline full upper denture		
	D6930 Recement fixed partial denture		
	PERIODONTICS/SURGERY	Tooth/Quad	
	D4341 Periodontal scaling and root planing,		
	per quadrant		
	Upper right		
	Upper left		
	Lower right		
	Lower left		
	D4210 Gingivectomy		
	D4240 Gingival flap		
	D4260 Osseous surgery		
	Upper right		
	Upper left		
	Lower right		
	Lower left		
	D7111 Extraction–Coronal remnant		
	D7140 Extraction–erupted tooth or exposed root		
	D7210 Surgical extraction		
	ADJUNCTIVE GENERAL SERVICES	Tooth #s	
	D9951 Occlusal adjustment–limited		
	OTHER		

Payments: $15 copay, check #1001   **Total charge:**

Remarks:

Collier Family Dental Care
Medical/Dental Arts Building
2890 Palm Avenue
Naples, FL 34104-8756
941-555-8900

PATIENT INFORMATION FORM

PERSONAL INFORMATION

Name (last, first): Ian McCubbin

Address: 20 Galleon Drive

Naples, FL 34110

Sex: [X] Male [ ] Female

Date of Birth: 10-1-1962

Social Security No.: 456-33-8763

Home Phone No.: (941) 555-5555

( )

Marital Status: [X] Married [ ] Single [ ] Separated [ ] Divorced [ ] Widowed

Employer: First Florida Bank

Address: 2400 Fifth Avenue

Naples, FL 34211

Work Phone No.: (941) 555-6666

Reason for visit: Restorative

Name of Referring Dentist

SPOUSE/PARENT INFORMATION

Name (last, first): Maryann McCubbin

Social Security No.: 347-55-8989

Employer: Fifth Avenue Clothiers

Address: 100 Fifth Avenue

Naples, FL 34211

EMERGENCY CONTACT

Name (last, first): Maryann McCubbin

Relationship: spouse

Phone No.: (941) 555-9999

INSURANCE INFORMATION

Insurance Company: DeltaDental PPO (since 1/1/2007)

Policy No.: 678222012R

Copayment: $15

Plan/Group No.: Plan RC/0021

Name of Responsible Party:

Relationship to Patient:

[X] Self [ ] Spouse [ ] Child [ ] Other

PHYSICIAN INFORMATION

Name (last, first):

Specialty:

Phone No.: ( )

Location/City:

PAYMENT INFORMATION

Check all that apply: [X] Insurance [ ] Cash [ ] Check [ ] Credit Card [ ] Other

Assignment and Release: I hereby authorize any insurance benefits to be paid directly to the dentist. I am financially responsible for the services provided, regardless of insurance coverage. I also authorize the dentist to release any information required.

Ian McCubbin

Patient's signature/Parent or guardian's signature

11/9/2007

Date

Collier Family Dental Care
Medical/Dental Arts Building
2890 Palm Avenue
Naples, FL 34104-8756
941-555-8900

Patient Name: Ian McCubbin **Chart Number:** MCCUBIAO **Dentist:** Dr. Miller **Date of Service:** 11/9/2007

	SERVICE DIAGNOSTIC/PREVENTIVE			FEE
	D1110 Prophylaxis – adult			
	D0120 Periodic oral evaluation			
	D0274 Bitewings – four X rays			
	D1120 Prophylaxis – child			
	D0210 Intraoral – complete series (including bitewings)			
	D0220 Intraoral – first X ray			
	D0230 Intraoral – each additional X ray			
	D0321 TMJ film			
	D0470 Diagnostic casts			

	ENDODONTICS		Tooth #s	
	D3310 Root canal 1			
	D3320 Root canal 2			
	D3330 Root canal 3			
	D3110 Pulp cap			
	D3220 Pulpotomy			
	D0460 Pulp vitality test			
	D2940 Sedative filling			

	RESTORATIVE Amalgam Restorations:	Surface	Tooth #s	
	D2140 One surface, primary or permanent			
	D2150 Two surfaces, primary or permanent			
	D2160 Three surfaces, primary or permanent			
	D2161 Four or more surfaces, primary or permanent			

	Resin-based Composite Restorations Anterior:	Surface	Tooth #s	
	D2330 One surface			
	D2331 Two surfaces			
	D2332 Three surfaces			
	D2335 Four or more surfaces			

	Posterior:	Surface	Tooth #s	
X	D2391 One surface	O	19	
X	D2392 Two surfaces	DO	21	
	D2393 Three surfaces			
	D2394 Four or more surfaces			

	Crown Restorations:		Tooth #s	
	D2740 Porcelain			
	D2750 Porcelain–metal			

Collier Family Dental Care
Medical/Dental Arts Building
2890 Palm Avenue
Naples, FL 34104-8756
941-555-8900

Patient Name: Ian McCubbin **Chart Number:** MCCUBIAO **Dentist:** Dr. Miller **Date of Service:** 11/9/2007

	Crown Restorations:	Tooth #s	
	D2920 Recement Crown		
	D2950 Core buildup		
	D2980 Repair		
	PROSTHETICS Complete Dentures:		
	D5110 Upper denture		
	D5120 Lower denture		
	D5130 Immediate upper denture		
	D5140 Immediate lower denture		
	Partial Dentures:		
	D5211 Upper partial denture–resin		
	D5212 Lower partial denture–resin		
	D5213 Upper partial denture–cast		
	D5214 Lower partial denture–cast		
	D5750 Reline full upper denture		
	D6930 Recement fixed partial denture		
	PERIODONTICS/SURGERY	Tooth/Quad	
	D4341 Periodontal scaling and root planing,		
	per quadrant		
	Upper right		
	Upper left		
	Lower right		
	Lower left		
	D4210 Gingivectomy		
	D4240 Gingival flap		
	D4260 Osseous surgery		
	Upper right		
	Upper left		
	Lower right		
	Lower left		
	D7111 Extraction–Coronal remnant		
	D7140 Extraction–erupted tooth or exposed root		
	D7210 Surgical extraction		
	ADJUNCTIVE GENERAL SERVICES	Tooth #s	
	D9951 Occlusal adjustment–limited		
	OTHER		

Payments: **Total charge:**

Remarks: $15 copay, check #1042

BCBS of Florida
700 State Way
Miami, FL 33101-3320

Collier Family Dental Care
Medical/Dental Arts Building
2890 Palm Avenue
Naples, FL 34104-8756

Practice ID: 76-5433310

Date Prepared: 11/8/2007   **RA Number:** 199391

Patient's Name	Dates of Service From – Thru	POS	Proc	Qty	Proc Charge	Amt Paid Provider
Arrez, Anthony	10-29-07 – 10-29-07	11	D2330	1	125.00	100.00
Arrez, Anthony	10-29-07 – 10-29-07	11	D2331	1	175.00	140.00
Jones, Susan	10-29-07 – 10-29-07	11	D4341-UR	1	225.00	180.00
Jones, Susan	10-29-07 – 10-29-07	11	D4341-UL	1	225.00	180.00

* * * * * * *   *Check #7642293 is attached in the amount of $600.00.*   * * * * * * * *

Collier Family Dental Care
Medical/Dental Arts Building
2890 Palm Avenue
Naples, FL 34104-8756
941-555-8900

| **Patient Name:** Diana Fondo | **Chart Number:** FONDODIO | **Dentist:** Dr. Miller | **Date of Service:** 11/12/2007 |

	SERVICE DIAGNOSTIC/PREVENTIVE		FEE
	D1110 Prophylaxis – adult		
	D0120 Periodic oral evaluation		
	D0274 Bitewings – four X rays		
	D1120 Prophylaxis – child		
	D0210 Intraoral – complete series (including bitewings)		
	D0220 Intraoral – first X ray		
	D0230 Intraoral – each additional X ray		
	D0321 TMJ film		
	D0470 Diagnostic casts		

	ENDODONTICS	Tooth #s	
	D3310 Root canal 1		
	D3320 Root canal 2		
	D3330 Root canal 3		
	D3110 Pulp cap		
	D3220 Pulpotomy		
	D0460 Pulp vitality test		
	D2940 Sedative filling		

	RESTORATIVE Amalgam Restorations:	Surface	Tooth #s
	D2140 One surface, primary or permanent		
	D2150 Two surfaces, primary or permanent		
	D2160 Three surfaces, primary or permanent		
	D2161 Four or more surfaces, primary or permanent		

	Resin-based Composite Restorations Anterior:	Surface	Tooth #s
	D2330 One surface		
	D2331 Two surfaces		
	D2332 Three surfaces		
	D2335 Four or more surfaces		

	Posterior:	Surface	Tooth #s
	D2391 One surface		
	D2392 Two surfaces		
	D2393 Three surfaces		
	D2394 Four or more surfaces		

	Crown Restorations:		Tooth #s
	D2740 Porcelain		
	D2750 Porcelain–metal		

Collier Family Dental Care
Medical/Dental Arts Building
2890 Palm Avenue
Naples, FL 34104-8756
941-555-8900

Patient Name: Diana Fondo   **Chart Number:** FONDODIO   **Dentist:** Dr. Miller   **Date of Service:** 11/12/2007

	Crown Restorations:	Tooth #s	
	D2920 Recement Crown		
	D2950 Core buildup		
	D2980 Repair		
	PROSTHETICS **Complete Dentures:**		
	D5110 Upper denture		
	D5120 Lower denture		
	D5130 Immediate upper denture		
	D5140 Immediate lower denture		
	Partial Dentures:		
	D5211 Upper partial denture–resin		
	D5212 Lower partial denture–resin		
	D5213 Upper partial denture–cast		
	D5214 Lower partial denture–cast		
	D5750 Reline full upper denture		
	D6930 Recement fixed partial denture		
	PERIODONTICS/SURGERY	Tooth/Quad	
X	D4341 Periodontal scaling and root planing,		
	per quadrant		
	Upper right		
	Upper left		
X	Lower right		
X	Lower left		
	D4210 Gingivectomy		
	D4240 Gingival flap		
	D4260 Osseous surgery		
	Upper right		
	Upper left		
	Lower right		
	Lower left		
	D7111 Extraction–Coronal remnant		
	D7140 Extraction–erupted tooth or exposed root		
	D7210 Surgical extraction		
	ADJUNCTIVE GENERAL SERVICES	Tooth #s	
	D9951 Occlusal adjustment–limited		
	OTHER		

Payments: $20 copay, check #3419   **Total charge:**

Remarks: Next appt. 1 week from today (11/19/07), 2:00 p.m., 30 minutes, with Dr. Miller

Collier Family Dental Care
Medical/Dental Arts Building
2890 Palm Avenue
Naples, FL 34104-8756
941-555-8900

| Patient Name: | Brad Walsh | Chart Number: | WALSHBRO | Dentist: | Dr. Miller | Date of Service: | 11/12/2007 |

	SERVICE DIAGNOSTIC/PREVENTIVE		FEE
	D1110 Prophylaxis – adult		
	D0120 Periodic oral evaluation		
	D0274 Bitewings – four X rays		
	D1120 Prophylaxis – child		
	D0210 Intraoral – complete series (including bitewings)		
X	D0220 Intraoral – first X ray		
X	D0230 Intraoral – each additional X ray		
	D0321 TMJ film		
	D0470 Diagnostic casts		

	ENDODONTICS	Tooth #s	
	D3310 Root canal 1		
	D3320 Root canal 2		
	D3330 Root canal 3		
	D3110 Pulp cap		
	D3220 Pulpotomy		
	D0460 Pulp vitality test		
	D2940 Sedative filling		

	RESTORATIVE Amalgam Restorations:	Surface	Tooth #s	
	D2140 One surface, primary or permanent			
	D2150 Two surfaces, primary or permanent			
	D2160 Three surfaces, primary or permanent			
	D2161 Four or more surfaces, primary or permanent			

	Resin-based Composite Restorations Anterior:	Surface	Tooth #s	
	D2330 One surface			
	D2331 Two surfaces			
	D2332 Three surfaces			
	D2335 Four or more surfaces			

	Posterior:	Surface	Tooth #s	
	D2391 One surface			
	D2392 Two surfaces			
	D2393 Three surfaces			
	D2394 Four or more surfaces			

	Crown Restorations:	Tooth #s	
	D2740 Porcelain		
	D2750 Porcelain–metal		

Collier Family Dental Care
Medical/Dental Arts Building
2890 Palm Avenue
Naples, FL 34104-8756
941-555-8900

Patient Name: Brad Walsh   **Chart Number:** WALSHBRO   **Dentist:** Dr. Miller   **Date of Service:** 11/12/2007

	Crown Restorations:	Tooth #s	
	D2920 Recement Crown		
	D2950 Core buildup		
	D2980 Repair		
	PROSTHETICS **Complete Dentures:**		
	D5110 Upper denture		
	D5120 Lower denture		
	D5130 Immediate upper denture		
	D5140 Immediate lower denture		
	Partial Dentures:		
	D5211 Upper partial denture–resin		
	D5212 Lower partial denture–resin		
	D5213 Upper partial denture–cast		
	D5214 Lower partial denture–cast		
	D5750 Reline full upper denture		
	D6930 Recement fixed partial denture		
	PERIODONTICS/SURGERY	**Tooth/Quad**	
	D4341 Periodontal scaling and root planing,		
	per quadrant		
	Upper right		
	Upper left		
	Lower right		
	Lower left		
	D4210 Gingivectomy		
	D4240 Gingival flap		
	D4260 Osseous surgery		
	Upper right		
	Upper left		
	Lower right		
	Lower left		
X	D7111 Extraction–Coronal remnant	29/LR	
	D7140 Extraction–erupted tooth or exposed root		
	D7210 Surgical extraction		
	ADJUNCTIVE GENERAL SERVICES	**Tooth #s**	
	D9951 Occlusal adjustment–limited		
	OTHER		

Payments: $207, check #3119   **Total charge:**

Remarks:

Collier Family Dental Care
Medical/Dental Arts Building
2890 Palm Avenue
Naples, FL 34104-8756
941-555-8900

PATIENT INFORMATION FORM

PERSONAL INFORMATION

Name (last, first): Stewart Schober

Sex: ☒ Male ☐ Female

Address: 65 Pineapple Lane
North Naples, FL 34110

Date of Birth: 4-29-1940

Social Security No.: 336-55-8765

Home Phone No.: (941) 555-8888
( )

Marital Status: ☐ Married ☐ Single ☐ Separated ☒ Divorced ☐ Widowed

Employer: Naples Performing Arts Center (part time)

Address: 43 Galleon Drive
Naples, FL 34111

Work Phone No.: (941) 555-6655

Reason for visit: Periodontal

Name of Referring Dentist

SPOUSE/PARENT INFORMATION

Name (last, first):

Social Security No.:

Employer:

Address:

EMERGENCY CONTACT

Name (last, first): Carlotta Lane

Relationship: daughter

Phone No.: (941) 333-9800

PHYSICIAN INFORMATION

Name (last, first):

Specialty:

Phone No.: ( )

Location/City:

INSURANCE INFORMATION

Insurance Company: BCBS of Florida

Policy No.: 444-009A

Copayment:

Plan/Group No.: Naples Arts / CFR-200

Name of Responsible Party:

Relationship to Patient:
☒ Self ☐ Spouse ☐ Child ☐ Other

PAYMENT INFORMATION

Check all that apply: ☒ Insurance ☐ Cash ☐ Check ☐ Credit Card ☐ Other

Assignment and Release: I hereby authorize any insurance benefits to be paid directly to the dentist. I am financially responsible for the services provided, regardless of insurance coverage. I also authorize the dentist to release any information required.

Stewart Schober

Patient's signature/Parent or guardian's signature

12/7/2007

Date

Collier Family Dental Care
Medical/Dental Arts Building
2890 Palm Avenue
Naples, FL 34104-8756
941-555-8900

Patient Name: Stewart Schober   **Chart Number:** SCHOBSTO   **Dentist:** Dr. Miller   **Date of Service:** 12/19/2007

	SERVICE DIAGNOSTIC/PREVENTIVE			FEE
	D1110 Prophylaxis – adult			
	D0120 Periodic oral evaluation			
	D0274 Bitewings – four X rays			
	D1120 Prophylaxis – child			
	D0210 Intraoral – complete series (including bitewings)			
	D0220 Intraoral – first X ray			
	D0230 Intraoral – each additional X ray			
	D0321 TMJ film			
	D0470 Diagnostic casts			

	ENDODONTICS		Tooth #s	
	D3310 Root canal 1			
	D3320 Root canal 2			
	D3330 Root canal 3			
	D3110 Pulp cap			
	D3220 Pulpotomy			
	D0460 Pulp vitality test			
	D2940 Sedative filling			

	RESTORATIVE Amalgam Restorations:	Surface	Tooth #s	
	D2140 One surface, primary or permanent			
	D2150 Two surfaces, primary or permanent			
	D2160 Three surfaces, primary or permanent			
	D2161 Four or more surfaces, primary or permanent			

	Resin-based Composite Restorations Anterior:	Surface	Tooth #s	
	D2330 One surface			
	D2331 Two surfaces			
	D2332 Three surfaces			
	D2335 Four or more surfaces			

	Posterior:	Surface	Tooth #s	
	D2391 One surface			
	D2392 Two surfaces			
	D2393 Three surfaces			
	D2394 Four or more surfaces			

	Crown Restorations:		Tooth #s	
	D2740 Porcelain			
	D2750 Porcelain–metal			

Collier Family Dental Care
Medical/Dental Arts Building
2890 Palm Avenue
Naples, FL 34104-8756
941-555-8900

Patient Name: Stewart Schober   **Chart Number:** SCHOBSTO   **Dentist:** Dr. Miller   **Date of Service:** 12/19/2007

	Crown Restorations:	Tooth #s	
	D2920 Recement Crown		
	D2950 Core buildup		
	D2980 Repair		
	PROSTHETICS Complete Dentures:		
	D5110 Upper denture		
	D5120 Lower denture		
	D5130 Immediate upper denture		
	D5140 Immediate lower denture		
	Partial Dentures:		
	D5211 Upper partial denture–resin		
	D5212 Lower partial denture–resin		
	D5213 Upper partial denture–cast		
	D5214 Lower partial denture–cast		
	D5750 Reline full upper denture		
	D6930 Recement fixed partial denture		
	PERIODONTICS/SURGERY	Tooth/Quad	
X	D4341 Periodontal scaling and root planing,		
	per quadrant		
X	Upper right		
	Upper left		
X	Lower right		
	Lower left		
	D4210 Gingivectomy		
	D4240 Gingival flap		
	D4260 Osseous surgery		
	Upper right		
	Upper left		
	Lower right		
	Lower left		
	D7111 Extraction–Coronal remnant		
	D7140 Extraction–erupted tooth or exposed root		
	D7210 Surgical extraction		
	ADJUNCTIVE GENERAL SERVICES	Tooth #s	
	D9951 Occlusal adjustment–limited		
	OTHER		

Payments: **Total charge:**

Remarks:

Collier Family Dental Care
Medical/Dental Arts Building
2890 Palm Avenue
Naples, FL 34104-8756
941-555-8900

Patient Name: Brad Walsh **Chart Number:** WALSHBRO **Dentist:** Dr. Wu **Date of Service:** 12/14/2007

	SERVICE			FEE
	DIAGNOSTIC/PREVENTIVE			
	D1110 Prophylaxis – adult			
	D0120 Periodic oral evaluation			
	D0274 Bitewings – four X rays			
	D1120 Prophylaxis – child			
	D0210 Intraoral – complete series (including bitewings)			
X	D0220 Intraoral – first X ray			
	D0230 Intraoral – each additional X ray			
	D0321 TMJ film			
	D0470 Diagnostic casts			
	ENDODONTICS		**Tooth #s**	
	D3310 Root canal 1			
	D3320 Root canal 2			
	D3330 Root canal 3			
	D3110 Pulp cap			
	D3220 Pulpotomy			
	D0460 Pulp vitality test			
	D2940 Sedative filling			
	RESTORATIVE Amalgam Restorations:	**Surface**	**Tooth #s**	
	D2140 One surface, primary or permanent			
	D2150 Two surfaces, primary or permanent			
	D2160 Three surfaces, primary or permanent			
	D2161 Four or more surfaces, primary or permanent			
	Resin-based Composite Restorations Anterior:	**Surface**	**Tooth #s**	
	D2330 One surface			
	D2331 Two surfaces			
	D2332 Three surfaces			
	D2335 Four or more surfaces			
	Posterior:	**Surface**	**Tooth #s**	
	D2391 One surface			
	D2392 Two surfaces			
	D2393 Three surfaces			
	D2394 Four or more surfaces			
	Crown Restorations:		**Tooth #s**	
	D2740 Porcelain			
	D2750 Porcelain–metal			

Collier Family Dental Care
Medical/Dental Arts Building
2890 Palm Avenue
Naples, FL 34104-8756
941-555-8900

| Patient Name: | Brad Walsh | Chart Number: | WALSHBRO | Dentist: | Dr. Wu | Date of Service: | 12/15/2007 |

	Crown Restorations:		Tooth #s	
	D2920 Recement Crown			
	D2950 Core buildup			
	D2980 Repair			
	PROSTHETICS **Complete Dentures:**			
	D5110 Upper denture			
	D5120 Lower denture			
	D5130 Immediate upper denture			
	D5140 Immediate lower denture			
	Partial Dentures:			
	D5211 Upper partial denture—resin			
	D5212 Lower partial denture—resin			
	D5213 Upper partial denture—cast			
	D5214 Lower partial denture—cast			
	D5750 Reline full upper denture			
X	D6930 Recement fixed partial denture	10		
	PERIODONTICS/SURGERY	**Tooth/Quad**		
	D4341 Periodontal scaling and root planing,			
	per quadrant			
	Upper right			
	Upper left			
	Lower right			
	Lower left			
	D4210 Gingivectomy			
	D4240 Gingival flap			
	D4260 Osseous surgery			
	Upper right			
	Upper left			
	Lower right			
	Lower left			
	D7111 Extraction—Coronal remnant			
	D7140 Extraction—erupted tooth or exposed root			
	D7210 Surgical extraction			
	ADJUNCTIVE GENERAL SERVICES		**Tooth #s**	
	D9951 Occlusal adjustment—limited			
	OTHER			

| Payments: $20, cash | Total charge: |

Remarks: Balance due ($90) to be paid on return visit, Dec. 21 (2:00 p.m.)

Collier Family Dental Care
Medical/Dental Arts Building
2890 Palm Avenue
Naples, FL 34104-8756
941-555-8900

Patient Name: Joshua Hersen   **Chart Number:** HERSEJ00   **Dentist:** Dr. Miller   **Date of Service:** 1/2/2008

	SERVICE DIAGNOSTIC/PREVENTIVE			FEE
	D1110 Prophylaxis – adult			
	D0120 Periodic oral evaluation			
	D0274 Bitewings – four X rays			
	D1120 Prophylaxis – child			
	D0210 Intraoral – complete series (including bitewings)			
	D0220 Intraoral – first X ray			
	D0230 Intraoral – each additional X ray			
	D0321 TMJ film			
	D0470 Diagnostic casts			
	ENDODONTICS		**Tooth #s**	
	D3310 Root canal 1			
	D3320 Root canal 2			
	D3330 Root canal 3			
	D3110 Pulp cap			
	D3220 Pulpotomy			
	D0460 Pulp vitality test			
	D2940 Sedative filling			
	RESTORATIVE Amalgam Restorations:	**Surface**	**Tooth #s**	
X	D2140 One surface, primary or permanent	M	4	
	D2150 Two surfaces, primary or permanent			
	D2160 Three surfaces, primary or permanent			
X	D2161 Four or more surfaces, primary or permanent	MODL	15	
	Resin-based Composite Restorations Anterior:	**Surface**	**Tooth #s**	
	D2330 One surface			
	D2331 Two surfaces			
	D2332 Three surfaces			
	D2335 Four or more surfaces			
	Posterior:	**Surface**	**Tooth #s**	
	D2391 One surface			
	D2392 Two surfaces			
	D2393 Three surfaces			
	D2394 Four or more surfaces			
	Crown Restorations:		**Tooth #s**	
	D2740 Porcelain			
	D2750 Porcelain–metal			

Collier Family Dental Care
Medical/Dental Arts Building
2890 Palm Avenue
Naples, FL 34104-8756
941-555-8900

Patient Name: Joshua Hersen   **Chart Number:** HERSEJ00   **Dentist:** Dr. Miller   **Date of Service:** 1/2/2008

		Tooth #s	
Crown Restorations:			
	D2920 Recement Crown		
	D2950 Core buildup		
	D2980 Repair		
PROSTHETICS	**Complete Dentures:**		
	D5110 Upper denture		
	D5120 Lower denture		
	D5130 Immediate upper denture		
	D5140 Immediate lower denture		
Partial Dentures:			
	D5211 Upper partial denture–resin		
	D5212 Lower partial denture–resin		
	D5213 Upper partial denture–cast		
	D5214 Lower partial denture–cast		
	D5750 Reline full upper denture		
	D6930 Recement fixed partial denture		
PERIODONTICS/SURGERY		**Tooth/Quad**	
	D4341 Periodontal scaling and root planing,		
	per quadrant		
	Upper right		
	Upper left		
	Lower right		
	Lower left		
	D4210 Gingivectomy		
	D4240 Gingival flap		
	D4260 Osseous surgery		
	Upper right		
	Upper left		
	Lower right		
	Lower left		
	D7111 Extraction–Coronal remnant		
	D7140 Extraction–erupted tooth or exposed root		
	D7210 Surgical extraction		
ADJUNCTIVE GENERAL SERVICES		**Tooth #s**	
	D9951 Occlusal adjustment–limited		
OTHER			

Payments: $20 copay, check #1291   **Total charge:**

Remarks:

Collier Family Dental Care
Medical/Dental Arts Building
2890 Palm Avenue
Naples, FL 34104-8756
941-555-8900

Patient Name: Juliet Schubert-Seku   **Chart Number:** SCHUBJUO   **Dentist:** Dr. Miller   **Date of Service:** 1/2/2008

	SERVICE DIAGNOSTIC/PREVENTIVE			FEE
X	D1110 Prophylaxis – adult			
X	D0120 Periodic oral evaluation			
	D0274 Bitewings – four X rays			
	D1120 Prophylaxis – child			
	D0210 Intraoral – complete series (including bitewings)			
	D0220 Intraoral – first X ray			
	D0230 Intraoral – each additional X ray			
	D0321 TMJ film			
	D0470 Diagnostic casts			
	ENDODONTICS		**Tooth #s**	
	D3310 Root canal 1			
	D3320 Root canal 2			
	D3330 Root canal 3			
	D3110 Pulp cap			
	D3220 Pulpotomy			
	D0460 Pulp vitality test			
	D2940 Sedative filling			
	RESTORATIVE Amalgam Restorations:	**Surface**	**Tooth #s**	
	D2140 One surface, primary or permanent			
	D2150 Two surfaces, primary or permanent			
	D2160 Three surfaces, primary or permanent			
	D2161 Four or more surfaces, primary or permanent			
	Resin-based Composite Restorations Anterior:	**Surface**	**Tooth #s**	
	D2330 One surface			
	D2331 Two surfaces			
	D2332 Three surfaces			
	D2335 Four or more surfaces			
	Posterior:	**Surface**	**Tooth #s**	
	D2391 One surface			
	D2392 Two surfaces			
	D2393 Three surfaces			
	D2394 Four or more surfaces			
	Crown Restorations:		**Tooth #s**	
	D2740 Porcelain			
	D2750 Porcelain–metal			

Collier Family Dental Care
Medical/Dental Arts Building
2890 Palm Avenue
Naples, FL 34104-8756
941-555-8900

Patient Name: Juliet Schubert-Seku   **Chart Number:** SCHUBJUO   **Dentist:** Dr. Miller   **Date of Service:** 1/2/2008

	Crown Restorations:	Tooth #s	
	D2920 Recement Crown		
	D2950 Core buildup		
	D2980 Repair		
	PROSTHETICS Complete Dentures:		
	D5110 Upper denture		
	D5120 Lower denture		
	D5130 Immediate upper denture		
	D5140 Immediate lower denture		
	Partial Dentures:		
	D5211 Upper partial denture–resin		
	D5212 Lower partial denture–resin		
	D5213 Upper partial denture–cast		
	D5214 Lower partial denture–cast		
	D5750 Reline full upper denture		
	D6930 Recement fixed partial denture		
	PERIODONTICS/SURGERY	**Tooth/Quad**	
	D4341 Periodontal scaling and root planing,		
	per quadrant		
	Upper right		
	Upper left		
	Lower right		
	Lower left		
	D4210 Gingivectomy		
	D4240 Gingival flap		
	D4260 Osseous surgery		
	Upper right		
	Upper left		
	Lower right		
	Lower left		
	D7111 Extraction–Coronal remnant		
	D7140 Extraction–erupted tooth or exposed root		
	D7210 Surgical extraction		
	ADJUNCTIVE GENERAL SERVICES	**Tooth #s**	
	D9951 Occlusal adjustment–limited		
	OTHER		

Payments: **Total charge:**

Remarks:

Collier Family Dental Care
Medical/Dental Arts Building
2890 Palm Avenue
Naples, FL 34104-8756
941-555-8900

Patient Name: Nancy Thompson   **Chart Number:** THOMPNAO   **Dentist:** Dr. Wu   **Date of Service:** 1/2/2008

	SERVICE			FEE
	DIAGNOSTIC/PREVENTIVE			
	D1110 Prophylaxis – adult			
	D0120 Periodic oral evaluation			
	D0274 Bitewings – four X rays			
	D1120 Prophylaxis – child			
	D0210 Intraoral – complete series (including bitewings)			
X	D0220 Intraoral – first X ray			
X	D0230 Intraoral – each additional X ray			
	D0321 TMJ film			
	D0470 Diagnostic casts			
	ENDODONTICS		**Tooth #s**	
X	D3310 Root canal 1		28	
	D3320 Root canal 2			
	D3330 Root canal 3			
	D3110 Pulp cap			
	D3220 Pulpotomy			
	D0460 Pulp vitality test			
X	D2940 Sedative filling		28	
	RESTORATIVE Amalgam Restorations:	**Surface**	**Tooth #s**	
	D2140 One surface, primary or permanent			
	D2150 Two surfaces, primary or permanent			
	D2160 Three surfaces, primary or permanent			
	D2161 Four or more surfaces, primary or permanent			
	Resin-based Composite Restorations Anterior:	**Surface**	**Tooth #s**	
	D2330 One surface			
	D2331 Two surfaces			
	D2332 Three surfaces			
	D2335 Four or more surfaces			
	Posterior:	**Surface**	**Tooth #s**	
	D2391 One surface			
	D2392 Two surfaces			
	D2393 Three surfaces			
	D2394 Four or more surfaces			
	Crown Restorations:		**Tooth #s**	
	D2740 Porcelain			
	D2750 Porcelain–metal			

Collier Family Dental Care
Medical/Dental Arts Building
2890 Palm Avenue
Naples, FL 34104-8756
941-555-8900

| Patient Name: | Nancy Thompson | Chart Number: | THOMPNAO | Dentist: | Dr. Wu | Date of Service: | 1/2/2008 |

	Crown Restorations:	Tooth #s	
	D2920 Recement Crown		
	D2950 Core buildup		
	D2980 Repair		
	PROSTHETICS Complete Dentures:		
	D5110 Upper denture		
	D5120 Lower denture		
	D5130 Immediate upper denture		
	D5140 Immediate lower denture		
	Partial Dentures:		
	D5211 Upper partial denture–resin		
	D5212 Lower partial denture–resin		
	D5213 Upper partial denture–cast		
	D5214 Lower partial denture–cast		
	D5750 Reline full upper denture		
	D6930 Recement fixed partial denture		
	PERIODONTICS/SURGERY	**Tooth/Quad**	
	D4341 Periodontal scaling and root planing,		
	per quadrant		
	Upper right		
	Upper left		
	Lower right		
	Lower left		
	D4210 Gingivectomy		
	D4240 Gingival flap		
	D4260 Osseous surgery		
	Upper right		
	Upper left		
	Lower right		
	Lower left		
	D7111 Extraction–Coronal remnant		
	D7140 Extraction–erupted tooth or exposed root		
	D7210 Surgical extraction		
	ADJUNCTIVE GENERAL SERVICES	**Tooth #s**	
	D9951 Occlusal adjustment–limited		
	OTHER		

| Payments: $15 copay, check #1022 | Total charge: |

Remarks:

Collier Family Dental Care
Medical/Dental Arts Building
2890 Palm Avenue
Naples, FL 34104-8756
941-555-8900

| Patient Name: | Myrna Walsh | Chart Number: | WALSHMY0 | Dentist: | Dr. Miller | Date of Service: | 1/2/2008 |

	SERVICE				FEE

DIAGNOSTIC/PREVENTIVE

	Service				Fee
	D1110 Prophylaxis – adult				
	D0120 Periodic oral evaluation				
	D0274 Bitewings – four X rays				
	D1120 Prophylaxis – child				
	D0210 Intraoral – complete series (including bitewings)				
	D0220 Intraoral – first X ray				
	D0230 Intraoral – each additional X ray				
	D0321 TMJ film				
	D0470 Diagnostic casts				

ENDODONTICS

				Tooth #s	
	D3310 Root canal 1				
	D3320 Root canal 2				
	D3330 Root canal 3				
	D3110 Pulp cap				
	D3220 Pulpotomy				
	D0460 Pulp vitality test				
	D2940 Sedative filling				

RESTORATIVE Amalgam Restorations:

		Surface	Tooth #s	
	D2140 One surface, primary or permanent			
	D2150 Two surfaces, primary or permanent			
X	D2160 Three surfaces, primary or permanent	MOD	4	
	D2161 Four or more surfaces, primary or permanent			

Resin-based Composite Restorations
Anterior:

		Surface	Tooth #s	
	D2330 One surface			
	D2331 Two surfaces			
	D2332 Three surfaces			
	D2335 Four or more surfaces			

Posterior:

		Surface	Tooth #s	
	D2391 One surface			
	D2392 Two surfaces			
	D2393 Three surfaces			
	D2394 Four or more surfaces			

Crown Restorations:

		Tooth #s	
	D2740 Porcelain		
X	D2750 Porcelain–metal	3	

Collier Family Dental Care
Medical/Dental Arts Building
2890 Palm Avenue
Naples, FL 34104-8756
941-555-8900

Patient Name: Myrna Walsh	**Chart Number:** WALSHMY0	**Dentist:** Dr. Miller	**Date of Service:** 1/2/2008

	Crown Restorations:	**Tooth #s**	
	D2920 Recement Crown		
	D2950 Core buildup		
	D2980 Repair		
	PROSTHETICS Complete Dentures:		
	D5110 Upper denture		
	D5120 Lower denture		
	D5130 Immediate upper denture		
	D5140 Immediate lower denture		
	Partial Dentures:		
	D5211 Upper partial denture–resin		
	D5212 Lower partial denture–resin		
	D5213 Upper partial denture–cast		
	D5214 Lower partial denture–cast		
	D5750 Reline full upper denture		
	D6930 Recement fixed partial denture		
	PERIODONTICS/SURGERY	**Tooth/Quad**	
	D4341 Periodontal scaling and root planing, per quadrant		
	Upper right		
	Upper left		
	Lower right		
	Lower left		
	D4210 Gingivectomy		
	D4240 Gingival flap		
	D4260 Osseous surgery		
	Upper right		
	Upper left		
	Lower right		
	Lower left		
	D7111 Extraction–Coronal remnant		
	D7140 Extraction–erupted tooth or exposed root		
	D7210 Surgical extraction		
	ADJUNCTIVE GENERAL SERVICES	**Tooth #s**	
	D9951 Occlusal adjustment–limited		
	OTHER		

Payments: $1,325, check #3219   **Total charge:**

Remarks:

Collier Family Dental Care
Medical/Dental Arts Building
2890 Palm Avenue
Naples, FL 34104-8756
941-555-8900

Patient Name: Georgette Foncet   **Chart Number:** FONCEGEO   **Dentist:** Dr. Miller   **Date of Service:** 1/2/2008

	SERVICE			FEE
	DIAGNOSTIC/PREVENTIVE			
	D1110 Prophylaxis – adult			
	D0120 Periodic oral evaluation			
	D0274 Bitewings – four X rays			
	D1120 Prophylaxis – child			
	D0210 Intraoral – complete series (including bitewings)			
	D0220 Intraoral – first X ray			
	D0230 Intraoral – each additional X ray			
	D0321 TMJ film			
	D0470 Diagnostic casts			
	ENDODONTICS		**Tooth #s**	
	D3310 Root canal 1			
	D3320 Root canal 2			
	D3330 Root canal 3			
	D3110 Pulp cap			
	D3220 Pulpotomy			
	D0460 Pulp vitality test			
	D2940 Sedative filling			
	RESTORATIVE Amalgam Restorations:	**Surface**	**Tooth #s**	
	D2140 One surface, primary or permanent			
	D2150 Two surfaces, primary or permanent			
	D2160 Three surfaces, primary or permanent			
	D2161 Four or more surfaces, primary or permanent			
	Resin-based Composite Restorations Anterior:	**Surface**	**Tooth #s**	
	D2330 One surface			
	D2331 Two surfaces			
	D2332 Three surfaces			
	D2335 Four or more surfaces			
	Posterior:	**Surface**	**Tooth #s**	
	D2391 One surface			
	D2392 Two surfaces			
	D2393 Three surfaces			
	D2394 Four or more surfaces			
	Crown Restorations:		**Tooth #s**	
	D2740 Porcelain			
	D2750 Porcelain–metal			

Collier Family Dental Care
Medical/Dental Arts Building
2890 Palm Avenue
Naples, FL 34104-8756
941-555-8900

| Patient Name: | Georgette Foncet | Chart Number: | FONCEGEO | Dentist: | Dr. Miller | Date of Service: | 1/2/2008 |

	Crown Restorations:	Tooth #s	
	D2920 Recement Crown		
	D2950 Core buildup		
	D2980 Repair		
	PROSTHETICS Complete Dentures:		
	D5110 Upper denture		
	D5120 Lower denture		
	D5130 Immediate upper denture		
	D5140 Immediate lower denture		
	Partial Dentures:		
	D5211 Upper partial denture–resin		
	D5212 Lower partial denture–resin		
X	D5213 Upper partial denture–cast		
X	D5214 Lower partial denture–cast		
	D5750 Reline full upper denture		
	D6930 Recement fixed partial denture		
	PERIODONTICS/SURGERY	**Tooth/Quad**	
	D4341 Periodontal scaling and root planing,		
	per quadrant		
	Upper right		
	Upper left		
	Lower right		
	Lower left		
	D4210 Gingivectomy		
	D4240 Gingival flap		
	D4260 Osseous surgery		
	Upper right		
	Upper left		
	Lower right		
	Lower left		
	D7111 Extraction–Coronal remnant		
	D7140 Extraction–erupted tooth or exposed root		
	D7210 Surgical extraction		
	ADJUNCTIVE GENERAL SERVICES	**Tooth #s**	
	D9951 Occlusal adjustment–limited		
	OTHER		

| Payments: | | Total charge: | |

Remarks:

Collier Family Dental Care
Medical/Dental Arts Building
2890 Palm Avenue
Naples, FL 34104-8756
941-555-8900

Patient Name: Paula Arrez **Chart Number:** ARREZPAO **Dentist:** Dr. Miller **Date of Service:** 1/2/2008

	SERVICE DIAGNOSTIC/PREVENTIVE		FEE
	D1110 Prophylaxis – adult		
	D0120 Periodic oral evaluation		
	D0274 Bitewings – four X rays		
	D1120 Prophylaxis – child		
	D0210 Intraoral – complete series (including bitewings)		
	D0220 Intraoral – first X ray		
	D0230 Intraoral – each additional X ray		
	D0321 TMJ film		
	D0470 Diagnostic casts		
	ENDODONTICS	**Tooth #s**	
	D3310 Root canal 1		
	D3320 Root canal 2		
	D3330 Root canal 3		
	D3110 Pulp cap		
	D3220 Pulpotomy		
	D0460 Pulp vitality test		
	D2940 Sedative filling		

	RESTORATIVE Amalgam Restorations:	Surface	Tooth #s	
	D2140 One surface, primary or permanent			
	D2150 Two surfaces, primary or permanent			
	D2160 Three surfaces, primary or permanent			
	D2161 Four or more surfaces, primary or permanent			

	Resin-based Composite Restorations Anterior:	Surface	Tooth #s	
	D2330 One surface			
	D2331 Two surfaces			
	D2332 Three surfaces			
	D2335 Four or more surfaces			
	Posterior:	Surface	Tooth #s	
	D2391 One surface			
	D2392 Two surfaces			
	D2393 Three surfaces			
	D2394 Four or more surfaces			
	Crown Restorations:		Tooth #s	
	D2740 Porcelain			
	D2750 Porcelain–metal			

Collier Family Dental Care
Medical/Dental Arts Building
2890 Palm Avenue
Naples, FL 34104-8756
941-555-8900

Patient Name:	Paula Arrez	Chart Number:	ARREZPAO	Dentist:	Dr. Miller	Date of Service:	1/2/2008

	Crown Restorations:	Tooth #s	
	D2920 Recement Crown		
	D2950 Core buildup		
	D2980 Repair		
	PROSTHETICS Complete Dentures:		
	D5110 Upper denture		
	D5120 Lower denture		
	D5130 Immediate upper denture		
	D5140 Immediate lower denture		
	Partial Dentures:		
	D5211 Upper partial denture–resin		
	D5212 Lower partial denture–resin		
	D5213 Upper partial denture–cast		
	D5214 Lower partial denture–cast		
	D5750 Reline full upper denture		
	D6930 Recement fixed partial denture		
	PERIODONTICS/SURGERY	**Tooth/Quad**	
	D4341 Periodontal scaling and root planing;		
	per quadrant		
	Upper right		
	Upper left		
	Lower right		
	Lower left		
	D4210 Gingivectomy		
	D4240 Gingival flap		
X	D4260 Osseous surgery		
	Upper right		
	Upper left		
X	Lower right		
	Lower left		
	D7111 Extraction–Coronal remnant		
	D7140 Extraction–erupted tooth or exposed root		
	D7210 Surgical extraction		
	ADJUNCTIVE GENERAL SERVICES	**Tooth #s**	
	D9951 Occlusal adjustment–limited		
	OTHER		

Payments:		Total charge:	

Remarks:

GLOSSARY

A

accounting cycle The flow of financial transactions in a business.

accounts receivable (AR) Monies that are flowing into a business.

ADA Dental Claim Form Authorized form for submitting dental insurance claims.

adjustments Changes to patients' accounts.

aging report A report that lists the amounts owed to the practice, categorized by the number of days late.

audit/edit report Response from a receiver to a sender regarding the status and completeness of a transmitted claim.

B

backup data An extra copy of data files made at a specific point in time that can be used to restore data to the system in the event the data in the system are accidentally lost or destroyed.

C

canines Two of the 32 permanent adult teeth.

capitated plan A managed care insurance plan in which payments are made on a regular basis to primary care providers for patients in the plan, regardless of whether the patients visit the provider during the time period covered by the payment.

capitation Advance payment to a provider that covers each plan member's health care services for a certain period of time.

capitation payments Payments made on a regular basis from an insurance carrier to a provider for providing services to plan members.

cases Groupings of transactions for visits to a dentist's office organized around a particular condition.

cement Hard connective tissue covering the tooth root.

charges The amounts a provider bills for services performed.

chart A folder that contains all records pertaining to a patient.

chart number A unique number that identifies a patient.

clearinghouse A service company that receives electronic/ paper claims from providers and transmits them in proper data format to carriers.

coinsurance Part of charges that an insured person must pay for health care services after payment of the deductible amount.

copayment Amount that an insured person must pay for each health care encounter.

Current Dental Terminology **(CDT-4)** American Dental Association publication containing a standardized classification system for reporting dental procedures and services.

D

database A collection of related facts.

day sheet A report that lists all transactions for a single day.

dental caries Common term for tooth decay.

dentin The hard material that fills 80 to 90 percent of the tooth.

Dentist's Pretreatment Estimate Dentist's estimate of needed dental work that is submitted to an insurance carrier before the service is performed.

Dentist's Statement of Actual Services Dental claim form that reports the services a dentist has performed for a patient.

E

e-commerce   The exchange of monies over the Internet.

electronic funds transfer (EFT)   A system that transfers monies electronically from one account to another.

electronic media claim (EMC)   An insurance claim that is sent by a computer over data communication lines.

enamel   The outer coating of the tooth.

encounter form   A list of the procedures and charges for a patient's visit.

endodontics   Dental specialty that treats disease and injuries of the pulp.

explanation of benefits (EOB)   Document from a payer that shows how the amount of a benefit was determined.

F

filter   A condition that data must meet to be included in a particular data group.

G

gingivae (sing., gingiva)   The gums.

guarantor   An individual who is a policyholder for a patient of the practice.

H

Health Insurance Portability and Accountability Act (HIPAA) of 1996   Federal government act that set forth guidelines for standardizing the electronic data interchange of administrative and financial transactions, exposing fraud and abuse in government programs, and protecting the security and privacy of health information.

health maintenance organization (HMO)   A managed health care system in which providers agree to offer health care to the organization's members for fixed periodic payments from the plan.

HIPAA Privacy Rule   Regulations for protecting individually identifiable information about a patient's past, present, or future physical or mental health or payment for health care that is created or received by a health care provider.

I

incisors   Four of the 32 permanent adult teeth; the cutting teeth.

indemnity plan   An insurance company's agreement to reimburse a policyholder for covered losses.

insurance carrier   A company that offers financial protection as a result of a specified event.

insurance payments   Payments made to the practice on behalf of a patient by an insurance carrier.

K

knowledge base   A collection of up-to-date technical information.

M

managed care   A type of insurance in which the carrier is responsible for both the financing and the delivery of health care.

mandible   Lower jaw bone.

maxilla   Upper jaw bone.

maxillofacial surgery   Surgical procedure related to the face and jaw.

MMDDCCYY format   A specific way in which dates must be keyed, in which "MM" stands for the month, "DD" stands for the day, "CC" stands for the century, and "YY" stands for the year; each day, month, century, and year entry must contain two digits and no punctuation.

molars   Six of the 32 permanent adult teeth; the grinding teeth.

MultiLink codes   A time-saving feature for entering multiple CDT codes under a single code; when the code for the MultiLink is entered, the other procedure codes in the group are entered automatically.

N

navigator buttons   In a dialog box, buttons that simplify the task of moving from one entry in a list to another.

O

occlusion   The contact between the upper and lower teeth.

Office Hours break   A block of time when a provider is unavailable for appointments with patients.

Office Hours schedule   A listing of time slots for a particular day for a specific provider.

oral cavity   Inner section of the mouth.

oral surgery   Surgical procedure related to the face and jaw.

orthodontics   Dental specialty that treats malocclusion of the teeth and their surrounding structures.

P

packing data   The deletion of vacant slots from a database.

palate   The hard and soft tissues that make up the roof of the mouth.

patient day sheet   A summary of the activity of patient accounts on any given day.

patient information form   Form that includes a patient's personal, employment, and insurance data needed to complete an insurance claim.

patient ledger   A listing of financial activity in a patient's account.

patient payments   Payments made to the practice from a patient or guarantor.

patient statement   A document that informs the patient of the amount owed to the provider.

payer   Private or governmental organization that insures or pays for health care on the behalf of beneficiaries.

payments   Monies received from patients and insurance carriers.

periodontics   Dental specialty that treats diseases of the supporting and surrounding tissues of the teeth.

policyholder   A person who buys an insurance plan; the insured.

practice analysis report   A report that shows the total revenue for each procedure performed during a specified time period.

preferred provider organization (PPO)   Managed care network of health care providers who agree to perform services for plan members at discounted fees.

premium   The periodic amount of money the insured pays to an insurance company for an insurance plan.

premolars   Four of the 32 permanent adult teeth; before the molars.

procedure   Work that is done by a provider for a patient.

procedure code   A code that identifies a dental service.

procedure day sheet   A list of all the procedures performed on a particular day.

prophylaxes (sing., prophylaxis)   Prevention of disease by removal of calculus, stains, and other extraneous materials from the teeth; cleaning of teeth by dentist or dental hygienist.

prostheses (sing., prosthesis)   Dental bridges and dentures.

pulp   The soft core of the tooth containing the nerves and blood vessels.

purging data   The process of deleting files of patients who are no longer seen by a provider in a practice.

R

rebuilding indexes   A process that checks and verifies data and corrects any internal problems with the data.

record of treatment and progress   A record containing a dentist's notes about a patient's condition and diagnosis.

referring provider   A dentist who recommends that a patient see another specific dentist.

remittance advice (RA)   An explanation of benefits transmitted by a payer to a provider.

removable media device   A device that stores data but is not a permanent part of a computer.

restorative services   Dental procedures that repair the surface of the tooth.

restoring data   The process of retrieving data from backup storage devices.

S

status bar help   Information provided in a series of messages that appear on the status bar as the mouse pointer is moved to certain items on the screen.

T

transactions   Charges, payments, and adjustments.

U

uvula   The cone-shaped structure at the end of the soft palate.

W

walkout receipt   A completed form a patient receives after an encounter that lists the services provided, fees, and payments received and due.

INDEX

searches for future dates, 163–164
shortcuts, 158–160
Office Hours break, 177
Office Hours schedule, 160
Open Report dialog box, 144–145, 221–222, 223
Options tab, 105–106
Oral cavity, 20
Oral surgery, 24
Orthodontic services, 24, 100
Other Information tab, 73–80

Packing data, 238–239
Palate, 20
Patient aging reports, 213–215, 264
Patient balances
finding, 262
recalculating, 241
remainder statements, 268–269
Patient data, 42, 68–81
accessing, 69–70
defined, 31
editing, 81, 248
entering new, 71–80, 248–252
organization of, 69–70
searching for, 70–71
Patient day sheets, 201–207, 202–203 (sample), 263–264
Patient/Guarantor dialog box, 71–80, 90
completing, 77–78
editing information through, 81
Name, Address tab, 71–73, 74, 77
Other Information tab, 73–80
Patient information form, 5, 6 (sample), 14, 36, 42
Patient ledgers, 216–218
Patient List button, 54
Patient List dialog box, 69–70, 81, 86–88
Close button, 88
Copy Case button, 87
Delete case button, 87
Edit case button, 86
New Case button, 87
Save button, 88
Patient medical/dental history form, 7 (sample), 7–8, 8 (sample)
Patient payments, 15, 139–143
applying, 140
entering, 139–143
printing walkout receipts, 144–145
Patient Recall Entry button, 54, 172–173
Patient Recall List dialog box, 172–176, 258
Patient statements, 218–222, 267
electronic, 33, 42, 194–197, 222
pretreatment, 221–222
remainder statements, 268–269
Payer, 13
Payments, 115
adjustments to, 115, 134, 135, 150–154
entering, 138–154
insurance carrier, 115, 134, 135, 139, 145–154, 255

patient, 15, 139–143, 144–145
reviewing and recording, 15, 135
Periodontal ligament, 22
Periodontic procedures, 24
Personal health information (PHI), 5–8
patient information form, 5, 6 (sample), 14, 36, 42
patient medical/dental history form, 7 (sample), 7–8, 8 (sample)
Personal tab, 89–91
Phone numbers
employer, 79
patient, 72–73, 76, 90, 162, 175
referring provider, 94
PINs (provider identification numbers), 96–97, 106, 108
Policy 1, 102–104, 134
Policy 2, 109, 134
Policy 3, 110, 134
Policyholders, 11, 102–103
POS (Place of Service), 121
Practice analysis reports, 15, 210–213, 211 (sample)
PractiSoft, 32–33
appointment scheduling in. See Office Hours
backup data, 43–44, 45–49, 61–65, 232–236
Claim Management. See Claim Management dialog box
databases, 42–43
deleting data, 59, 87, 127
described, 42
editing data. See Editing data
entering data. See Entering data
exercises, 176
exiting, 54, 61–63
Help options, 59–61
Menu bar, 49–52
recall lists, 172–176, 258
saving data, 59, 88, 163, 176
setting up practice, 32
student data disk, 43–49
Toolbar, 53–55
utility features, 231–241
Preferred provider organization (PPO), 13
Premiums, 11
Premolars, 21
Pretreatment Claim Management button, 54
Pretreatment Plan/Estimate dialog box, 127–128, 193–194
Pretreatment statements, 221–222
Pretreatment Transaction Entry button, 54
Preventive services, 23–24
Preview
of Office Hours schedules, 179–180
Report, 204–207
Printing, 200–228
appointment lists, 179–180, 263
custom reports, 201, 219–220, 223–228
electronic media claims, 195–196, 222, 268
exercises, 207, 210, 212–213, 214, 217–218, 220–222, 224–225, 226–228